Cytopathology of Pulmonary Disease

Monographs in Clinical Cytology

Vol. 11

Editor
George L. Wied, Chicago, Ill.

Co-Editors
Emmerich von Haam, Columbus, Ohio
Leopold G. Koss, New York, N.Y.
James W. Reagan, Cleveland, Ohio

KARGER

Basel · München · Paris · London · New York · New Delhi · Singapore · Tokyo · Sydney

Cytopathology of Pulmonary Disease

Dorothy L. Rosenthal, MD, F.I.A.C.
Department of Pathology, Cytology Service, Center for the Health Sciences, University of California, Los Angeles, Calif., USA

106 figures, of which 18 are in color, 24 tables, 1988

KARGER

Basel · München · Paris · London · New York · New Delhi · Singapore · Tokyo · Sydney

Monographs in Clinical Cytology

Library of Congress Cataloging-in-Publication Data
　　Rosenthal, Dorothy L.
　　Cytopathology of pulmonary disease.
　　(Monographs in clinical cytology; vol. 11)
　　Bibliography: p.
　　Includes index.
　　1. Lungs – Cytopathology.　2. Lungs – Diseases – Diagnosis.　I. Title.　II. Series.
　　[DNLM: 1. Cytodiagnosis.　2. Lung Diseases – pathology.
　　W1 M0567KF v. 11 / WF 600 R815c]
　　RC711.R57　1988　616.2′4071　88–670
　　ISBN 3–8055–4740–4

Bibliographic Indices
　　This publication is listed in bibliographic services, including Current Contents® and Index Medicus.

Drug Dosage
　　The author and the publisher have exerted every effort to ensure that drug selection and dosage set forth in this text are in accord with current recommendations and practice at the time of publication. However, in view of ongoing research, changes in government regulations, and the constant flow of information relating to drug therapy and drug reactions, the reader is urged to check the package insert for each drug for any change in indications and dosage and for added warnings and precautions. This is particularly important when the recommended agent is a new and/or infrequently employed drug.

All rights reserved.
　　No part of this publication may be translated into other languages, reproduced or utilized in any form or by any means, electronic or mechanical, including photocopying, recording, microcopying, or by any information storage and retrieval system, without permission in writing from the publisher.

©　　Copyright 1988 by S. Karger AG, P.O. Box, CH– 4009 Basel (Switzerland)
　　Printed in Switzerland by Thür AG Offsetdruck, Pratteln
　　ISBN 3–8055–4740–4

Contents

Dedication VII
Acknowledgements VIII
Introduction IX

I. Anatomy and Functional Histology 1
   Anatomy 1
   Histology 2

II. Variations among Benign Cellular Elements in Exfoliated and Aspirated Material 13
   Benign Cells in Sputum Samples 13
   Fiberoptic Bronchoscopic Specimens 18
   Fine Needle Aspirate Samples 19
   Bronchoalveolar Lavage 20

III. Cell Changes Currently *not* Associated with Neoplasia 23
   Cytologic Changes Specific to Cell Types 23
   Noncellular Elements 36

IV. Infectious Diseases 42
   Introduction 42
   Tuberculosis and Sarcoidosis 42
   Major Fungi Causing Granulomatous Inflammation in the Lung 44
      Histoplasmosis 46
      Coccidioidomycosis 47
      Cryptococcosis 51
      North American Blastomycosis 52
   Invasive Fungal Pneumonias 56
      Aspergillosis 58
      Mucormycosis (Phycomycosis) 62
   Fungi Variably Producing Disease 62
      Candidiasis 64
      Actinomycosis 64
      Nocardiosis 65
      Pneumocystis 67

Contents VI

    Viral Infections 72
    Specific Viral Infections 76
        Herpes Virus Type I 76
        Cytomegalovirus 78
        Varicella-Zoster Virus 80
        Measles Virus 82
        Adenovirus 82
        Respiratory Syncytial Virus 84
        Influenza Virus 84
    Bacterial Infections 84
    Infectious Rarities 85

V. Probable Preneoplastic Lesions and Their Role in Carcinogenesis
    of Lung Cancer 86

VI. Neoplasms of the Lung 93
    General Considerations 93
    Classification of Lung Tumors 95
        Squamous (Epidermoid) Carcinoma 96
        Adenocarcinoma 107
        Small Cell 'Oat Cell' Carcinoma 132
        Large Cell Undifferentiated Carcinoma 150
        Carcinoid Tumors 152
        Other Primary Lung Tumors 153
        Lymphomas and Leukemia 156
        Miscellaneous and Rare Tumors 162
        Metastatic Carcinoma to the Lungs 169
    Comparative Cytologic Criteria for Lung Tumors 169

VII. Diagnostic Accuracy of Pulmonary Cytology 189
    Historic Background 191
    Sputum Cytology 191
    Fiberoptic Bronchoscopy 195
    Fine Needle Aspiration of the Lung 197
    Bronchoalveolar Lavage 198
    Accuracy of Cell Typing 199

VIII. Into the Future (circa 1987) 203

IX. Appendix: Preparatory and Staining Procedures 207

    References 213

    Subject Index 229

Dedication

Once again, my children, Ann, James and Larry, waited patiently while this monograph took shape. It is living testimony to the lesson that my parents stressed: Nothing is impossible!

To all of them, for their love and understanding, this effort is dedicated.

Acknowledgements

I am fortunate that I have practiced cytology only since the invention of the fiberoptic bronchoscope. I cannot imagine life without it! To those who came before, I salute their skill in dealing with more art than science. To all those at UCLA who believe in cytodiagnosis of lung disease, my sincere thanks. Particular gratitude is owed to Dr. Donald Tierney, Chief of Pulmonary Disease at UCLA, and his flexible bronchoscopists, first Dr. Fouad Ben-Isaac, and now Dr. Henry Gong. Their productive collaboration is reflected in these pages; without them and the Pulmonary Fellows, this book would not have been possible. To the cytotechnologists on the UCLA Cytology Service, my special thanks for their care in the preparation and interpretation of the challenging specimens we receive on a daily basis.

A cytology text is only as good as its illustrations. Carol Appleton's skills in developing the negatives are obviously superb, and are only exceeded by her patience at my demands. The secretarial efforts of Rochelle Greenwald and Giok Brandt are much appreciated. Denise Greder and her editorial staff at Karger paid meticulous attention to the details which make a scientific text readable. My thanks to the UCLA pathology residents who humorously tolerated the time that this work stole from their education; my collective experience with them is in large part responsible for the final product. Finally, to Dr. George L. Wied and Mr. Thomas Karger, who convinced me that *another* book on respiratory cytology was needed, I hope this volume affirms their conviction.

Introduction

Respiratory cytology has assumed a primary diagnostic place in the order of the work-up for the patient with pulmonary disease. The importance placed upon the cytologic diagnosis has resulted from a cumulative experience of the past 25 years [115, 118, 130, 131, 139, 285]. The early years of cytology, from the 1940s through the 1950s, were devoted to samples from the female genital tract, and definitely established the discipline as diagnostically reliable. The simplicity and low cost of cytologic sampling made the technique attractive for other body sites. The coincidence of the now obvious world-wide epidemic of carcinoma of the lung, and the development of the fiberoptic bronchoscope [103, 228] accelerated the experience of cytopathologists with samples from the lower respiratory tract. Today, such specimens constitute the second most popular body site in most cytopathology laboratories which deal with both gynecologic and nongynecologic samples.

Although there are scattered early reports of diagnosis of lung cancer based on cell samples from expectorated sputum, it was not until the past quarter century that the need for screening of patients at risk for lung cancer saw the establishment of mass population screening programs, utilizing sputum cytologies. The great hope that such programs would effect the diagnosis of early lesions and thus improve the dismal salvage rate, did not prove true, and most of the general lung cancer screening projects have folded.

In current protocols for the work-up of patients with pulmonary disease, especially lung cancer, sputum cytology still plays a major role, and the diagnostic yield from sputum cytology alone in a patient with clear evidence of a lung neoplasm can be as high as the yield from bronchoscopically obtained specimens, depending on the cell type [113]. Sample adequacy is enhanced if the specimens are induced [185].

However, current practice has established the immediate use of the fiberoptic bronchoscope [37; 118, p. 8; 234] when a patient with evidence of pulmonary disease, either benign or neoplastic, presents to the pulmonologist. The overall diagnostic yield of fiberoptic bronchoscopy is too great to delay the procedure, waiting for diagnosis of a sputum sample. With cost-effectiveness being the keystone to medical survival, this technique is definitely one whose time is *now*.

While cancer diagnosis automatically comes to mind when considering respiratory cytodiagnosis, numerous infectious diseases can be definitely diagnosed or strongly suspected based on samples recovered either via fiberoptic bronchoscopy, bronchoalveolar lavage, or transthoracic needle aspiration. As the patient population becomes more complex, including the numerous immunocompromised patients from whatever cause, the need for astute non-neoplastic/infectious diagnosis is a mandate that the cytopathology laboratory cannot ignore. While special stains are a classic crutch, the portions of this book devoted to infectious disease will hopefully convince the reader that much information, frequently definitive, can be gained from material stained in the standard Papanicolaou manner. This allows treatment to begin within a few hours of collection of the diagnostic sample, with minimal expense.

When all factors are considered, the role of the cytotechnologist and cytopathologist in the management of patients with respiratory disease is key to the successful outcome of these patients. The high diagnostic yield of pulmonary cytodiagnosis is, without question, the result of a team approach. From our experience at UCLA, we strongly and enthusiastically emphasize the importance of close collaboration of the cytology staff with the bronchoscopy team and the thoracic radiologists. The excellent and highly diagnostic specimens which illustrate this book are the result of this cooperative effort.

I. Anatomy and Functional Histology

Anatomy

Numerous excellent texts exist which thoroughly describe the anatomy of the respiratory tract. The points covered below are those considered pertinent to a complete understanding of the types of specimens and their cellular components which are retrieved from the respiratory tract.

Although the upper airway is not the focus of this monograph, its subdivisions, and especially the epithelial lining of the upper respiratory tract must be considered. Cellular elements from there can contaminate specimens from the lower respiratory tract, either because the upper respiratory tract was inadvertently sampled during expectoration or bronchoscopy, or because these cells gravitated downward contaminating the specimen from the tracheobronchial tree.

The subdivisions of the upper respiratory tract include the nasal cavity, the oral cavity, the pharynx, and the larynx. The nasal cavity is the only portion which is covered by alternate areas of squamous and ciliated columnar epithelium, the latter containing occasional goblet cells. The oral cavity, the mesopharynx and hypopharynx are lined by stratified squamous epithelium, nonkeratinized in the healthy state. The laryngeal epithelium is a combination of ciliated columnar and stratified squamous [118, p. 31]. A very thorough and graphic description of the anatomy of the lower respiratory tract can be found in the *Atlas of Early Lung Cancer* [166], and salient features are extracted here.

Rather than assign names to the intrasegmental airways according to their size, which varies with the phase of inspiration or expiration, the airways are best named by their sequence distally from the trachea. The first order, the bronchi, have support cartilage, which can be demonstrated in any cut plane along the bronchus. More peripherally, cartilage is less frequent and may be missed in histologic sections. Once the cartilage plates disappear, the airways are termed bronchioles. The ciliated lining epithelia of the bronchioles is occasionally interrupted by alveoli and are the so-called respiratory bronchioli. This is the most proximal site of gaseous exchange and is also the beginning of the ciliary 'escalator'. The basic respiratory unit of the lung consists of a single terminal bronchiolus, usually three orders of respiratory bronchioles, and 2–9 alveolar ducts. Attached to these alveolar ducts are the alveolar sacs and together form an acinus which is approximately 1 cm across; this latter anatomic unit is the basic respiratory unit of the lung [24, p. 3].

Each of the bronchial branches and its accompanying pulmonary parenchyma constitutes an independent unit. This concept is most important when localization of a lesion, especially an occult lesion, is attempted by the bronchoscopist. With the skills of the fiberoptic bronchoscopist, 5th and 6th generation bronchial branches can be visualized and samples recovered directly from areas in question. Until recently, direct sampling was confined to the bronchial branches, but with the use of bronchoalveolar lavage (BAL), no segment of the respiratory tract is excluded from the probing eye of the cytopathologist.

Histology

To fully appreciate the fine points of respiratory histology, the reader is referred again to the *Atlas of Early Lung Cancer,* or other cited histology texts [26, 275]. The practicing cytologist must have a clear understanding of the cell population within the various compartments of the respiratory tract, appreciating the range of benign change before attempts at diagnosis of disease can be made (fig. 1).

The cells lining the various parts of the upper respiratory tract should be anticipated as they will be found from time to time in lower respiratory tract specimens. Fortunately, the epithelia are similar, except for the exaggerated length of the specialized ciliated columnar cells lining the nasopharynx.

The mouth, oropharynx, and hypopharynx shed mature stratified squamous epithelial cells, closely resembling those from the female genital tract, except that under normal conditions, true keratinization is not present. When such keratinization occurs, as in areas of chronic irritation from dentures or other trauma, the thick epithelium will become white and have the clinical appearance of 'leukoplakia'. Such cells must not be mis-

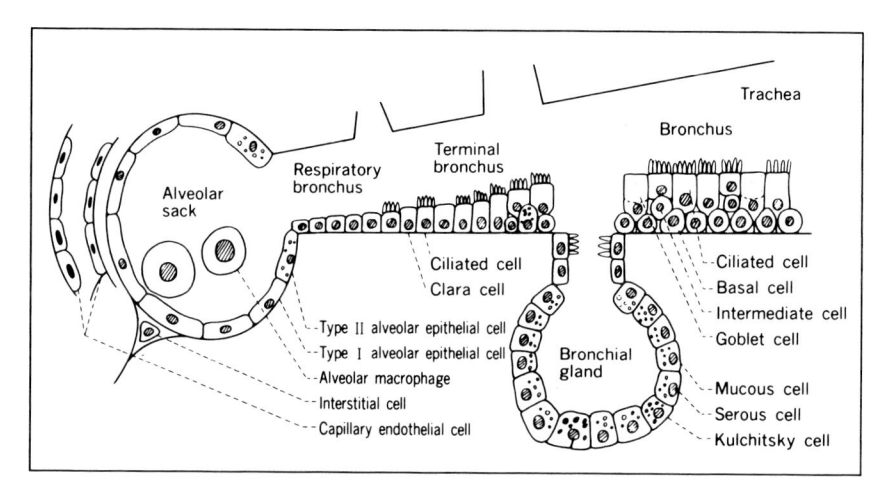

Fig. 1. Schematic of histologic structures and cell types in the lower respiratory tract [118]. Reproduced with permission of the authors and publishers.

taken for keratinizing squamous carcinoma either in the local area, or from the lower respiratory tract. More will be discussed of this pitfall when squamous carcinoma of the lung is the topic.

Submucosal Glands

Mucus-secreting glands are found from the larynx to the small bronchi, i.e. wherever supportive cartilage is present in the airway wall. Approximately 4,000 glands are present in the human trachea and, after birth, no new glands are formed. However, each gland unit is capable of cell proliferation to increase the size of the unit in response to disease such as chronic bronchitis [24, p.11].

Lymphoid Tissue

Such tissue within the lung can be categorized into three groups: (1) lymph nodes; (2) bronchus-associated lymphoid tissue (BALT); (3) lymphoreticular aggregates. Additionally, free lymphocytes, plasma cells, and mast cells may be scattered through the walls of the bronchi of disease-free adults [24, pp. 12–16].

Lymph nodes are situated in relation to large bronchi in the parabronchial tissue. They, therefore, do not directly contact the respiratory epithelium. They may be found as far out as the pleura.

BALT are aggregates of lymphoid tissue, which closely resemble Peyer's patches of the small intestines, and are most frequently found at airway bifurcations, probably in defense of the greatest concentration of inhaled antigens. BALT may be found anywhere within the bronchial mucosa. A distinctive overlying epithelium, lymphoepithelium, is formed by flattened nonciliated epithelial cells which may be infiltrated by lymphocytes. Although lymphatics have not been identified in BALT, postcapillary venules are present in the parafollicular region.

Lymphoreticular aggregates are small collections of lymphocytes, and scattered plasma cells and eosinophils which are widely distributed throughout the lung, especially around the bronchi, in the interlobular septa and in the pleura. These aggregates form the origin of pulmonary lymphatics, and monitor fluid and cells draining from the alveolar tissue. Alveolar macrophages carry particles not only out through the airway, but also into these aggregates for transport to the lymph nodes and beyond.

Pulmonary dust sumps are formed when macrophages phagocytize and condense dust from heavy atmospheric pollution in these lymphoreticular aggregates [24, p. 16].

Respiratory Epithelium

The trachea and bronchi are lined by a pseudostratified epithelium which consists of 4–5 principal cell types: basal or reserve cells, intermediate cells, goblet cells, and columnar cells with or without cilia. The term pseudostratified implies that all the cells rest on the basement membrane, but not all reach the airway lumen [24, p. 5].

Basal cells are rarely recovered in spontaneously exfoliated specimens, but can be seen in brushings and when there is rapid turnover of the epithelium. They are small cells, measuring 10–12 µm in diameter, with an irregularly round or oval nucleus, a conspicuous but small nucleolus, and scanty cytoplasm. These give rise to the other cell types. Turnover of respiratory epithelium is slow, with 1% of cells in division in the normal adult at any given time. Stimuli such as tobacco smoke will increase the mitotic index [24, p. 9].

Dense-core granulated cells are rare and usually basal in position, but thin cytoplasmic projections may reach the lumen. The demonstration of biogenic amines and peptides such as bombesin provides evidence of their regulatory function on the smooth muscle of blood vessels and bronchi, ciliary activity, and mucus secretion [24, p. 7].

Intermediate cells can be found just above the basal cell layer, being derived from them, and are slightly larger with more cytoplasm. These cells in turn give rise to either the ciliated columnar cells or mucus-secreting cells of the mature respiratory epithelium.

Ciliated columnar cells comprise approximately 85% of the respiratory epithelium. They extend from the basement membrane to the luminal surface. Nuclei are oval, slightly larger than the nuclei of the basal cells and in the resting epithelium, i.e. nonstimulated, are basally placed. Basal and intermediate cells will compress the apical end of the cell which is attached to the basement membrane and lift the nucleus toward the center of the cell, providing the pseudostratified appearance. The thick terminal bar at the luminal surface supports the cilia. Cilia are considered the hallmark of a benign respiratory epithelial cell, and any ciliated cell, no matter how anaplastic appearing, should be categorized as benign. Each of the 200–300 cilia per cell beats at approximately 1,000 times per minute to propel substances rostrally. The terminal bar of the respiratory mucosa prevents excess fluid movement across the epithelium. However, after tobacco smoke or ether exposure the epithelium appears to become permeable to molecular weight substances of approximately 40,000 molecular weight.

Nonciliated columnar cells are less common and are usually found more frequently toward the more peripheral radicals of the bronchial tree. Although they have surface microvilli, these are not appreciable by light microscopy. Interspersed at a ratio of 1:5–6 [118, p. 32] are *mucus* or *goblet cells,* which compose approximately 15% of the total columnar epithelial cells. They are similar in appearance to the ciliated columnar cells but their cytoplasm adjacent to the lumen contains an acid mucin, a product correct in viscosity and amount to maintain mucociliary clearance, which can easily be moved by cilia and/or cough. The number of such cells increases in disease or by exogenous irritants such as tobacco smoke and sulfur dioxide [24, p. 7]. These cells can increase in number, so-called mucus metaplasia (goblet cell hyperplasia), if an altered physiologic state so demands (see p. 30).

As the terminal bronchioles are approached, goblet cells disappear as well as cilia. *Clara cells* are now encountered for the first time in the very small bronchioles. These are nonciliated cells, which present a bulging appearance, and although their function has not been well established, they probably play a role in the production of surfactant. They may behave as stem cells in the absence of basal cells. At the end of the respiratory bronchioles, the duct divides into two or more alveolar ducts and then opens into alveolar sacs and alveoli. The respiratory lining at the bronchiole level measuring 0.5 mm or less in diameter is nonciliated cuboidal epithelium with occasional retained cilia.

Pulmonary Alveoli

The major functional units of the lung, concerned with gas exchange, are the pulmonary alveoli. These are separated from each other by the alveolar walls, consisting of a supportive connective tissue framework, the interstitium, in which pulmonary capillaries course. The alveolar walls are covered by a continuous thin alveolar epithelium which sometimes fuses with the endothelial basement membrane resulting in an extremely short distance between alveolar gas and capillary blood [24, pp. 19–20].

The *alveolar epithelium* is a simple continuous sheet, composed of two cell types, type 1 and type 2 pneumocytes (syn: 1 and 2, a and b, small and large, nonvacuolated and vacuolated, membranous [squamous] and granular, respectively). The junction between the cuboidal epithelium lining the bronchioles and the pneumocytes is sometimes abrupt, although, embryologically, all of the epithelium of the respiratory tract is derived from the primitive endodermal lung bud. The basement membrane is continuous throughout the entire respiratory tract supporting both the respiratory ciliated epithelium and the alveolar epithelium.

Type 1 pneumocytes cover the greater area of the alveolar walls in a monolayer. Their thinness, no more than 0.2 µm, facilitates rapid gas exchange. They contain few organelles, e.g. mitochondria, and are very sensitive to damage by a variety of agents.

Type 2 pneumocytes are taller, more numerous than type 1, but cover less of the alveolar septa. They are commonly found at the corners of alveoli and are frequently covered over by type 1 pneumocytes, except for a small free surface which has blunt microvilli. The cytoplasm contains numerous organelles, mitochondria, rough endoplasmic reticulum, Golgi apparatus, and the secretory vacuoles of pulmonary surfactant, i.e. osmiophilic lamellar structures.

Following injury, type 2 cells will replace the easily destroyed type 1 pneumocytes, providing evidence that the type 2 cell behaves as a stem cell for both. An intermediate cell between the type 1 and type 2 cell provides further evidence to this theory, and can be seen following alveolar wall damage. Animal studies have demonstrated the turnover time of type II cells to be 25 days; transformation of type 2 to type 1 cells occurs in 2 days. This cell is the site of active transport of solutes across the gas-blood barrier [29].

Anatomy and Functional Histology

Alveolar capillary walls play an important role in the blood-gas barrier when the endothelium is fused to the alveolar epithelium to form a single membrane of approximately 0.15 µm thick. In other places, the interstitial tissue separates the two layers to produce an air-blood barrier up to 12 µm thick. Weibel and Knight [273] demonstrated that the air-blood barrier consists of the alveolar epithelium (30%), the interstitium (40%), and the capillary endothelium (30%).

Alveolar Interstitium
The supporting framework of the alveolar wall is the alveolar interstitium, which contains collagen and elastin fibers, unmyelinated axons with two types of nerve endings, and interstitial cells. This interstitium is the termination of the peribronchial connective tissue also attached to the connective tissue of the interlobular septa, and the pleural connective tissue. Lymphatics are not present in the alveolar interstitium, but fluid flows from the alveolar spaces to the more proximal interstitium of the peribronchial connective tissue, where the lymphatics begin. In addition to the above cells, mast cells and a cell intermediate between blood monocytes and alveolar macrophages have been demonstrated. The latter may be the origin of alveolar macrophages [24, p. 21].

Alveolar Macrophages
These cells are the hallmark of a 'deep cough' sputum specimen. The origin of alveolar macrophages (fig. 2) is controversial and under intense investigation. All research considered together, the data suggest that the origin of new alveolar macrophages is bone-marrow-derived monocytes under normal conditions. Under an inflammatory stimulus, cells already in the lung (stem cells and macrophages) have been seen to divide, and are probably the origin of the increased numbers of alveolar macrophages needed in inflammatory conditions. The differences in the morphologic characteristics between the blood monocyte and the alveolar macrophage are probably environmental [24, p. 122].

Alveolar macrophages are probable mediators of immune responses in the lung. They also provide enormous phagocytic capabilities, an important defense against inhaled bacteria and other harmful elements. Phagocytosis is enhanced by surfactant, which, once exhausted, is then removed by the alveolar macrophage.

The visual appearance of the macrophage is greatly dependent upon which of its roles it is performing. When containing particulate matter, the cytoplasm is the more prominent portion of the cell, and reflects the material contained therein. When activated in response to an immune situation, the nucleus becomes more prominent and nucleoli are activated and conspicuous.

Multinucleated giant cells are produced by fusion of alveolar macrophages in response to a macrophage fusion factor released from mitogen-stimulated lymphocytes. Lymphokines will also induce macrophage aggregation, migration, and inhibition.

After surviving approximately 7 days in the alveoli, alveolar macrophages exit the lung via the pharynx by ciliary transport, and are either swallowed or expectorated. Approximately 5 million macrophages take this journey every hour. Except for migration into dust sumps, macrophages are not thought to re-enter the pulmonary interstitium [24, p. 22]. The pulmonary macrophages are also responsible for the ingestion, digestion and clearing of neutrophil infiltrates. This process is no doubt responsible for the often observed phenomenon of an intense neutrophilic infiltrate initially, with no residual damage to the underlying lung.

Neutrophils

Although neutrophils are considered to be the hallmark of acute inflammation, and thus an abnormal situation within the pulmonary parenchyma, recent work has convincingly demonstrated that a small number of neutrophils can be found in alveoli at all times, and represent approximately 2% of cells found in BALs (fig. 3). The source of these neutrophils is no doubt the peripheral blood where they are located at the margins of the capillaries adherent to the endothelium. This position allows them to be rapidly released through the interstitium of the lung into the alveolar spaces in response to inflammatory stimuli [24, p. 121]. The mechanism of passage of neutrophils into the alveolar spaces is not clearly understood. Several researchers have suggested that neutrophils as well as

---

Fig. 2. Pulmonary macrophages (bronchial wash): These cells are found in streams of mucus in sputa, in which they are the hallmark of a deep cough, and in bronchoscopy specimens. Their cytoplasm is variable, opaque to finely vacuolated, and cytoplasmic rims are usually distinct. Nuclei are most commonly eccentrically placed, bean-shaped, with finely to coarsely granular chromatin and inconspicuous nucleoli. If many lipid-laden macrophages are present (*b*), a lipid pneumonia can be suspected. Papanicolaou. $a = \times 360; b = \times 900$.

Anatomy and Functional Histology

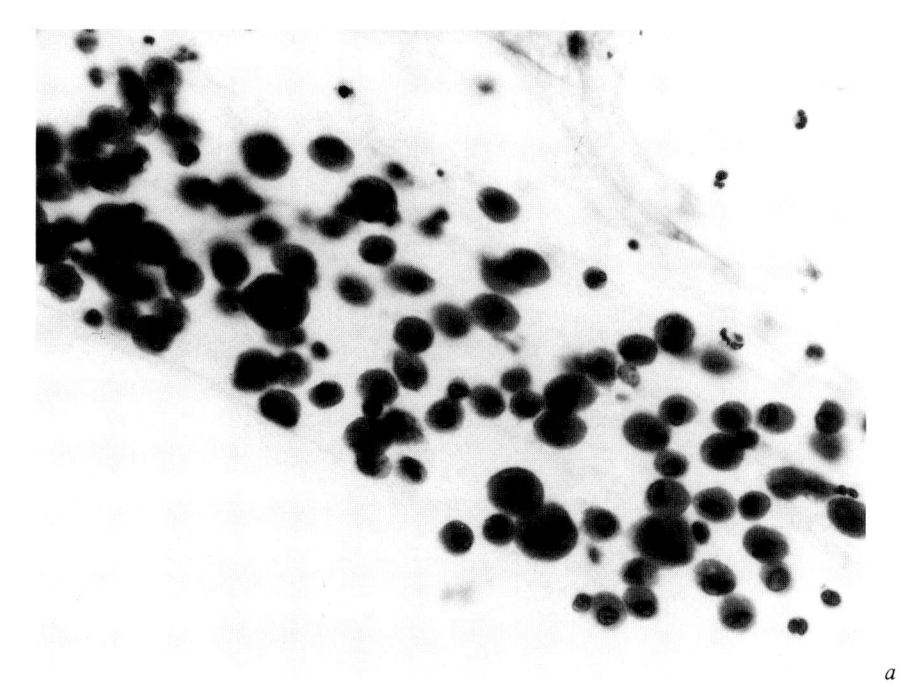

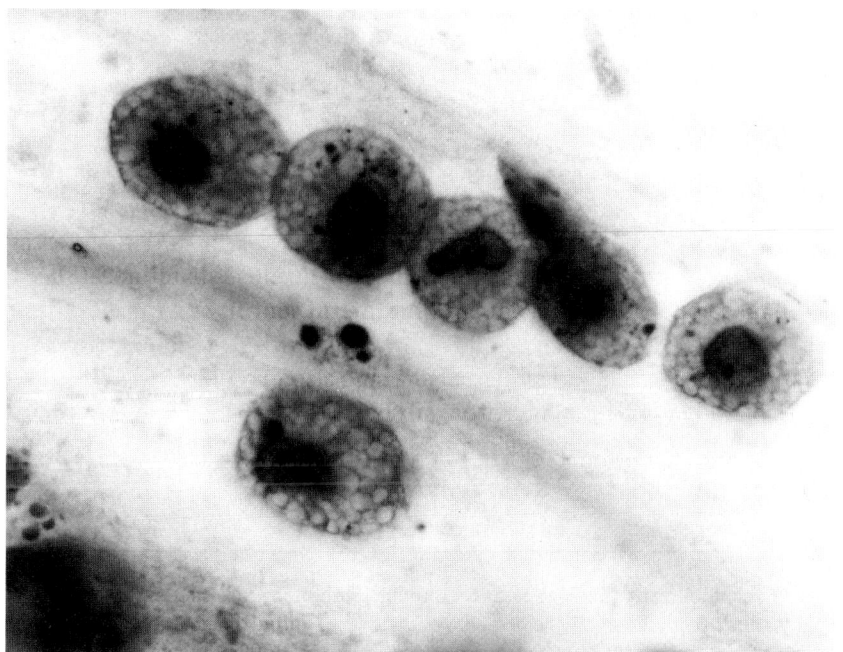

a

b

metastatic tumor cells are capable of proteolytically digesting a path through capillary basement membranes [24, p. 126].

Neutrophils in excessive numbers within the lung can be both protective as well as destructive. A neutrophil-filled lung in pneumococcal pneumonia can resolve with proper treatment with no residual damage. Conversely, neutrophil-derived proteinases are considered the probable cause of the destruction seen in emphysema and neutrophil-derived oxygen radicals are undergoing intense investigation and implication as inducers of pulmonary fibrosis [24, p. 129]. Neutrophils die after performing their function, resulting in abundant cellular debris. Such cell death with release of organelles could well be an initiator of a clean-up and repair process. Pulmonary macrophages ingest the end product of neutrophils and carry them up through the airway as described above [24, p. 133].

Lymphocytes

Lymphocytes make up approximately 10% of the bronchoalveolar cell population. In smokers, the relative percentage of lymphocytes is decreased, but the absolute lymphocyte count is elevated about 2–3 times; the largest increase in smokers is in total number of macrophages.

T, B, and null cells can be identified, as in peripheral blood, based on surface marker studies. The proportion of T and B lymphocytes studied from BALs closely approximates the proportion in the peripheral blood. T lymphocytes comprise 60–70% found in normal BAL fluid; 10–15% can be identified as B cells. A smaller proportion can be categorized as null cells. This latter group of cells is curious because of the greater proportion in the lung when compared with peripheral blood. Speculation suggests that killer or cytotoxic lymphocytes may be part of this cell group [24, p. 167].

The functions of these lymphocytes are similar to that found within peripheral blood lymphocytes, i.e. T lymphocytes are involved with cell mediated immunity, form rosettes with sheep red blood cells, and can be subdivided into T-helper and T-suppressor cells. In small and preliminary studies, the percentages of these two subgroups are identical to those found in peripheral blood [102].

Fig. 3. Pulmonary macrophages (BAL): The predominant cell in a BAL, the macrophage frequently contains particulate matter in its cytoplasm, the most common being carbon pigment. Papanicolaou. $a = \times 180$; $b = \times 360$.

Anatomy and Functional Histology

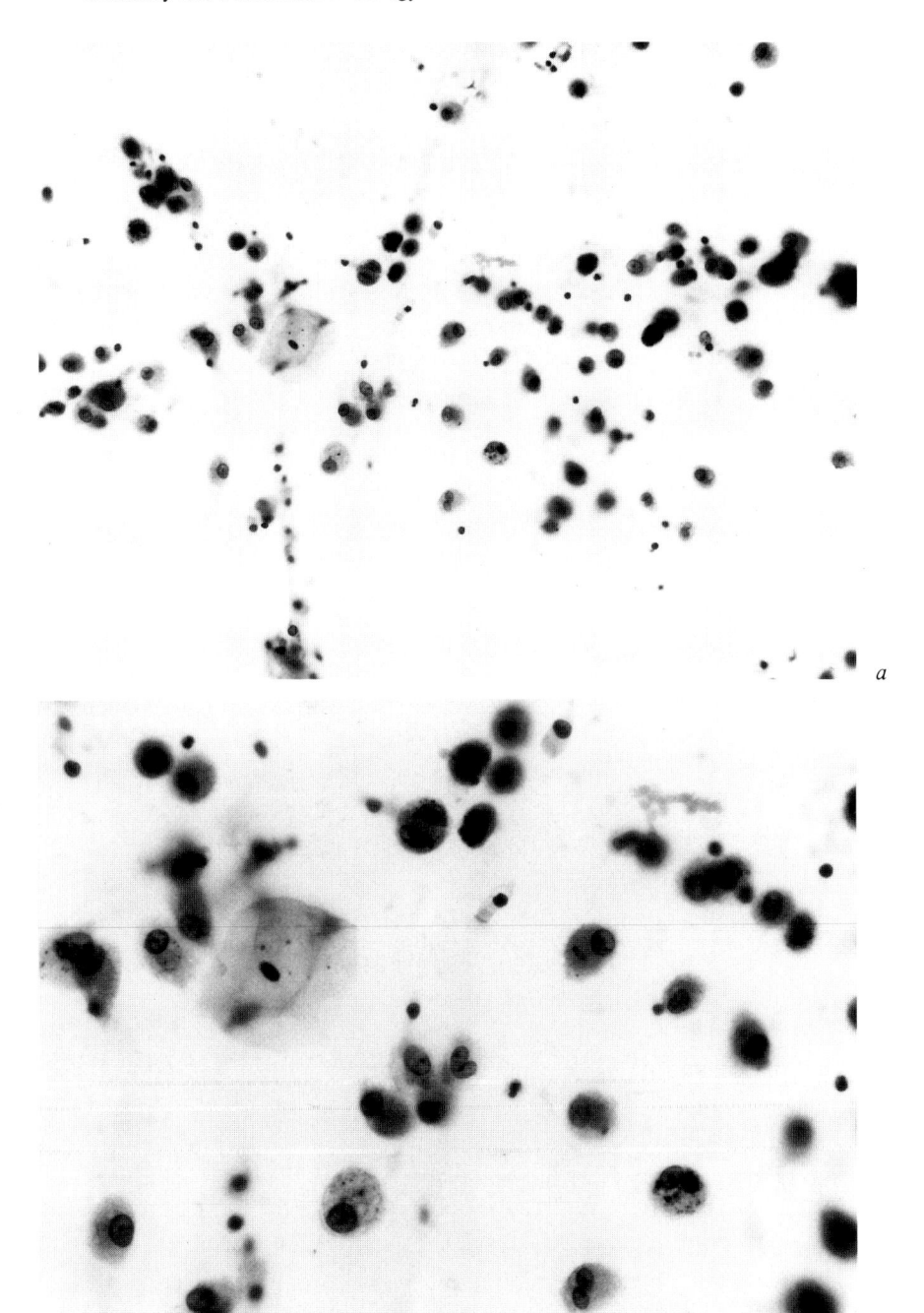

a

b

Eosinophils

Pulmonary eosinophilia is associated with numerous clinical disorders; the description is far beyond the scope of this monograph. As in general disease processes, the identification of eosinophilia immediately calls to mind helminthic infections, hypersensitivity reactions, vascular disease, granulomas, and in the case of the lungs, specifically, bronchogenic carcinoma. In addition to biologic properties similar to the general category of neutrophils, eosinophilic granules possess a specific destructive agent within the large crystalloid granules. Such destruction is classically aimed at helminthic larvae. The cells are also invariably seen in chronic bronchial asthma. The place of eosinophils in IgE-mediated allergic disease may be linked to its capacity to inactivate mast cell mediators. A more attractive current theory is that eosinophils are mistakenly recruited to fight allergic disease in which the allergens have been confused with parasitic worms [24, p. 151].

II. Variations among Benign Cellular Elements in Exfoliated and Aspirated Material

The expected cellular elements found in a cytologic specimen from the respiratory tract will vary somewhat depending upon the method of obtaining the specimen. Cells exfoliated spontaneously, retained in pulmonary secretions, and expectorated or suctioned after an unknown period of time will display degenerative changes, whereas specimens obtained from a needle aspiration of a tumor or infectious material will contain extremely fresh cells whose characteristics will be somewhat different from degenerated cells. To the novice, fine needle aspirate samples can present diagnostic difficulties if the observer is depending upon the traditional criteria learned on exfoliated material [27, 90]. This is especially true of the less-well-differentiated neoplasms of the lung. In general, if criteria learned on spontaneously exfoliated material are applied to freshly acquired, i.e. brushed or aspirated cell samples, the microscopist must remember to allow for the differences between dying cells and freshly obtained cells.

Benign Cells in Sputum Samples

Cells recovered in sputum samples consist of both epithelial and non-epithelial cells. The epithelial cells usually are from the mouth and lower respiratory tract, but occasional contamination by nasopharyngeal cells also occurs. Cells from the mouth are of the squamous type, occasionally including parabasal cells (not to be confused with metaplastic cells of the respiratory epithelium), intermediate and superficial squamous cells, with prekeratin formation. True keratinization will not be encountered unless an area of leukoplakia or hyperkeratosis from a fungal infection is present. Extensive keratinization must be a warning that an underlying squamous carcinoma may be present.

Cells from the lower respiratory tract include ciliated columnar cells, goblet cells, and rarely basal cells. Basal cells will be found in tight clusters, so-called reserve cell hyperplasia, if a stimulating factor is present. In addition to epithelial cells, alveolar macrophages, lymphocytes and neutrophils can be noted. The hallmark of a deep cough specimen is the *alveolar mac-*

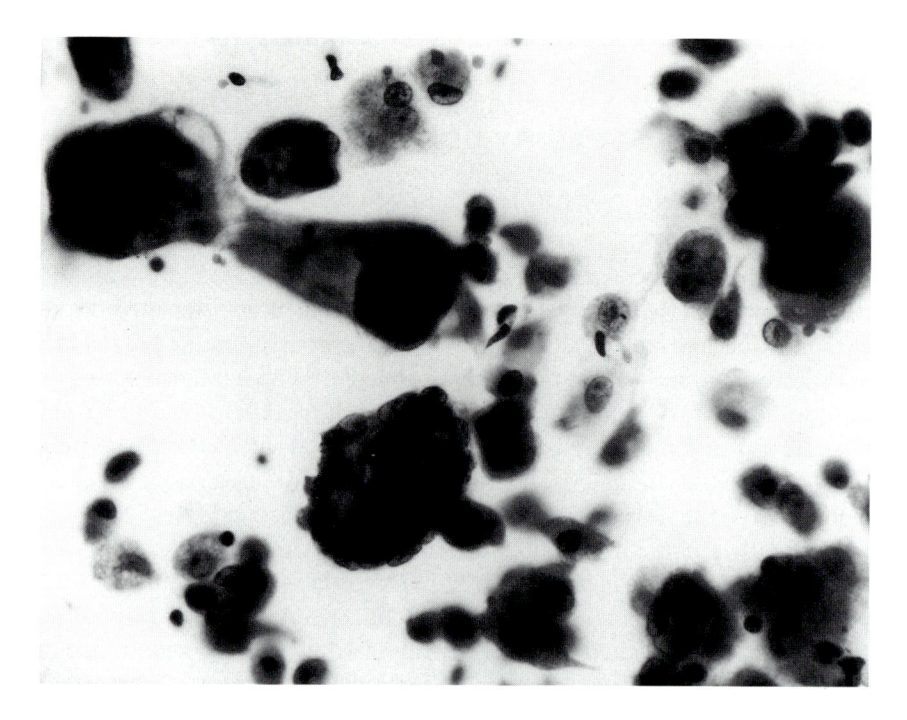

Fig. 4. Multinucleated histiocytes (BAL): An occasional giant cell in a sputum, wash, or BAL may be insignificant or raise the question of a granuloma. However, this presentation demands a search for granulomatous disease. The patient has biopsy-proven sarcoidosis. Papanicolaou. × 360.

rophage (fig. 3), usually containing varying amounts of intracytoplasmic pigment or 'dust'. This cell is frequently bi- or multinucleated, and can be found either in streams, or aggregates, if the deep cough is a good one. Lipid may indicate a lipid pneumonia [200]. Increased amounts of carbon pigment may suggest the patient has pneumoconiosis [126]. Numbers of multinucleated giant cells may indicate granulomatous disease (fig. 4) or

Fig. 5. a Benign lymphocytes (sputum): A stream of small mononuclear round cells can be appreciated as lymphocytes. They are detached cells with no relationship to each other, except that they are suspended in a shared stream of mucus. Compare with *b*. Papanicolaou stain. × 400. *b* Lymphoma (sputum): A similar configuration of cells is seen compared to those benign lymphocytes in figure 5a, except that the cells are larger, vary in size within the group, and have convoluted nuclear outlines. Papanicolaou. × 340.

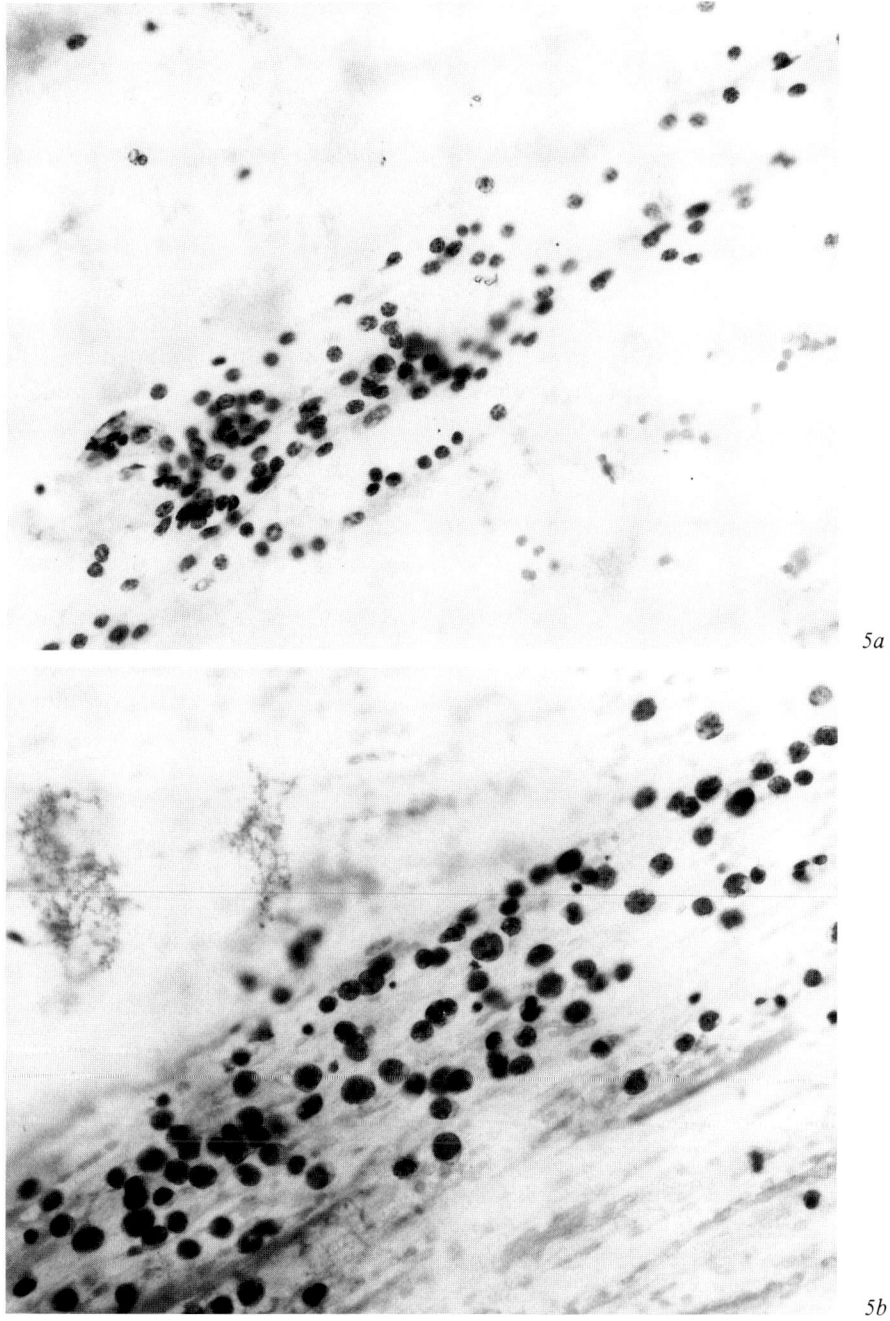

Variations among Cellular Elements in Exfoliated and Aspirated Material 15

5a

5b

giant interstitial pneumonia [255]. Hemosiderin is frequently seen in macrophages of patients with embolism and/or infarct [233].

Lymphocytes (fig. 5a) in small numbers can be ignored, but if streams or clusters are found, the differential diagnosis should include chronic infection, such as fungal disease, sarcoidosis, or tuberculosis; leukemia/lymphoma (fig. 5b), which should have an accompanying history of same; or host response to a cancer, which should also be noted in the patient's history.

Columnar cells (fig. 6) can be found singly and in clusters in routine sputum samples, but most have lost their cilia, with only the blunt, slightly thickened terminal plate remaining. Occasionally, tufts of cilia attached to fragments of cytoplasm can be seen, so-called ciliacytophthoria, a seldom used term, probably because of its difficult pronunciation, and even harder spelling. The nucleus of columnar cells, located toward the pointed or apical end of the cell, is round with a finely granular chromatin. Nucleoli will be either inconspicuous or prominent depending upon the stage of activity of the cell, and occasional multinucleation can be seen in a rapidly reproducing cell.

Goblet cells, cousins to the ciliated columnar cells, but without cilia, are infrequently encountered in spontaneous sputa. The cytoplasm of these cells is distended by mucous vacuoles, and the nucleus, which is essentially identical to the ciliated columnar cell, is frequently compressed or displaced by such vacuoles.

Basal cells are rarely found in sputum samples, and have circular shapes, large round nuclei possessing fine granular chromatin, and high nuclear-cytoplasmic ratios. Small nucleoli are usually noted. If such cells are numerous or appear in clusters, basal cell hyperplasia should be considered, and the cause sought. Basal cells should be distinguished from small cell carcinoma, carcinoid tumor, and lymphocytes as well as squamous metaplastic cells from either the mouth or respiratory epithelium.

Fig. 6. Ciliated respiratory epithelial cells (bronchial brush): These columnar cells have specialized cilia, which are attached to a distinct terminal plate. At the opposite end of the cell, the nucleus contains finely to coarsely granular chromatin with inconspicuous nucleoli. Goblet cells can be found interspersed among the ciliated cells. If the cytoplasm is attenuated, as in *b*, the cell is most likely from the nasopharynx. Cilia can still be seen if the cells are very fresh. Papanicolaou. *a, b* = × 900.

a

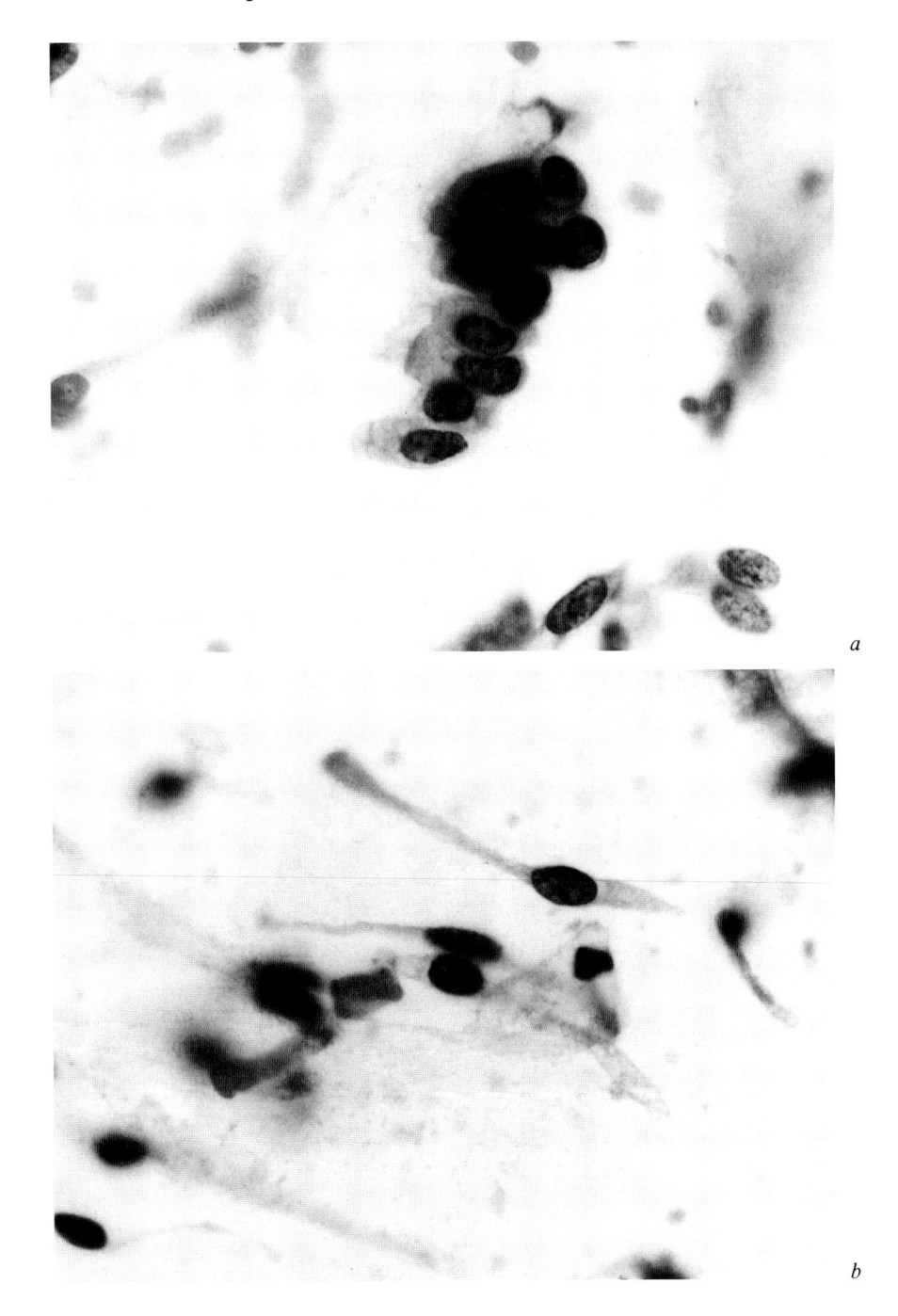

b

Fiberoptic Bronchoscopic Specimens

Cells obtained in *washings* at fiberoptic bronchoscopy (not BAL specimens) have cells quite similar to those found in sputum specimens, except that the degree of degeneration is usually considerably less. Clusters of respiratory epithelium, with intact cilia, and numerous macrophages and inflammatory cells are usually found in washing specimens. If the bronchial biopsy has been performed, then varying amounts of fresh blood will be found in the specimen. If, however, fibrinated blood and/or blood pigment within macrophages are present, then previous bleeding can be assumed.

By far, the freshest, and most diagnostic specimen of the exfoliative type is the *bronchial brushing*. Even before the advent of the fiberoptic bronchoscope, brushing samples were obtained using a polyethylene catheter through which a tiny brush was threaded. These were fluoroscopically directed, but the brushing was done relatively blindly [23, 256]. With the fiberoptic bronchoscope, the brush can be visually directed at any suspicious area and usually excellent diagnostic material can be recovered. The real trick of getting optimal sampling is the way in which the material is transferred from the brush to the slide. With any delay, or smearing too thinly, the material will air-dry, resulting in the usual disastrous results. Our advice to clinicians is to manipulate the brush quickly, have the fixative bottle open and nearby, and, using a circular and rolling motion, transfer the mucoid material from the brush to the slide in an area the size of a nickel (2 cm). If more material is obtained than can easily fit in this area, a second slide should be utilized.

The major difference between brushed and washed or exfoliated cells resides in the phenomenon of cells rounding up when in liquid media. In a brushing sample, rounding up does not occur: the material is spread, hopefully not with too much pressure or too thinly, so that the architecture of cell fragments can be appreciated, and intercellular relationships preserved. Therefore, 'mini-biopsies' of benign epithelium or tumor will be represented in a good brushing. Hyperplasia of respiratory epithelium is a good example of a benign condition easily appreciated on a brushing. When tumors are discussed, the reader will appreciate the amount of information that can be derived from a brush sampling, essentially as diagnostic as a tissue biopsy. One of the pitfalls for the inexperienced with brushings is the same as that for the inexperienced observer of fine needle aspirates, i.e. misinterpreting the degree of differentiation of a tumor because of the freshness of the sample. This same mistake is usually not a problem when dealing with benign samples. The only possibility that comes to mind is misinterpreting basal cell or reserve cell hyperplasia for an oat-cell carcinoma. If the material is well presented on the slide, the cytoplasmic framework of the basal cell hyperplasia can be contrasted with the inconspicuous amount of cytoplasm and lack of adherence of the cells of an oat-cell carcinoma.

Fine Needle Aspirate Samples

All that can be said about brushing samples applies to fine needle aspirates, especially concerning the freshness of the cells. With good preservation, and adequate sampling, such specimens essentially replace a tissue biopsy. The major consideration is to confirm that the material aspirated was definitely from the area assumed to be sampled. In other words, if a negative non-neoplastic sample is obtained, is this sample definitely representative of the target area? This is a difficult question to answer, but several guidelines are helpful.

First, the microscopist is reliant on the aspirator, either radiologist, or bronchoscopist. If the needle aspirate has been obtained via the bronchoscope, the area in question has usually been visualized, the needle seen piercing the mucosa or entering the lesion, so that the material aspirated is localized with a high degree of confidence. Sometimes, however, the needle may penetrate the respiratory mucosa, but not truly enter a lesion, and recover only respiratory epithelium, or lymphoid material from BALT. If the lesion is surrounded by a mantle of fibrosis, the needle aspiration may be even more difficult and less likely productive. Therefore, if only respiratory epithelium is seen on a needle aspirate of a transbronchial approach, the specimen should be considered inadequate.

Different parameters should be used when evaluating a fine needle aspirate from the transthoracic approach. Once again, the radiologist should be queried as to the position of the needle in the lesion. Ideally, the microscopic interpreter should be in the room at the time of the aspiration to verify the location of the needle, as well as to immediately ascertain that sufficient material has been obtained for interpretation.

Microscopically, mesothelial cells can present a real hazard, for their interpretation as intraparenchymal epithelial cells, i.e. tumor, should be avoided at all costs. Remembering the classic appearance of mesothelial cells, even the highly reactive ones, can prevent such an overcall. Alveolar macrophages and respiratory epithelial cells from small bronchioles should also be sought, to identify that the needle was actually within the lung. Encountering multinucleated histiocytes should not lull the diagnostician into calling the lesion a granuloma, unless this type of lesion is high on the diagnostic differential list. Such granulomatous reaction can be seen surrounding a tumor, especially squamous cell carcinoma (fig. 7). These giant histiocytes are no doubt in reaction to the 'foreign body' that is the tumor. In addition to the cells mentioned, chunks of fibrous tissue and muscle can be aspirated and should be identified reliably. Unexpected materials such as sequestered exogenous material from an aspiration pneumonia should be considered if plant (vegetable) cells are encountered [46].

Bronchoalveolar Lavage

In order to study the components of the immune system found within the small airways and in alveolar air spaces the technique of BAL has been used recently with encouraging results [102]. Even with access to the peripheral lung parenchyma by the fiberoptic bronchoscope, the usual sampling by washing, brushing, and forceps biopsy has not provided samples which truly reflect the cellular components of the alveolar air spaces. In addition to its usefulness in research, BAL can provide reliable diagnoses of reaction to pollutants [160], interstitial lung diseases, and opportunistic pulmonary infections [51], such as pneumocystis (fig. 8), CMV and herpes [254]. Its safety and patient acceptance enable repeat performances to provide a longitudinal evaluation of the patient.

The method: the patient is premedicated into a relaxed state and topical anesthesia to the nasopharynx and trachea is applied. The broncho-

Fig. 7. Multinucleated histiocyte, benign, from a case of squamous cell carcinoma (FNA): This multinucleated giant histiocyte is indeed benign, and is no doubt from a granulomatous reaction to the keratin produced by a squamous cell carcinoma. Such is a common reaction to tumor within the lung, especially squamous cell carcinoma, as the keratin behaves as a foreign body. Note the globs of opaque cytoplasm (arrows), derived from the tumor adjacent to the giant cell. Papanicolaou. × 340.

Fig. 8. Pneumocystis (BAL): Even on very low power, the spongy aggregates of organisms provide definitive diagnosis in this specimen from the alveoli. See figures 37 and 38. Papanicolaou. × 170.

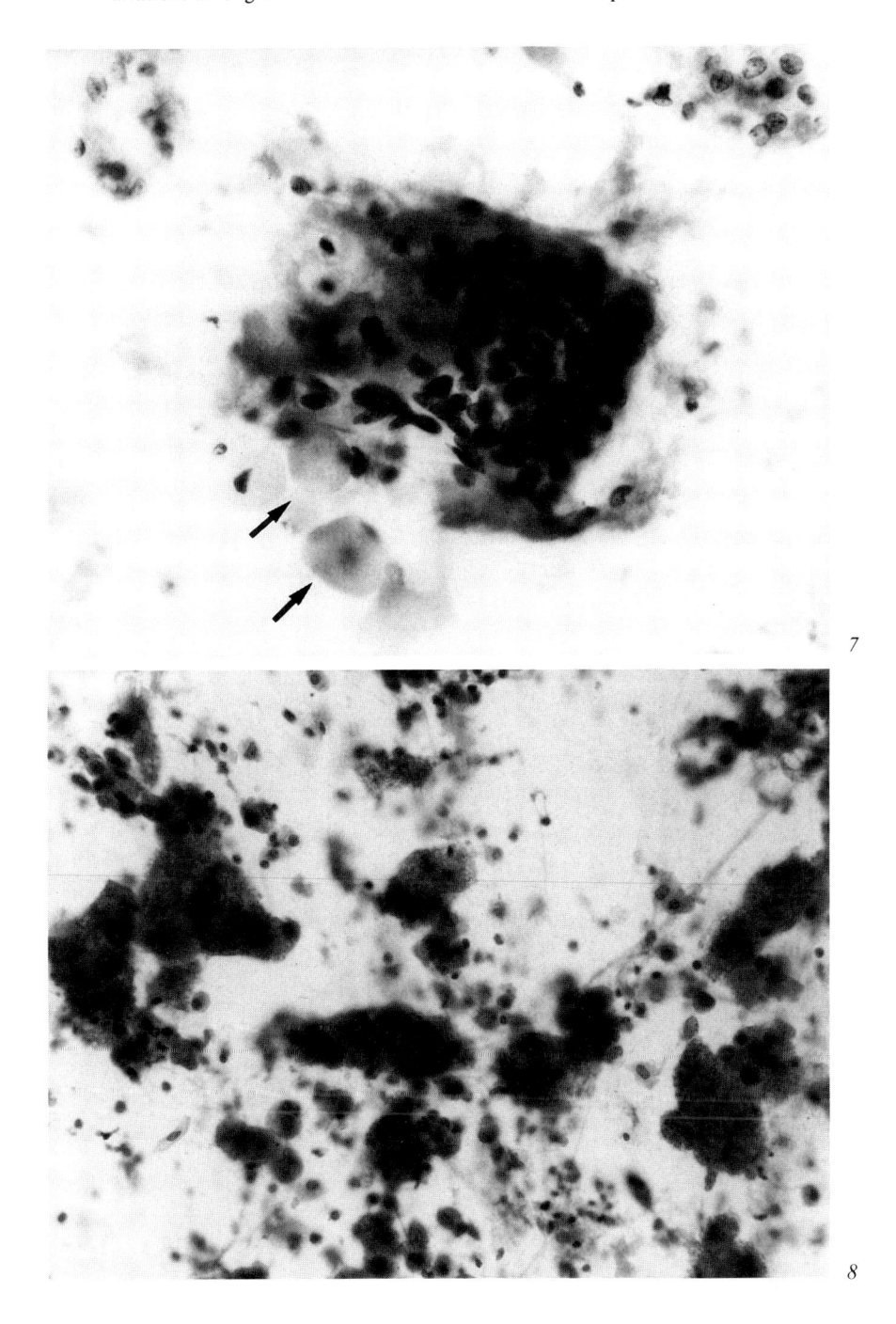

Variations among Cellular Elements in Exfoliated and Aspirated Material 21

scope is passed in the usual manner into the airways and wedged into a convenient third or fourth bronchial segment. Three hundred milliliters of sterile isotonic saline is instilled in 50-ml aliquots and aspirated with a suitable syringe. Approximately 50–75% of the wash can be recovered and contains cellular components as well as noncellular substances, primarily proteins or lipids (surfactant). The proteins can be studied in relation to their role in the immune response [102].

To the cytologist, the cellular constituents are of great interest. The cell elements are centrifuged at 500 g into a pellet which is resuspended and washed in a balanced salt solution. A numeric estimate of inflammatory and respiratory cells is accomplished with a hemocytometer and a Wright stain. Macrophages can be readily identified with the use of neutral red dye or dyes for esterase. Viability of the cells can be verified by their ability to exclude Trypan blue or other nonvital dye [24, p. 164]. The expected lavage of a normal nonsmoker contains 10–20 million respiratory cells. Approximately 90% of the cells in a BAL are alveolar macrophages. The remaining cells are usually lymphocytes with only a small number of neutrophils. Eosinophils and basophils are rare. Smokers yield many more cells (4–5 × normal) than nonsmokers with a relative decrease in lymphocytes but a finite increase [102]. This increase correlates roughly with the extent and duration of the smoking history.

Considerable work is accumulating to describe disease patterns reflected by the differential counts of the cells recovered in BAL specimens. This is particularly true with the granulomatous and nongranulomatous interstitial lung diseases [44], whose diagnoses previously relied upon open lung biopsy. The accurate diagnosis of opportunistic infectious disease by the same method is increasing the popularity of the BAL and will be discussed in chapter IV. The simplicity of the procedure, the low cost, the minor morbidity and the ability to follow a disease with a minimally invasive procedure makes BAL a technique with a promising future [24, p. 164].

III. Cell Changes Currently *not* Associated with Neoplasia

The components of the lung, like all other biologic entities, react to stimuli in a limited variety of ways in order to restore homeostasis. Frost et al. [166, p. 40] eloquently summarize responses of the lung 'resulting from chronic inflammation and irritation, hypersensitivity, irradiation, drug therapy or chemotherapy, and viral diseases. Although lung tissues react to their environment in only a few basic ways, combinations of changes can produce a wide range of morphologic abnormalities that may be mistaken for cancer.

'Normally functioning cells display rounding and regularity of the nucleus with predictable configuration of nuclear chromatin, chromatinic rim, parachromatin, and nucleoli.

'Increased cellular activity, including stimulation, repair and replication, is characterized by increased undulation of the nuclear membrane, chromatin granularity, parachromatin clearing, prominent nucleoli, mitosis, multinucleation, and cytoplasmic immaturity.

'Decreased cellular activity secondary to injury, aging, degeneration, or death produces blurring of the nuclear chromatin, clumping, alteration of chromasia, cytoplasmic acidophilia, fragmentation, and loss of cell borders.

'Mixtures of these three levels of cellular activity may cause structural abnormalities closely resembling cancer. However, true malignant disease exhibits additional morphologic characteristics that are specifically associated with cancer.'

Cytologic Changes Specific to Cell Types

With the above guidelines in mind, general changes of specific benign cell types will be described in the following pages, but those changes thought to precede true malignancy, i.e. the metaplasias, will be covered in chapter V.

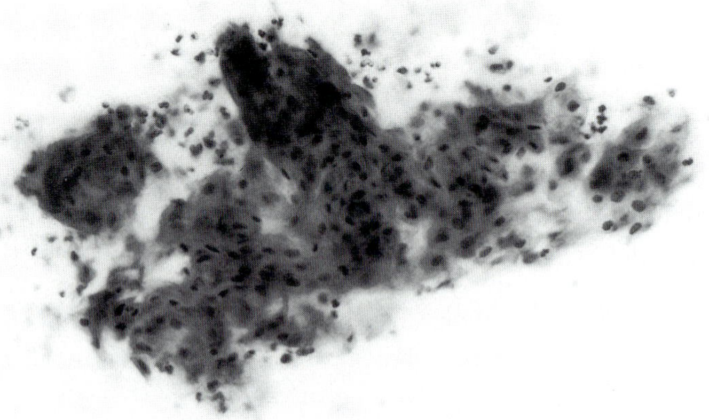

Fig. 9. Squamous metaplasia and keratosis (sputum): From an area of squamous metaplasia, this hyperkeratotic fragment could be either from the mouth, especially in a patient with oral candidiasis, or from the lower respiratory tract. Papanicolaou. × 180.

Benign Squamous Cells

Squamous cells from the mouth respond to irritants in the same manner that squamous cells from the female genital tract respond to infection and irritation, i.e. with accelerated maturation. Therefore, if dentures or other appliances irritate a squamous focus, hyperkeratinization will occur and will be reflected by true keratin formation in *large* squamoid cells (fig. 9). Since there is no squamocolumnar junction in the same sense as in the uterine cervix, smaller metaplastic cells are usually not encountered in the mouth, unless ulceration with healing has occurred, and basal cells have become dyskeratotic.

Fungi, especially Candida, will become pathogenic under certain circumstances, grow in the squamous epithelium (fig. 10), and produce a dramatic hyperkeratosis. Such lesions should be investigated thoroughly, including a full thickness biopsy, to exclude squamous carcinoma. These

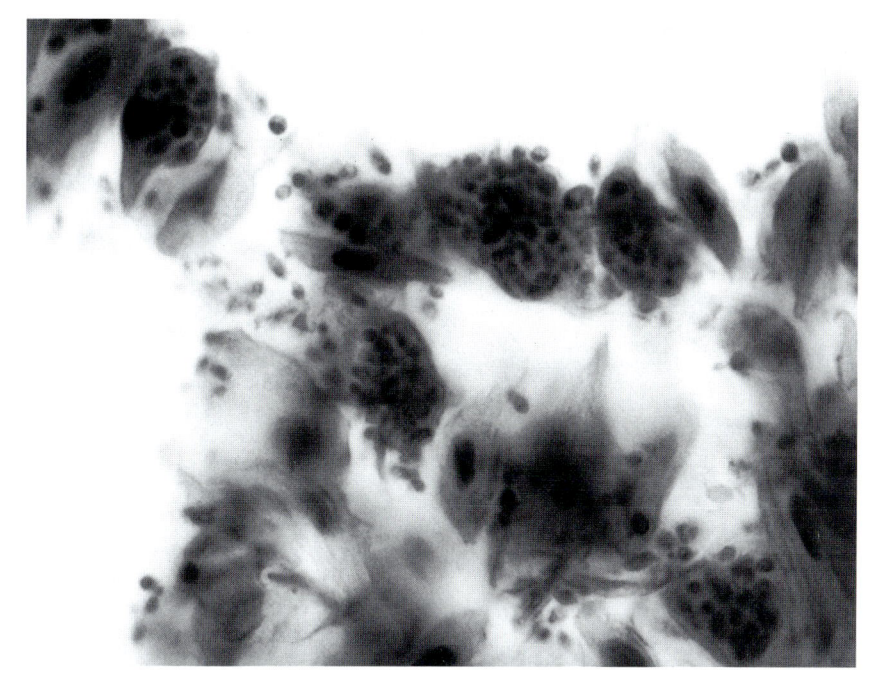

Fig. 10. Candidiasis (sputum): Although usually from the mouth, such specimens can be retrieved from lesions in the lower respiratory tract. The metaplastic epithelium is a response to colonization of the epithelium by the spores. Papanicolaou. × 900.

squamous cells can contaminate sputum specimens, but their large size will avoid attributing these changes from the mouth to the lower respiratory tract.

'Repair' Cells

Cousins to large squamous cells, repair cells in the respiratory tract are similar to such cells seen within the female genital tract. They are characterized by cohesive sheets of polyhedral cells, having attenuated cytoplasmic connections, semiopaque cytoplasm, enlarged nuclei with delicate nuclear chromatin, and usually prominent and sometimes irregular nucleoli (fig. 11). Multinucleation also can be seen. Such cells can be found from the mouth following a mucosal ulceration, but can be diagnostically treacherous when they actually come from the lower respiratory tract. They are a frequent consequence of respiratory epithelial abrasion, from

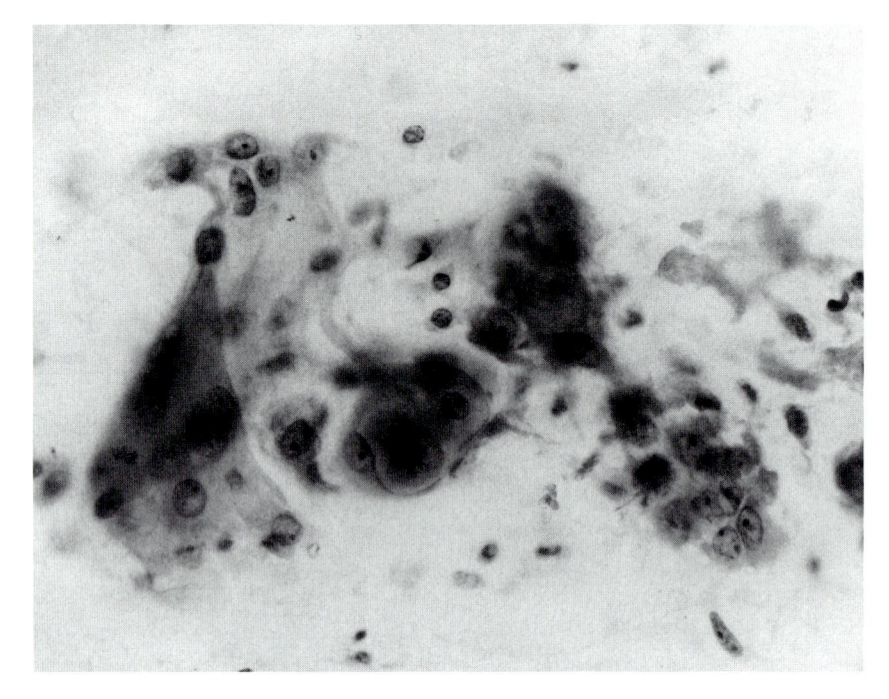

Fig. 11. Repair (bronchial brushing): Large fragments of squamous epithelium from the lower respiratory tract indicate either a metaplasia, repair process, or squamous carcinoma. The cohesion of the cells and the fine chromatin pattern provide a benign diagnosis. Patient had recently undergone bronchial biopsy. Papanicolaou. × 340.

therapeutic or diagnostic instrumentation or from radiation or thermal injury [30, 43], following a pulmonary infarct or embolus [233], or lining a granulomatous cavity (see fig. 26) and can be confused with squamous carcinoma cells. Careful attention to cohesiveness of the cell groups, uniform thinness of the nuclear membrane, and delicacy of the nuclear chromatin will attest to their benign nature (fig. 12). When in doubt, a careful history to detect prior instrumentation and/or biopsy, and a period of watchful waiting with repeat studies will usually clarify the issue.

Benign Metaplastic Cells

When a columnar epithelium, including the respiratory type, becomes sufficiently irritated as from cigarette smoke or other toxic inhalents, squamous metaplasia is the unavoidable result. Such cells are smaller than

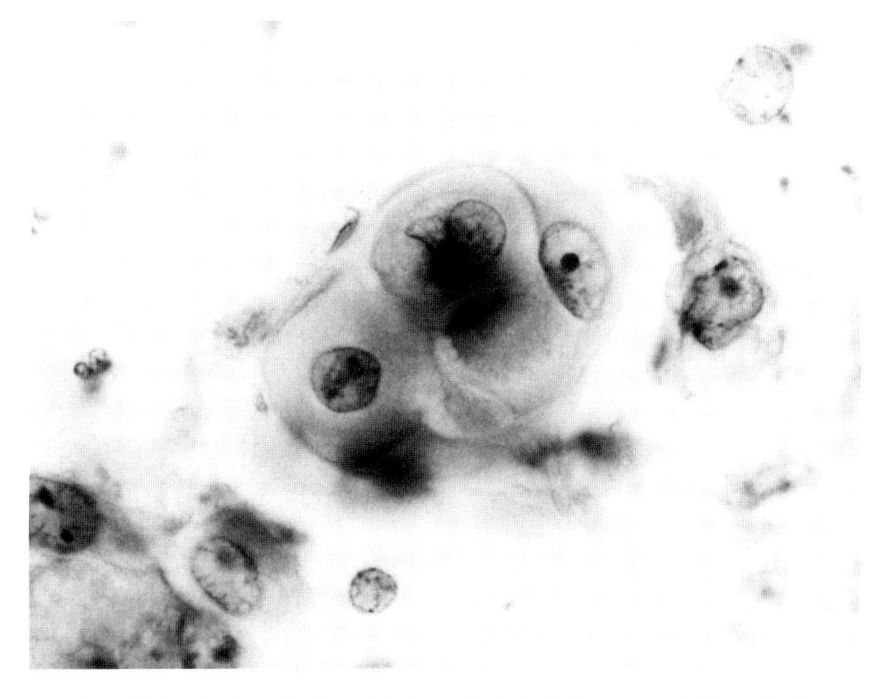

Fig. 12. Atypical repair (bronchial brushing): A higher power of figure 11 shows a benign chromatin pattern, but prominent nucleoli and irregular nuclear outlines. Careful evaluation of such a specimen with complete clinical history is important to avoid an overdiagnosis. See figure 57 from the same patient. Papanicolaou. × 900.

those from the mouth or from repair, have a mosaic appearance, and are essentially the same as those found in the uterine cervix (fig. 13). To be considered totally benign, they should have uniform nuclear size, delicate chromatin, and small round nucleoli. Nuclear-cytoplasmic ratios should be constant. These cells will be discussed further in the chapter on preneoplastic lesions. They can be confused with plant cells; a double refractile wall on such identify them as inanimate.

Columnar Cells

Columnar cells respond to stress by either individual nuclear enlargement or multinucleation in response to the need to increase the cell population, unless they undergo squamous metaplasia. The pattern of cell change seen will depend upon the specific cell type which is stimulated to respond.

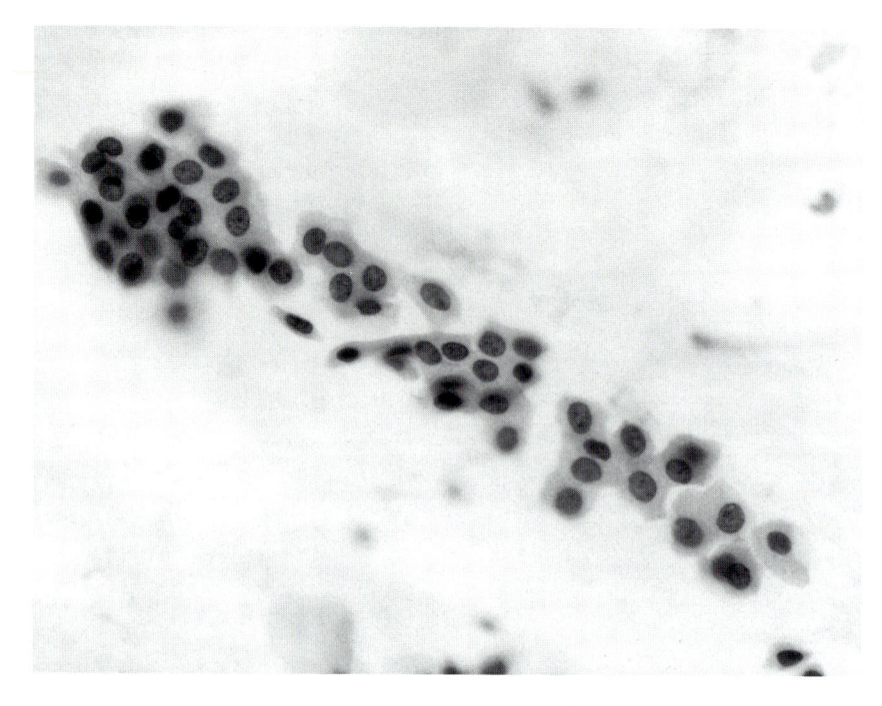

Fig. 13. Squamous metaplasia (sputum): Groups of uniform size metaplastic cells are frequently seen in benign lung disease, such as pneumonia, bronchiectasis, and asthma. The uniform nuclear size and chromatin distribution attest to their benign nature. Careful search for more severe changes is imperative. Papanicolaou. × 340.

Ciliated columnar cells usually respond by an overall increase in cell size, increase in nuclear size with some coarsening of the chromatin and accentuation of nucleoli. If the need for more cells is present, then multinucleation of cell groups will result (fig. 14). If only occasional multinucleated columnar cells are observed, their presence no doubt reflects a benign response to such situations as viral infection, or postinstrumentation (within 42–72 h). However, Chalon et al. [34] studied bronchial aspirate smears from 955 patients with a wide variety of tumors, against controls matched for age, sex and smoking history. 'Patients with all types of invasive and non-invasive carcinomas had approximately 2.3 times greater percentage-incidence of high degree multinucleation ($\geq 2.5\%$) than in the controls (39 and 17%, respectively).' The authors advise that in any negative respiratory specimens with obvious columnar cell multi-

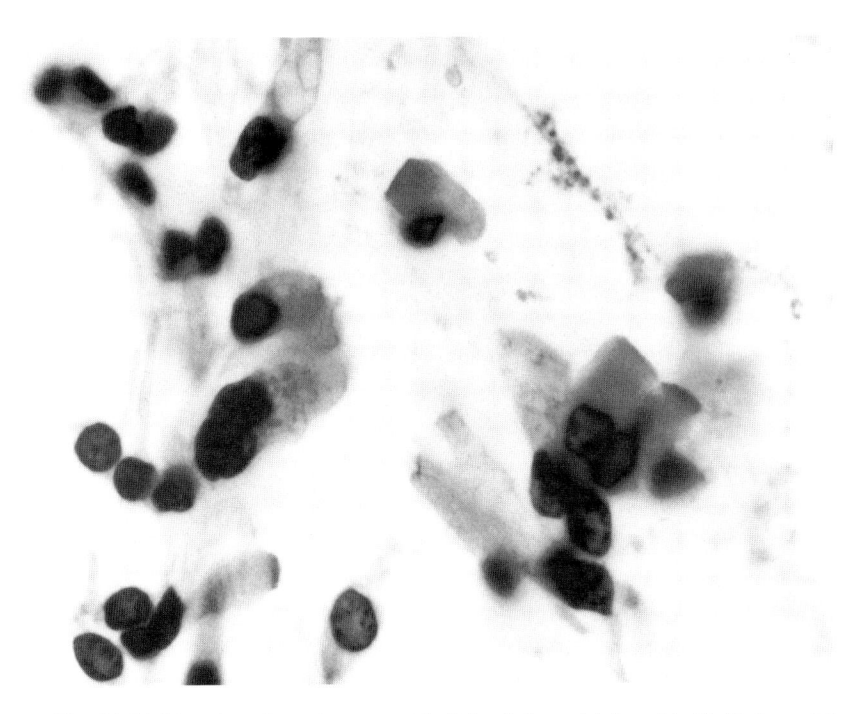

Cell Changes Currently *not* Associated with Neoplasia 29

Fig. 14. Multinucleated respiratory epithelial cell (bronchial wash): Multiple nuclei within a columnar cell indicate a reactive process. Many such cells need further investigation to search for possible neoplasm. Papanicolaou. × 900.

nucleation, careful search or repeat specimens be done to exclude an occult carcinoma.

When such hyperplastic cell groups exfoliate and are recovered in a sputum, they can appear curled, like a caterpillar, and can be mistaken for a fragment of an adenocarcinoma [168] (fig. 15). So-called Creola bodies [167], their benign nature is verified by the presence of cilia. These groups are most abundant in patients with asthma, and are seen in other chronic bronchial diseases.

In all cases, cilia are retained if the specimen is fresh, and the benign nature of the cells is assured. Degenerative changes can mimic reactive coarsening of chromatin, but the nuclear membrane in a degenerated cell will be interrupted, providing evidence that the changes are degenerative and not reactive.

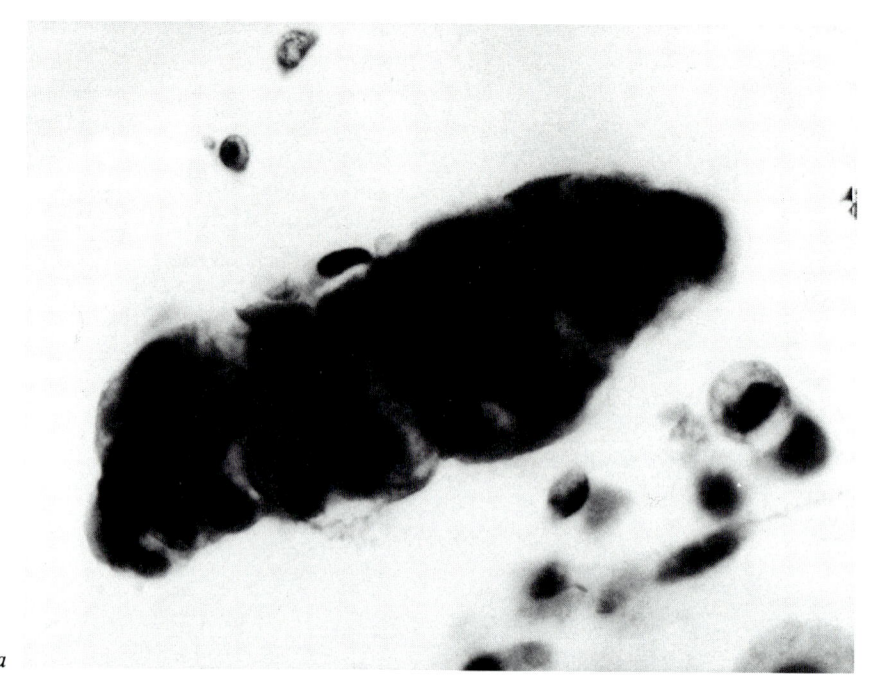

Fig. 15. Columnar epithelial groups (*a* = Creola body; *b* = Creola body, *c* = adenocarcinoma of the colon) (all sputa): Figure *a* is a typical Creola body, a fragment of benign respiratory epithelium, the surface of which contains cilia. Compare figures *b* and *c* together, figure *b* being a lower power of a Creola body, and figure *c* a group of adenocarcinoma cells at the same magnification. Figure *c* has no cilia on the surface of the fragment, and the nuclei are distinctly larger and more hyperchromatic than those in figure *b*. Papanicolaou. *a* = ×900; *b*, *c* = ×340.

If the cells are *nonciliated goblet cells,* the response to irritants is an increase in mucus within single cells, and an increase in number of the mucus containing cells. Goblet cell hyperplasia (fig. 16) commonly results from cigarette smoke, and reflects chronic obstructive pulmonary disease, emphysema, and chronic bronchitis [16]. Especially in a brushing, goblet cell hyperplasia can be seen by focusing through groups of epithelial cells and appreciating the increased number of 'holes' within the epithelial sheet (fig. 16a). Remember that the usual ratio of goblet cells to ciliated respiratory epithelial cells is approximately 1:5–6. The nuclear changes in such cells are similar to the ciliated cell changes.

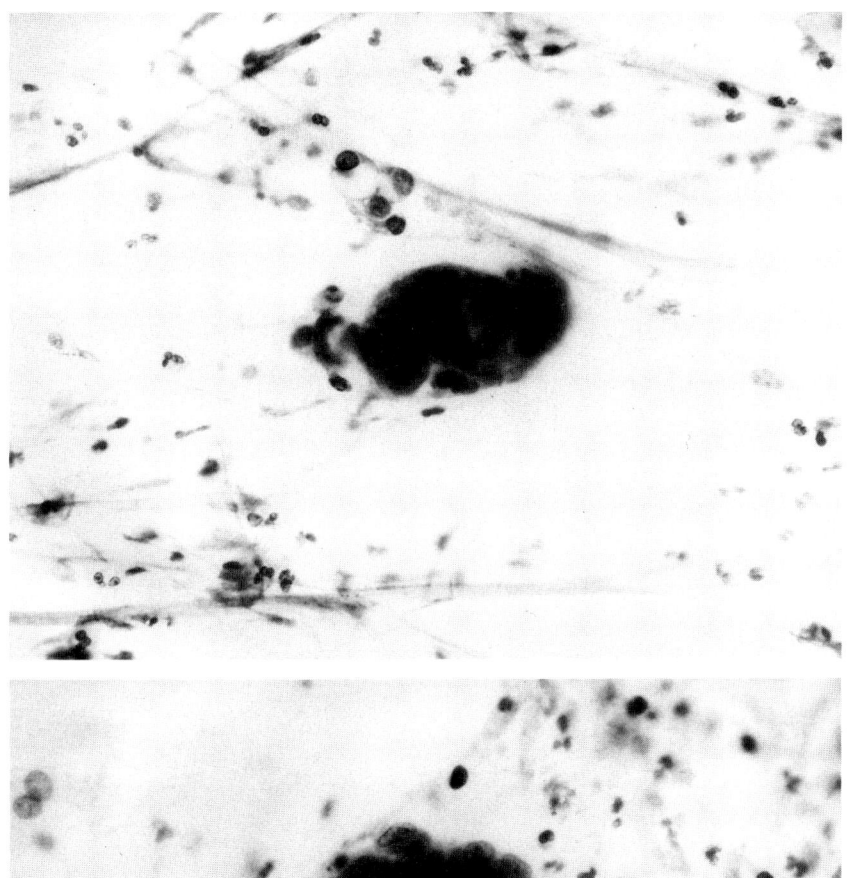

Cell Changes Currently *not* Associated with Neoplasia 31

b

c

a

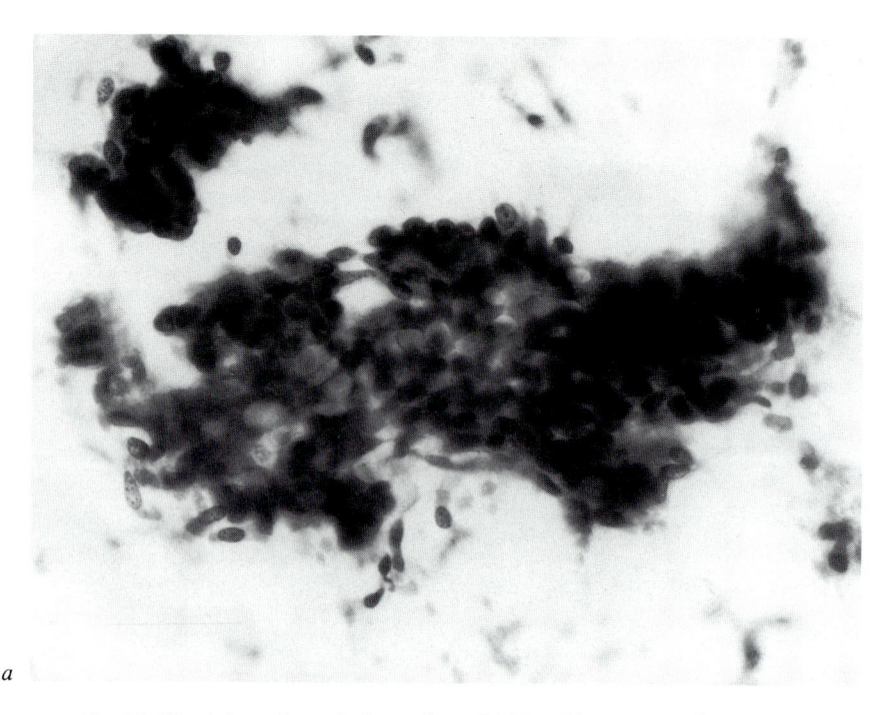

Fig. 16. Glandular cell atypia (*a–c* = bronchial brushings): *a* and *b* represent goblet cell hyperplasia, an increased number of goblet cells in fragments of benign respiratory epithelium (the ratio of normal respiratory epithelium is one goblet cell to 5–6 ciliated cells). The 'holes' correspond to the mucous vacuoles in the cytoplasm of goblet cells. Note the small nuclear size and cilia (arrow). *c* demonstrates columnar cell atypia which was provoked by a pneumonia. Note the increased size of the nuclei and irregular nuclear outlines. The fine chromatin and lack of prominent nucleoli provide benign criteria. Careful search for more severe changes which could indicate an adenocarcinoma is necessary. Papanicolaou. *a* = × 340; *b, c* = × 900.

Clara cells are nonciliated mucus-producing cells of the bronchioles. Like goblet cells, they respond to stimuli by becoming hyperplastic (fig. 16b). If such proliferation involves immature mucus-secreting cells, precursors of both goblet and Clara cells, a glandular hyperplasia can result, perhaps a precursor of bronchioloalveolar carcinoma. When such a proliferative process is accompanied by diffuse fibrosis, the end result may be Hamman-Rich syndrome. A localized fibrous nodule may be the ground-work of a 'scar' adenocarcinoma. None of these cancer precursor states has been proven.

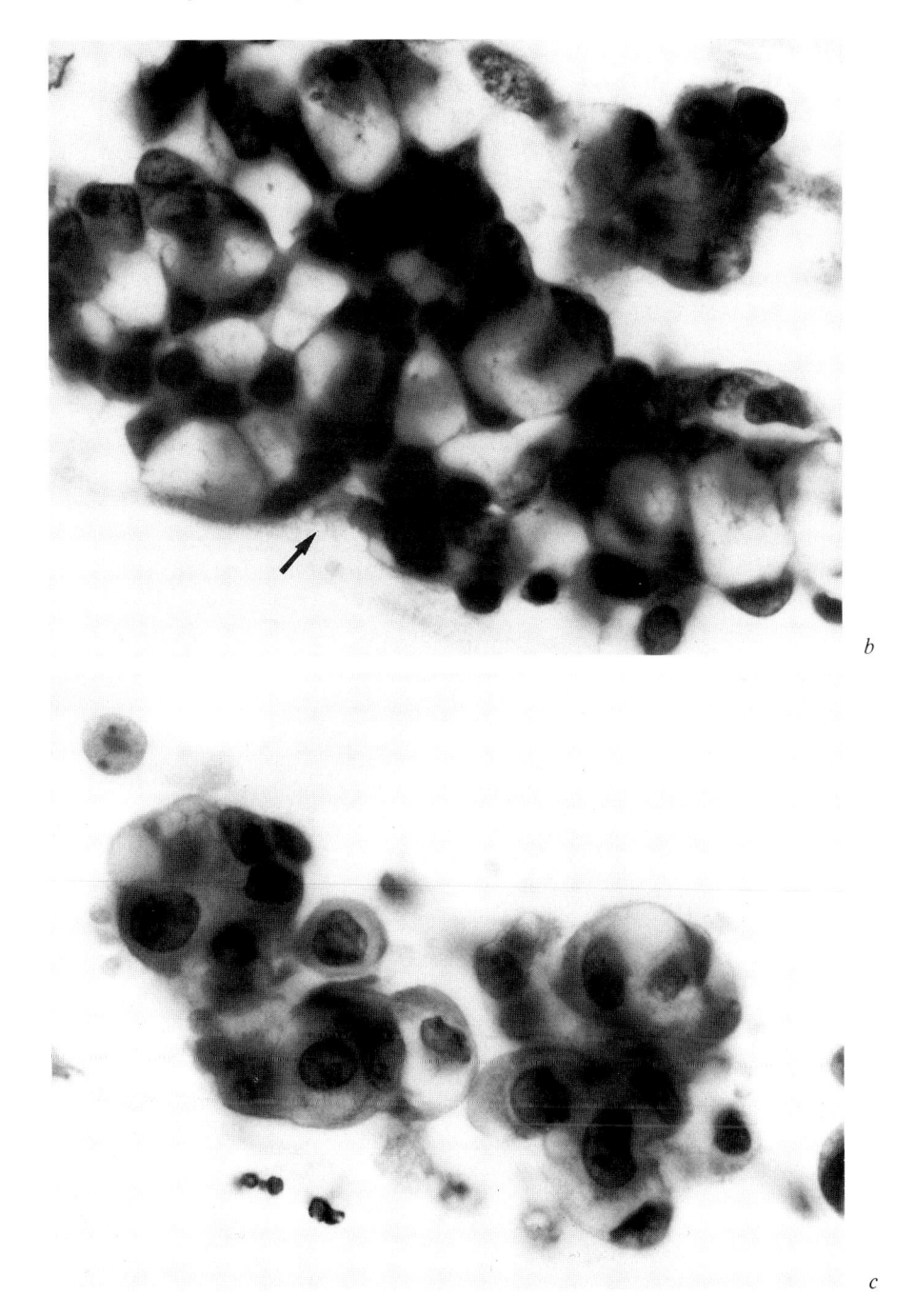

Cell Changes Currently *not* Associated with Neoplasia

33

b

c

Basal Cell or Reserve Cell Hyperplasia

These germinal cells respond as do germinal cells throughout the body by an increase in mitotic activity to increase the numbers of second and third generation cells. These cells are usually shed in groups, and will be seen in dense aggregates in a brushing or an aspirate (fig. 17a). Their hyperchromasia can suggest neoplasia, but careful attention to their regular small size, cohesiveness and visible cytoplasm, as well as regular fine chromatin will convince the observer that they are benign (fig. 17b). The most common pitfall is to mistake them for oat-cell carcinoma. The latter can be distinguished by their almost invisible cytoplasm, coarser 'salt and pepper' chromatin, and clearly discernable molding yet disconnected appearance.

Pneumocytes are commonly divided into type I and type II. The type I pneumocyte is so fragile that it is rarely seen in any preparations for light microscopy. Type II pneumocytes are hardy and dramatically respond to stimuli, especially to toxic and viral injury. They are characteristically large epithelial cells, with squamoid cytoplasm, large nuclei, huge nucleoli, often indistinguishable from viral inclusions (which they frequently are) (fig. 18). Electron microscopy is necessary to definitely identify the type of pneumocyte and the presence and kind of viral particles. Additional causes of alveolar epithelial atypia are listed in table 1, compiled by Bedrossian et al. [16].

Table 1. Causes of cytologic atypia affecting distal air spaces [16]

Infections	Chemotherapy	Radiation therapy
Viruses	Bleomycin	
Mycoplasma	Busulfan	Miscellaneous
Pneumocystis	Methotrexate	Hamman-Rich syndrome
	Cytoxan	Scleroderma
Inhalants	BCNU	Rheumatoid arthritis
Oxygen	Melphalan	Old granulomas
Nitrogen dioxide	Chlorambucil	Asbestosis
Smoke (from fire)		

Fig. 17. Reserve cell hyperplasia (bronchial brushing): A large fragment of small, tightly clustered columnar cells should not be mistaken for an adenocarcinoma, or small cell carcinoma. The cohesion of the cells, the obvious cytoplasm, and small size of the cells when compared with nearby inflammatory cells, indicate their benign nature. Papanicolaou. $a = \times 360; b = \times 900$.

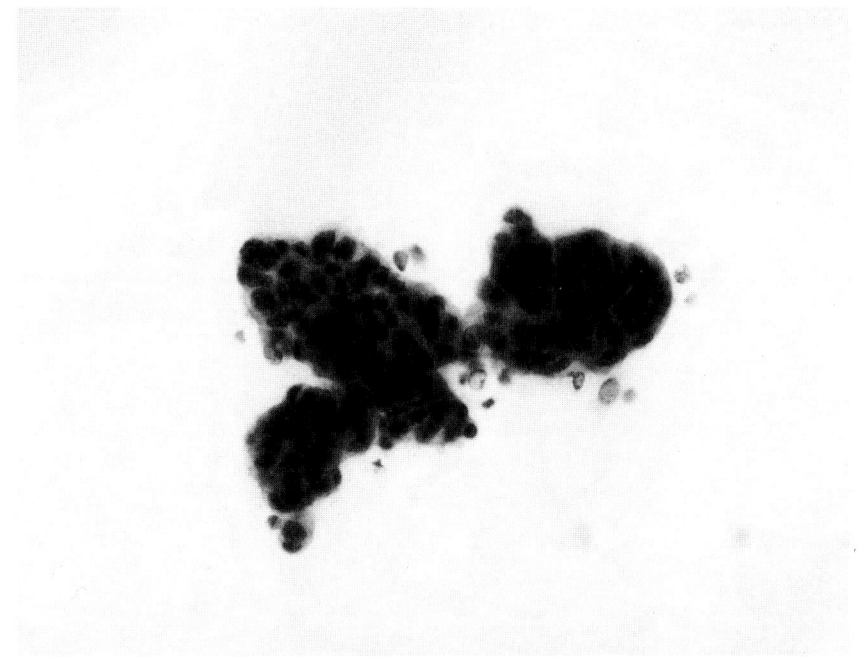

Cell Changes Currently *not* Associated with Neoplasia 35

a

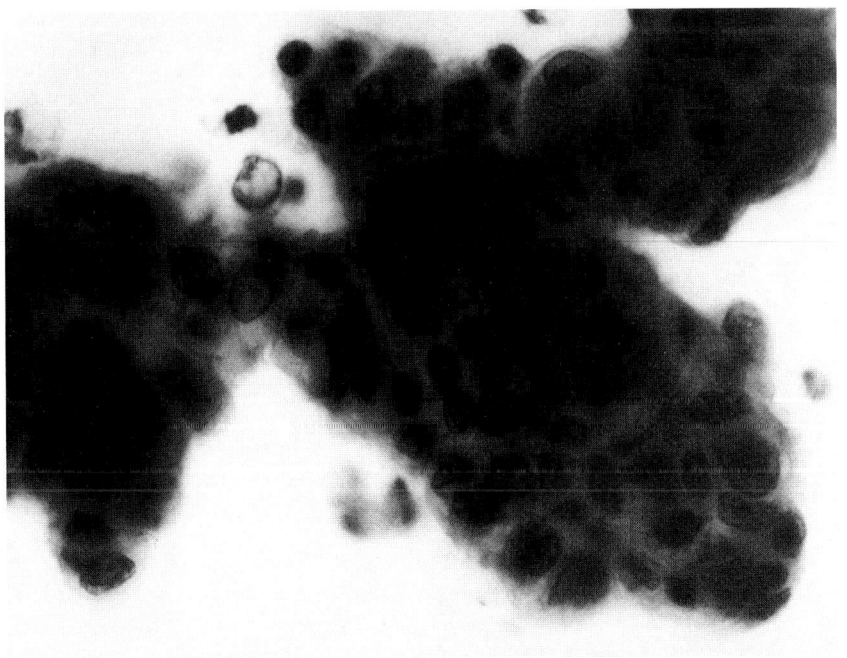

b

Megakaryocyte nuclei, filtered out of the blood, can be mistaken for tumor cells. The lack of cytoplasm and rarity add clues to their identity. Repeat sputa will provide evidence for absence of neoplasm.

Noncellular Elements

Curschmann's spirals are produced when inspissated mucus accumulates in the terminal bronchioles, partially solidifies, and then is coughed up. The central string-like axis stains purple with hematoxylin (fig. 19a), and is often covered by an outer semitransparent sheath in which a helix is appreciated [259] (fig. 19b). Such spirals can be only a few millimeters long or as long as several centimeters. Their presence indicates a patient with some form of obstructive lung disease.

Charcot-Leyden crystals are most frequently seen in the sputa of patients with asthma, and are thought to derive from crystallized fragments of degenerated eosinophils. They are difficult to appreciate in Papanicolaou stain; toluidine blue demonstrates them well in a fresh specimen.

Asbestos bodies, or more properly, *ferruginous bodies,* result from the impregnation of a filament of asbestos or other mineral fiber by iron-protein pigment [211] (fig. 20a). Generally, the central fiber itself cannot be recognized unless oil immersion is used or the fiber is especially thick

---

Fig. 18. Pneumocytes (touch prep of lung): Epithelioid in character, pneumocytes are derived from the alveolar lining, and when seen in BALs or other respiratory samples, are undoubtedly type II pneumocytes. Their usually opaque cytoplasm can sometimes be vacuolated and cytoplasmic borders are sharp. They are considerably larger than macrophages and other inflammatory cells and contain large vesicular nuclei with very prominent nucleoli. If the disease is possibly viral, the pneumocytes should be searched for viral inclusions, both intranuclear and intracytoplasmic. $a = \times 340$, Papanicolaou. $b = \times 170$, MGG.

Fig. 19. Curschmann's spiral (sputa): *a* is a well-defined Curschmann's spiral, more prominent than usual, whereas *b* is more typical. Note the coiling, and the association of inflammatory cells. Such spirals are usually seen in patients with chronic lung disease. Papanicolaou. $\times 180$.

Fig. 20. Ferruginous ('asbestos') body (sputum): Usually formed by asbestos, but potentially any inert mineral can become coated with iron, hence the name. The irregular layer over the thin filament produces the bamboo or string-of-beads effect. Papanicolaou. $a = \times 360$; $b = \times 850$.

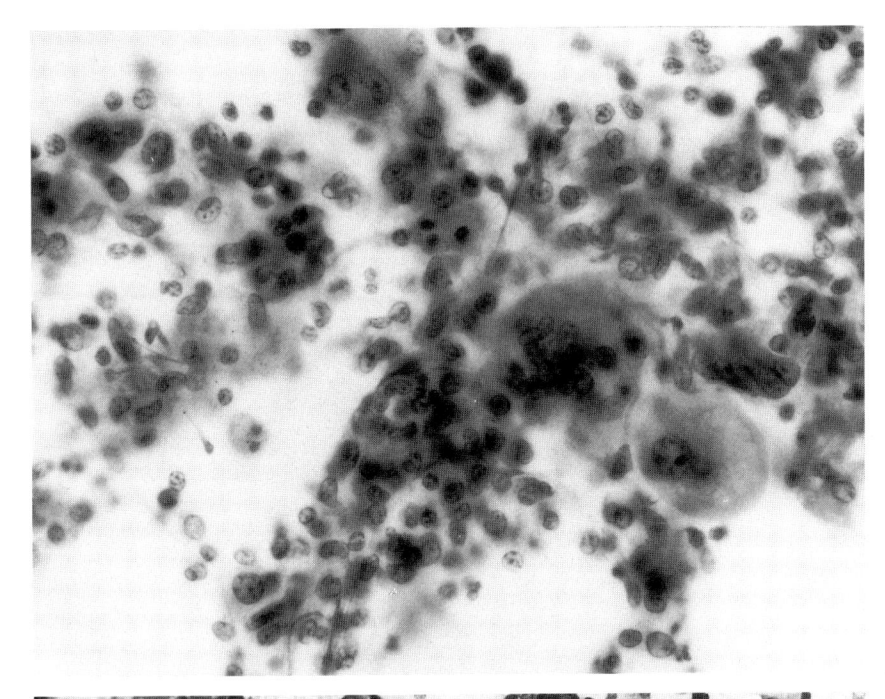

Cell Changes Currently *not* Associated with Neoplasia

18a

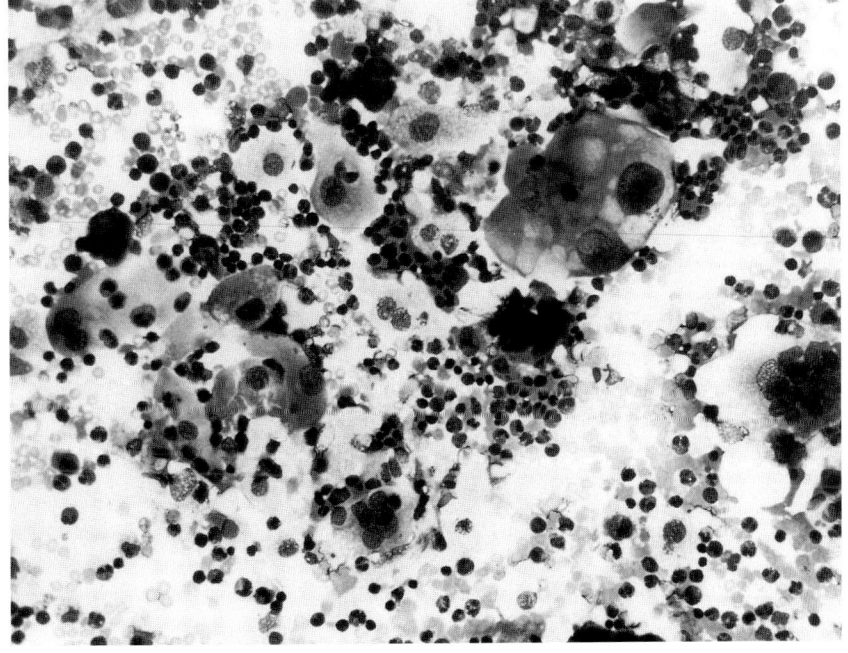

18b

Cytopathology of Pulmonary Disease 38

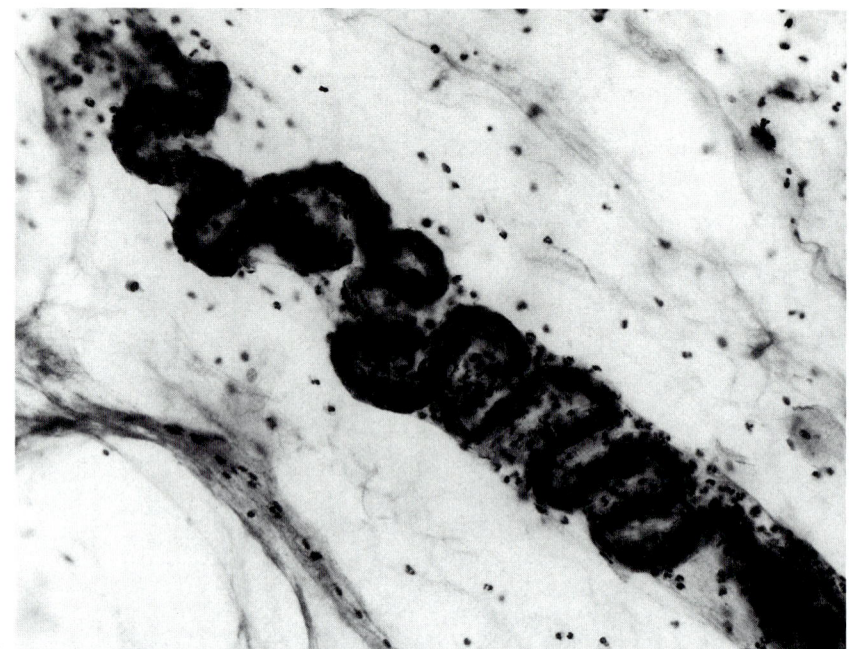

19a

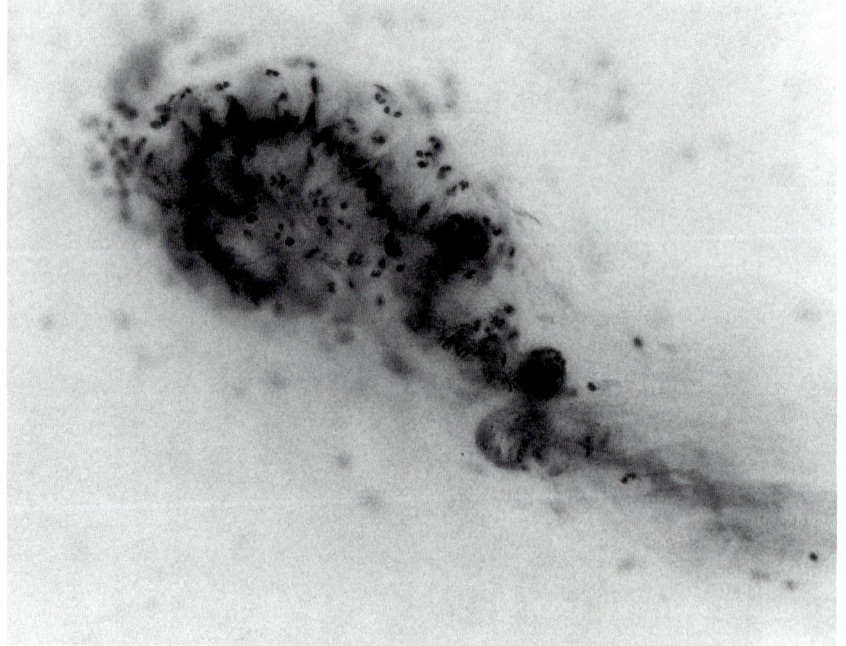

19b

(For legend see p. 36.)

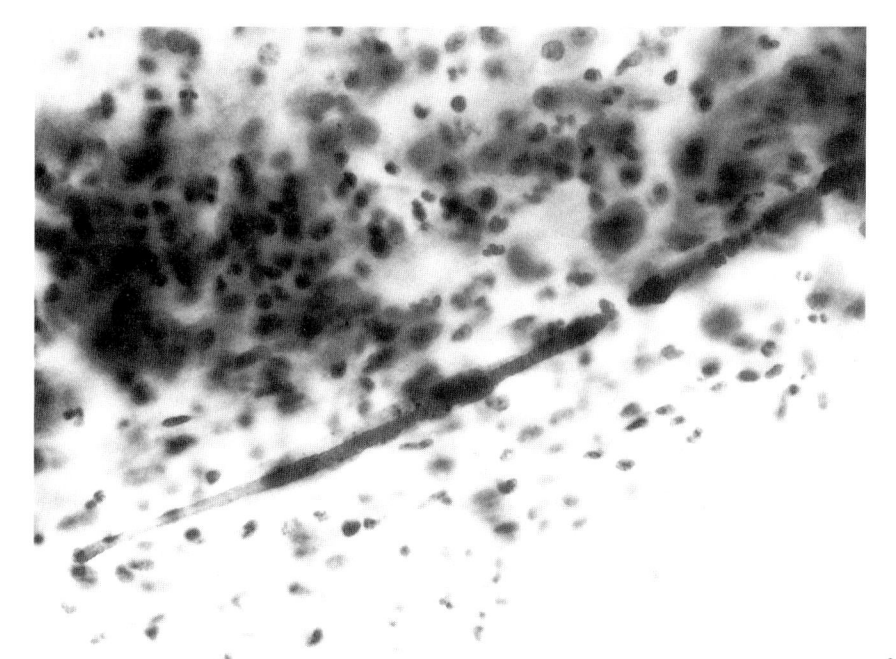

Cell Changes Currently *not* Associated with Neoplasia

20a

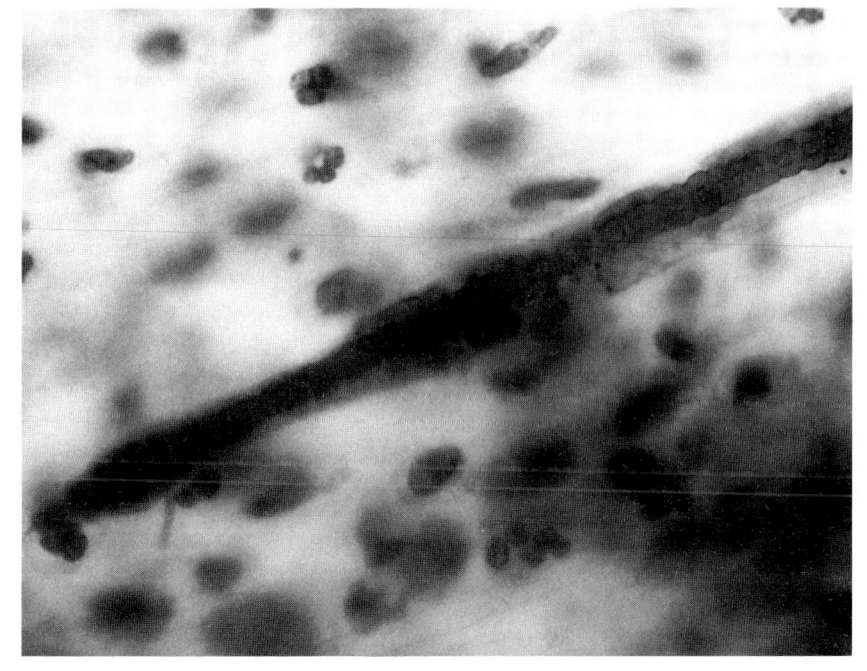

20b

(For legend see p. 36.)

Cytopathology of Pulmonary Disease

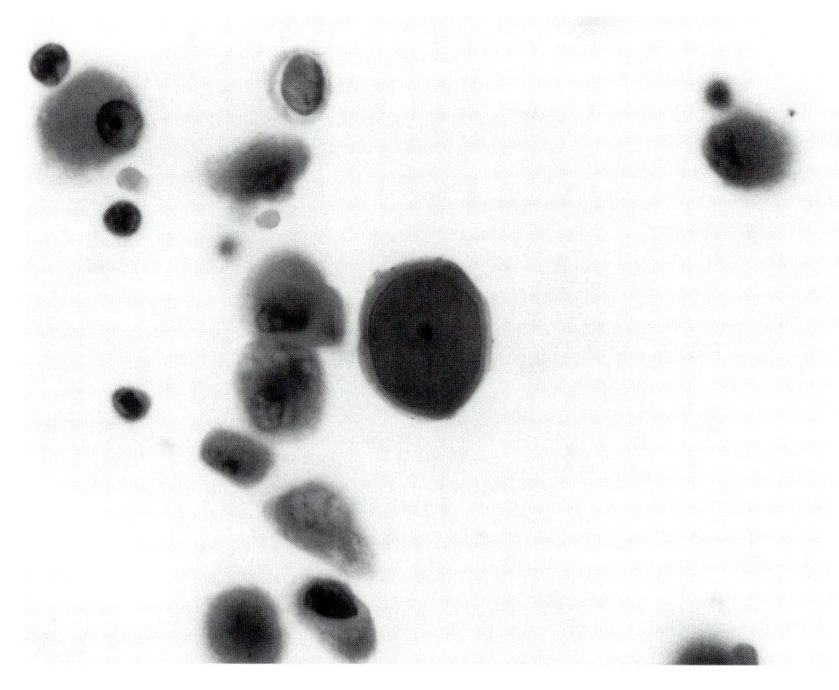

Fig. 21. Pollen (sputum): Noncellular material can mimic cells of diagnostic significance. Pollen from the air, psammoma bodies from tumors, and concretions from inspissated mucus are all round. This pollen has a characteristic thick, refractile wall, which needs be distinguished from potentially pathogenic fungi. Pollen usually stains a golden brown, whereas fungi stain pink with the Papanicolaou stain. Papanicolaou. × 850.

(fig. 20b). Ferruginous bodies usually measure between 5 and 200 µm in length, and will appear either yellow, gold, or black. The ends of the bodies can assume either a branching, attenuated, or rounded appearance, and the intervening rod usually is segmented to look like a string of beads or segments of bamboo. Ferruginous bodies can be recovered with difficulty from lungs of approximately 90% of the population [208], but their presence is pathogenically significant in only a small percentage of the population [157], and usually reflects prolonged exposure [63, 276]. Their association with mesothelioma and bronchogenic carcinoma is now well established [115; 130, p. 661].

Concretions of both amorphous mucus and accumulations of edema fluid proteins, so-called *corpora amylacea,* may occasionally be observed in sputa and will stain medium to dark purple.

Calcific concretions may be seen in patients with chronic pulmonary disease such as tuberculosis. A rare entity, alveolar microcalcinosis could also be indicated by such concretions, especially if they are present in significant numbers [130, pp. 546–547].

Amyloid has rarely been described in respiratory specimens. The disease can present as tumor but on smears appears as amorphous, waxy eosinophilic material. Special stains confirm [36].

Psammoma bodies should alert the microscopist to the strong possibility of a pulmonary adenocarcinoma [86], either primary or from thyroid or ovary or other adenocarcinoma, which classically produces them. A single case report describes psammoma bodies associated with a small cell carcinoma of the lung [14].

Vegetable material, while cellular, is obviously not of human origin. However, some vegetable groups may be mistaken for various degrees of human pathology, such as metaplasia or adenocarcinoma. Most often, such cells represent oral contamination, but an inhaled 'foreign body' [39] or aspirated/regurgitated gastric contents can be the source. When such is the case, *meat fibers* complete with cross-striations may also be seen. A superbly illustrated article by Weaver et al. [271] describes the 'cytologic' appearance of common vegetables.

Pollen stains golden to amber, usually has a double-wall and homogeneous center (fig. 21); be careful not to confuse pollen with pathogenic fungi.

Talc used to powder gloves can be identified by its Maltese cross appearance with polarized light.

IV. Infectious Diseases

Introduction

What commonly was seen only in the surgical pathology laboratory can now be encountered in the cytology case-load due to the accessibility of all lesions by fine needle aspiration [22, 27, 195] and bronchoalveolar lavage [174]. Until a short time ago, only bronchial and peribronchial infections were the concern of the cytologist. Now the pattern of parenchymal lesions is of vital interest in order to identify the diagnostic possibilities [25, 121, 198]. The diseases in the next few sections will therefore be grouped not only according to the type of infectious organism, but also according to the disease pattern that the organism produces.

The incidence of such diseases will vary depending upon the geographic location of the receiving laboratory. A word of caution, however; in this world of fast-moving jets, unexpected diseases may present themselves, especially in cities with transient populations. As has been witnessed with the incredible epidemic of AIDS patients, previously unencountered diseases suddenly become a daily occurrence [159]. All of these factors make the once banal benign diseases extremely fascinating and challenging [214].

The infectious organisms whose hallmarks can be recognized by Papanicolaou stain or inferred by cytologic features can be divided into two categories: those which create a pneumonic process, and those which result in a granulomatous infection. Of the latter, tuberculosis, the prototype of granulomatous infections, and sarcoidosis, have no pathognomonic features recognizable in Papanicolaou stained material, but can be suspected by the patterns of cellular and noncellular material.

Tuberculosis and Sarcoidosis

Tuberculosis (TB), a disease of historic significance and protean manifestations, is still to be found worldwide. Although classically an infection of the impoverished, TB is not a respecter of class or caste; it should be considered an ubiquitous disease, and always be part of the differential diagnosis of pulmonary lesions.

Infectious Diseases

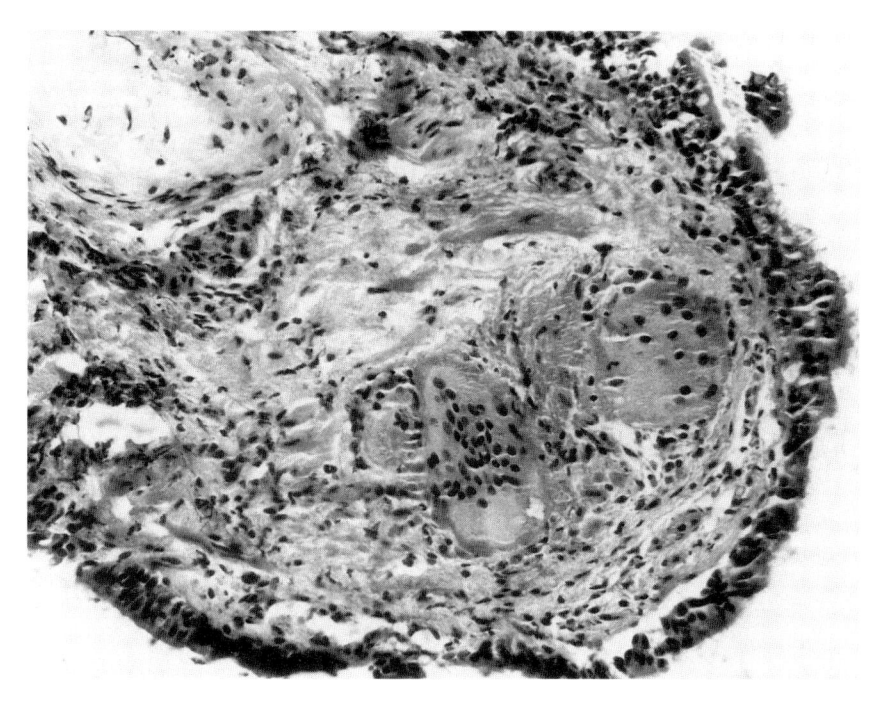

Fig. 22. Sarcoidosis (transbronchial biopsy): The classical noncaseating granuloma is produced by sarcoid, a disease of obscure etiology. Easily diagnosed on transbronchial biopsy specimens, these lesions are usually submucosal, therefore accessible to the bronchoscope. However, their products in cytologic samples from bronchoscopy are rare. See figures 4 and 23. HE. × 170.

TB has not been a common consideration for the cytologist because of the paucity of diagnostic material retrievable in routine cytologic specimens, e.g. sputa, bronchial washings, and brushings. Occasionally, Langhans' type giant cells will be recovered in these specimens; in such instance TB should be high on the list of diagnoses [163, 207]. A single case report describes two pulmonary tumorlets, cytologically mistaken for cancer, associated with tuberculomas in 2 patients [146]. However, pulmonary FNA provides material directly from the granuloma. The TB organism cannot be identified by Papanicolaou stain, but the contents of the granulomatous complex is sufficiently characteristic to prompt search for visible organisms, i.e. the fungi described later, or to stain for mycobacteria; cultures are necessary for positive identification of the infectious agents.

The cytologic features of all aspirated granulomas, regardless of the cause, are similar; however, more amorphous debris can be expected from caseous centers of TB lesions. In all granulomas, clusters or confluent sheets of epithelial cells, necrotic debris, calcified particles, lymphocytes and multinucleated Langhans' type giant cells [9, 231] are sufficient clues to strongly suggest the diagnosis. For the mycobacteria, special stains (Fites or auramine-rhodamine) are necessary to locate and tentatively identify them. As will be illustrated below, the granuloma-producing fungi are readily seen on Papanicolaou stained material.

Sarcoidosis has always been a diagnosis of exclusion, as no causative agent has yet been associated with this multisystem disease. Diagnosis has traditionally been made by open lung biopsy and more recently by transbronchial biopsy (TBB) via the fiberoptic bronchoscope, as most of the lesions are central. Rarely the disease will present as a solitary nodule [177]. Infrequent reports have documented the appearance of classic Schaumann or asteroid bodies in multinucleated histiocytes recovered in sputa [3; 130, p. 573]. We recently reviewed bronchoscopic specimens from a patient with suspected sarcoidosis, in which the TBB and brushing contained noncaseating granulomas. While finding diagnostic material in a TBB was expected (fig. 22), the cytologic features of a non-caseating granuloma in a bronchial brushing were a surprise (fig. 23).

Major Fungi Causing Granulomatous Inflammation in the Lung

Table 2 characterizes the four most common fungi to produce significant granulomatous disease in the lung. Their incidence, as noted above, will vary depending upon geographic location, with blastomyces commonly occurring in the southeast United States, histoplasma in the middle-west, coccidioides in the southwest, and cryptococcus being an ubiquitous and frequent second invader following another debilitating disease.

Fig. 23. Sarcoidosis (bronchial brushing): This excellent cytologic sample of granulomatous inflammation was obtained from the same patient as figure 22. Note the multinucleated giant cell in *a*, the tangle of monocytes, fibroblasts, and macrophages mixed with chronic inflammatory cells and scattered lymphocytes. If caseation is present, then the diagnosis of tuberculosis or fungal infection should be considered over sarcoidosis, which is devoid of necrosis. Papanicolaou. $a = \times 180$; $b = \times 340$.

Infectious Diseases

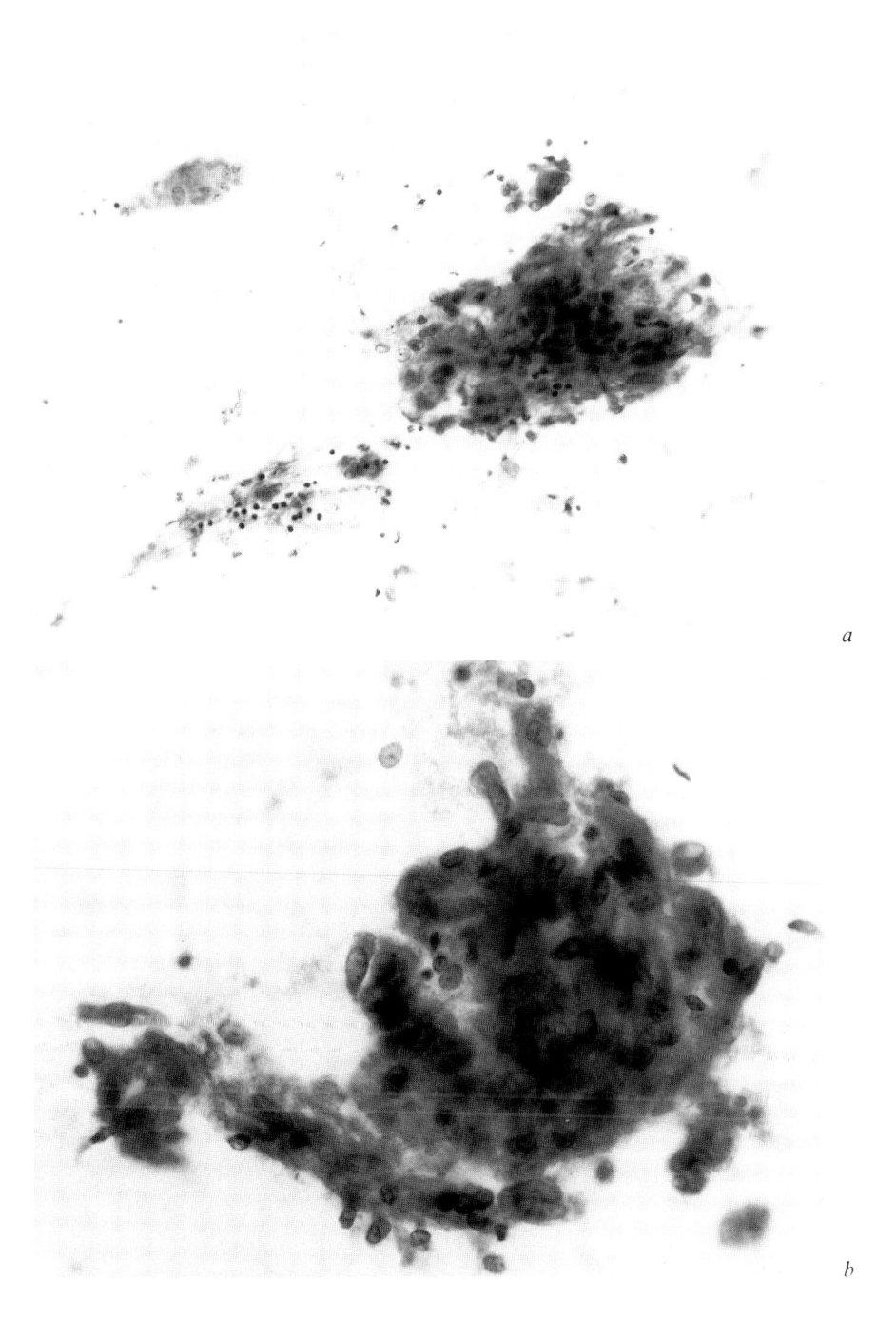

a

b

Table 2. Contrasting morphologic features of major fungi causing granulomatous inflammation in the lung [121]

	Histoplasma	Coccidioides	Cryptococcus	Blastomyces
Average size	3 μm (range: 1–5 μm)	30–60 μm (spherules); 2–5 μm (endospores)	4–7 μm (range: 2–15 μm)	8–15 μm (range: 2–30 μm)
Morphologic features	oval, budding yeast	spherules, endospores; no budding forms	round, budding yeast; fragmented forms	round, budding yeast
Distinguishing structural features (HE)	single nucleus, perinuclear clear zone (intracellular organisms only)[1]	thick wall, central basophilic endospores (spherule only)	pale, thin cell wall; extracellular clear zone	thick cell wall, basophilic protoplasm, multiple nuclei
Mucicarmine staining	–	–	+	–
Type of granulomas	caseating	caseating; early lesions, suppuration	caseating, noncaseating	necrotizing with suppuration

[1] Intracellular organisms are seen only in disseminated histoplasmosis. Histoplasma cannot be visualized within caseous necrosis in lung granulomas in HE-stained sections.

Histoplasmosis

Histoplasma capsulatum is found throughout the Middle Western United States in the soil, especially in areas with large amounts of bird droppings. The mycelial form in nature is transformed to the yeast phase at body temperature.

The clinical syndrome is quite variable and usually benign in its outcome. The initial infection is usually asymptomatic but occasional outbreaks, including fever and cough, will announce a minor epidemic. Hilar and mediastinal nodal enlargement and patchy parenchymal infiltrates characterize the chest X-ray. The result is either a resolved disease or occasional dissemination. A variant of the primary disease form is a dramatic flu-like syndrome as a result of inhalation of large numbers of spores.

The chest X-ray will show patchy soft infiltrates. This is usually self-limited, with no debilitating residual disease.

Disseminated histoplasmosis can occur in both healthy and immunocompromised people, with approximately one-third of the patients being less than a year old. This form of the disease affects not only the lung but multiple organs, in which marked histiocytic proliferation is the predominant finding. These histiocytes will contain the organisms which can be demonstrated by silver stains. Necrotizing granulomas are usually absent and interstitial lung infiltrates will be apparent on X-ray.

Chronic histoplasmosis will occur in patients with long-standing lung disease and for years was the confusing mimic of tuberculosis. In fact, many midwestern tuberculosis sanitariums contained a significant percentage of patients with histoplasmosis and/or tuberculosis. Both infiltrative and cavitary lesions characterize the chest X-ray. Sputum and FNA cultures for the organisms are the definitive test although lung biopsies may be necessary if cultures are negative.

Histoplasmomas are the lesions most likely to be misinterpreted as neoplasms, for they appear radiographically as well-circumscribed lesions which may enlarge gradually. These are usually chest X-ray findings in an otherwise healthy individual. The lesions are traditionally excised to exclude the possibility of neoplasm; the diagnosis could well be made by FNA [121, p. 261].

This is the one fungus of the four in this section in which the Papanicolaou stain is the least helpful, although the small (2–5 µm) intracytoplasmic yeasts can be suggested in the cytoplasm of multinucleated histiocytes (fig. 24). The amorphous center of histoplasmomas is the same as in caseating granulomas caused by the mycobacteria. Special stains are needed to clearly visualize the organisms.

Coccidioidomycosis
Coccidioides immitis is a saprophytic fungus also occurring in the soil. A dimorphic fungus, the natural growth form is a mold, but in man the spherule contains the endospores which are the infective components. The diagnostic spherules are large round structures measuring 30–60 µm, and are thick walled. Spherules may be empty or contain numerous endospores, 2–5 µm (fig. 25).

Lung involvement is usually asymptomatic or mildly symptomatic, with chest X-ray revealing patchy, hazy infiltrates. Known as 'valley fever', after the San Joaquin Valley (California), the endemic area, the disease

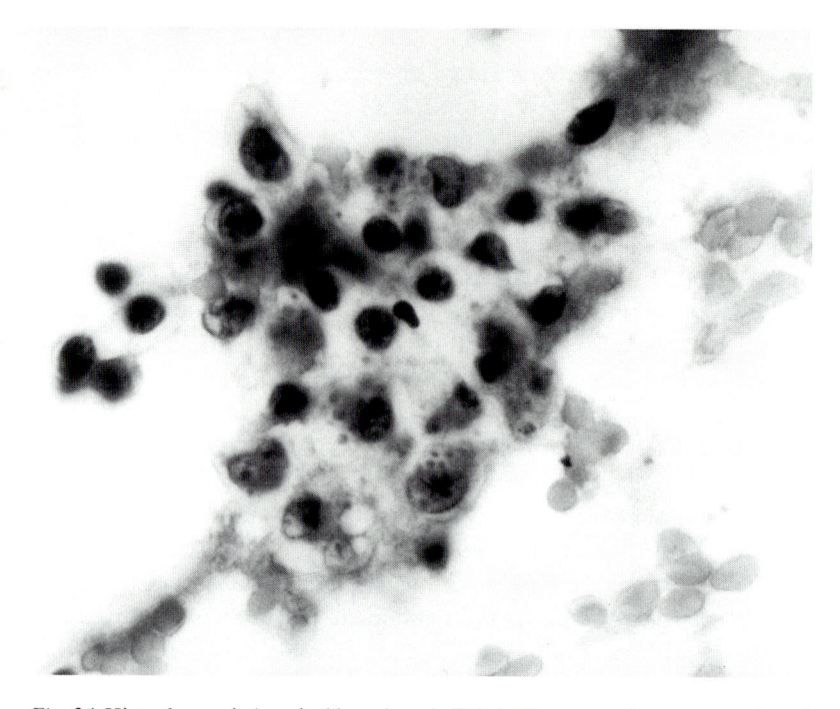

Fig. 24. Histoplasmosis (cervical lymph node FNA): These organisms were aspirated from the cervical node of a patient with pulmonary histoplasmosis. The organisms are quite small, and always found within cytoplasm of macrophages. Giemsa and PAS stains are usually preferred, but the Papanicolaou stain can reveal the organisms. Papanicolaou. × 900.

consists of a symptom complex of erythema nodosum, erythema multiforme, and arthralgias. Usually self-limited, it clears in 2–3 weeks. If the disease persists for more than 6–8 weeks, persistent pneumonia and miliary dissemination may ensue. These patients may have a severe illness of fever, chest pain, cough and longstanding pulmonary infiltrates. A less common form, chronic progressive pneumonia, closely resembles tuberculosis. Occasionally, a cavity or coccidioidoma may result which will be

Fig. 25. Coccidioidomycosis (BAL): Scattered throughout the specimen, containing predominantly macrophages, are large spherules containing the spores of coccidioidomycosis. Note the thick wall of the spherule and the small nuclei of the organisms. Empty spherules can also be seen in such specimens. Papanicolaou. a = × 340; b = × 900.

Infectious Diseases

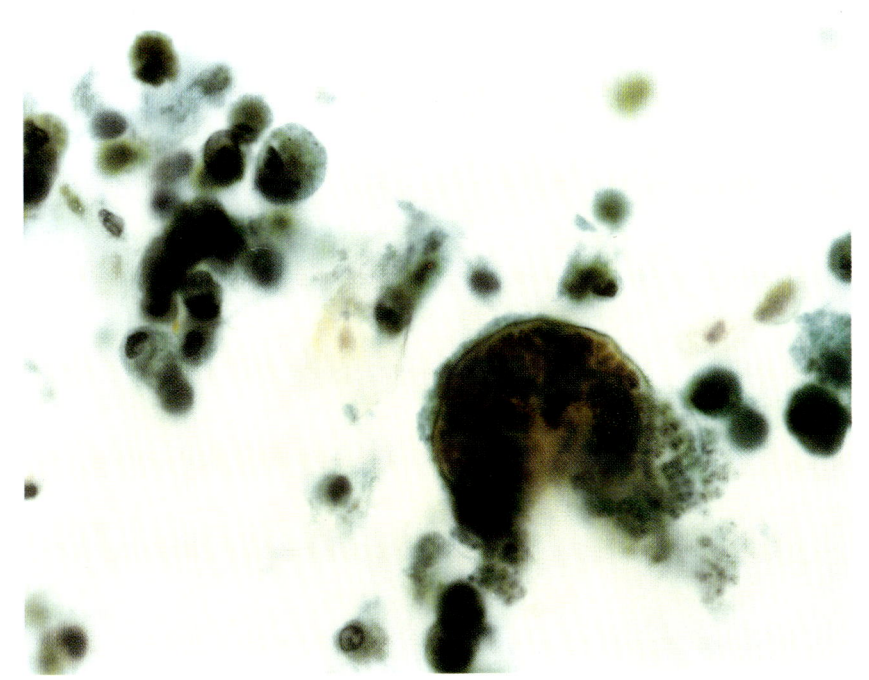

25a

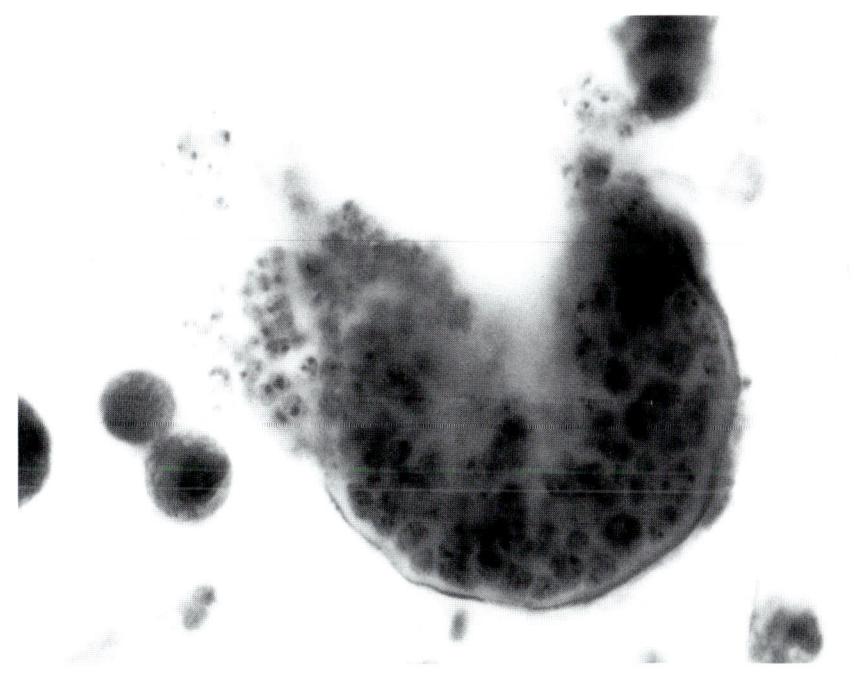

25b

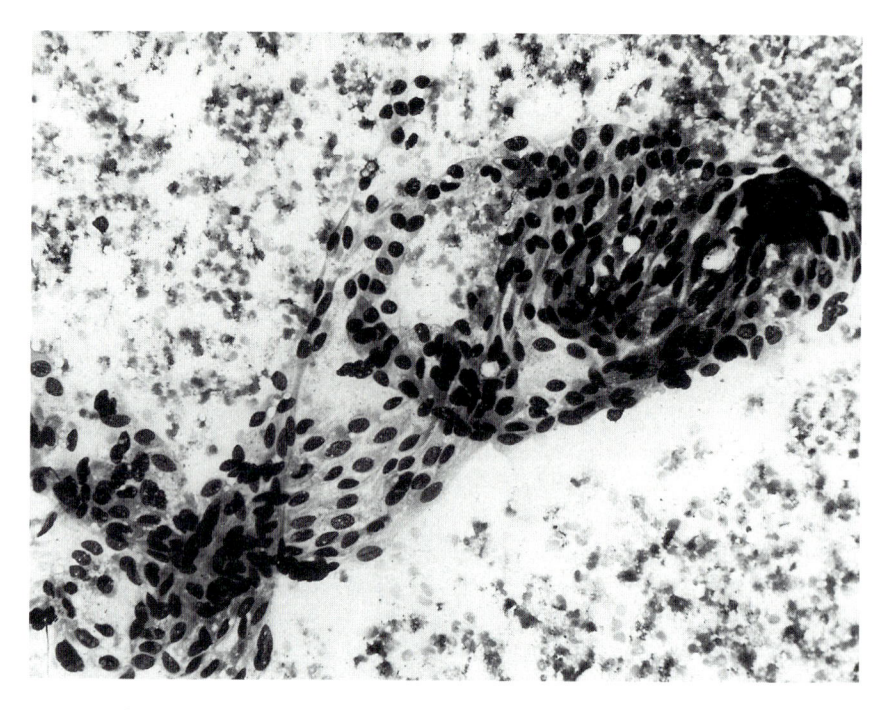

Fig. 26. Coccidioidomycosis (FNA): This squamous epithelium was aspirated from the lining of a mycetoma cavity containing coccidioidomycosis. Amorphous debris in the background, and the uniform pattern of the epithelium, provide the benign diagnosis. Beware that a squamous carcinoma can lurk in benign cavities. Careful examination of the entire specimen is mandatory. See figure 58. MGG. × 170.

detected on routine chest X-ray, the lining of which resembles 'repair' or metaplastic epithelium (fig. 26). Disseminated disease is rare but is more common in immunocompromised patients, pregnant women, blacks, Mexicans and Filipinos [121, p. 263].

The cytologic features are best appreciated in a fine needle aspirate of a lung lesion which may be cystic. The spherules are readily identified in Papanicolaou stain and the endospores, if present within the spherules, are also easy to recognize [130, p. 581]. Empty, sometimes collapsed spherules are also apparent. Small endospores can be distinguished from Histoplasma and Cryptococcus because the endospores of 'Cocci' do not bud. Not only will the granulomatous reaction be obvious (fig. 27), but an acute inflammatory reaction is thought to be provoked by the endospores, so the pattern will be a combined granulomatous and acute inflammatory re-

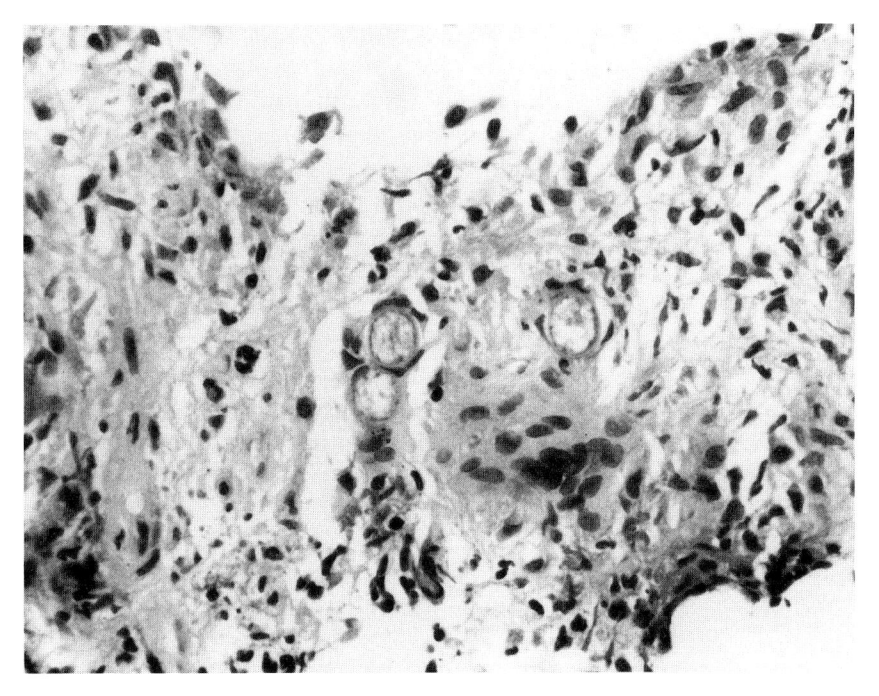

Fig. 27. Coccidioidomycosis (transbronchial biopsy): Coccidioidomycosis can also be diagnosed on transbronchial biopsy if the lesion is close to the major bronchi. The spherules are readily seen, and are adjacent to, if not within, the cytoplasm of a multinucleated histiocyte. Special stains are not necessary. HE. × 340.

sponse. According to Johnston and Frable [115] and in our experience, the spherules of Cocci may be seen frequently in the sputum of infected patients; BAL is an excellent means of recovering these organisms (fig. 28).

Cryptococcosis

Cryptococcus neoformans is an ubiquitous yeast, found in soil, especially that which is rich in pigeon droppings. The budding organism has a thick mucinous capsule and a widely variable size, averaging 4–7 μm, with a range of 2–15 μm. The organism can produce primary disease, or can be a secondary invader in an immunocompromised host [78]. The yeast can be found not only in bronchial material but in urine and cerebrospinal fluid. Cryptococcosis, when it affects the lung, can be asymptomatic [260];

approximately one-third of the patients present with a range of symptoms from mild cough and low-grade fever to a life-threatening infection. Radiographically, single or multiple nodules are noted, with 10–15% cavitating. Segmental pneumonias or miliary dissemination can occur. A primary complex, such as seen in tuberculosis, has been rarely described.

The infectious pattern varies depending upon the immune status with granulomatous reaction occurring in otherwise healthy individuals. These granulomas contain numerous intracellular organisms, and can be caseating or noncaseating [230, 277]. Organisms can be identified on both HE and Papanicolaou stain but are most characteristically developed by silver stain. Cryptococcus can be distinguished from Histoplasma by its larger size, thicker cell wall and budding [81]. The thin isthmus of the bud distinguishes Cryptococcus from the broader-based bud of Blastomycosis. Most patients that are immunocompromised, approximately 10%, may not manifest a granulomatous pattern, but will have sheets of organisms within the alveolar spaces with little cellular response other than macrophages. This is similar to the nonresponse seen in cerebrospinal fluid.

Cytologically, in a Papanicolaou stained specimen the budding yeast can have a darkened birefringent center, which resembles a mounting-medium artefact, or may appear simply as a pale pink round or budding structure with a thick outer rim and central density [88, 196] (fig. 29). While no special stains other than the Papanicolaou stain are needed, silver stains and the periodic acid-Schiff (PAS) stain will clearly define the organism. The India ink preparation is also another diagnostic method which will clearly demonstrate the thick capsule.

North American Blastomycosis

Blastomycosis is caused by *Blastomyces dermatitidis*, a dimorphic fungus which grows as mycelia at room temperature, and as yeasts, the usual infectious form, at body temperature. These round yeasts vary in size usually from 8 to 15 μm, but can grow up to 30 μm in diameter. The cell is surrounded by a thick refractile wall and contains multiple nuclei. These

---

Fig. 28. Coccidioidomycosis (BAL): The background of this BAL contains very coarsely granular material. On closer inspection (*b*), these round, approximately 2 μm diameter organisms, are identified as cocci. They can be found within spherules, within the cytoplasm of macrophages, and loosely in the background. Papanicolaou. *a* = × 340; *b* = × 900.

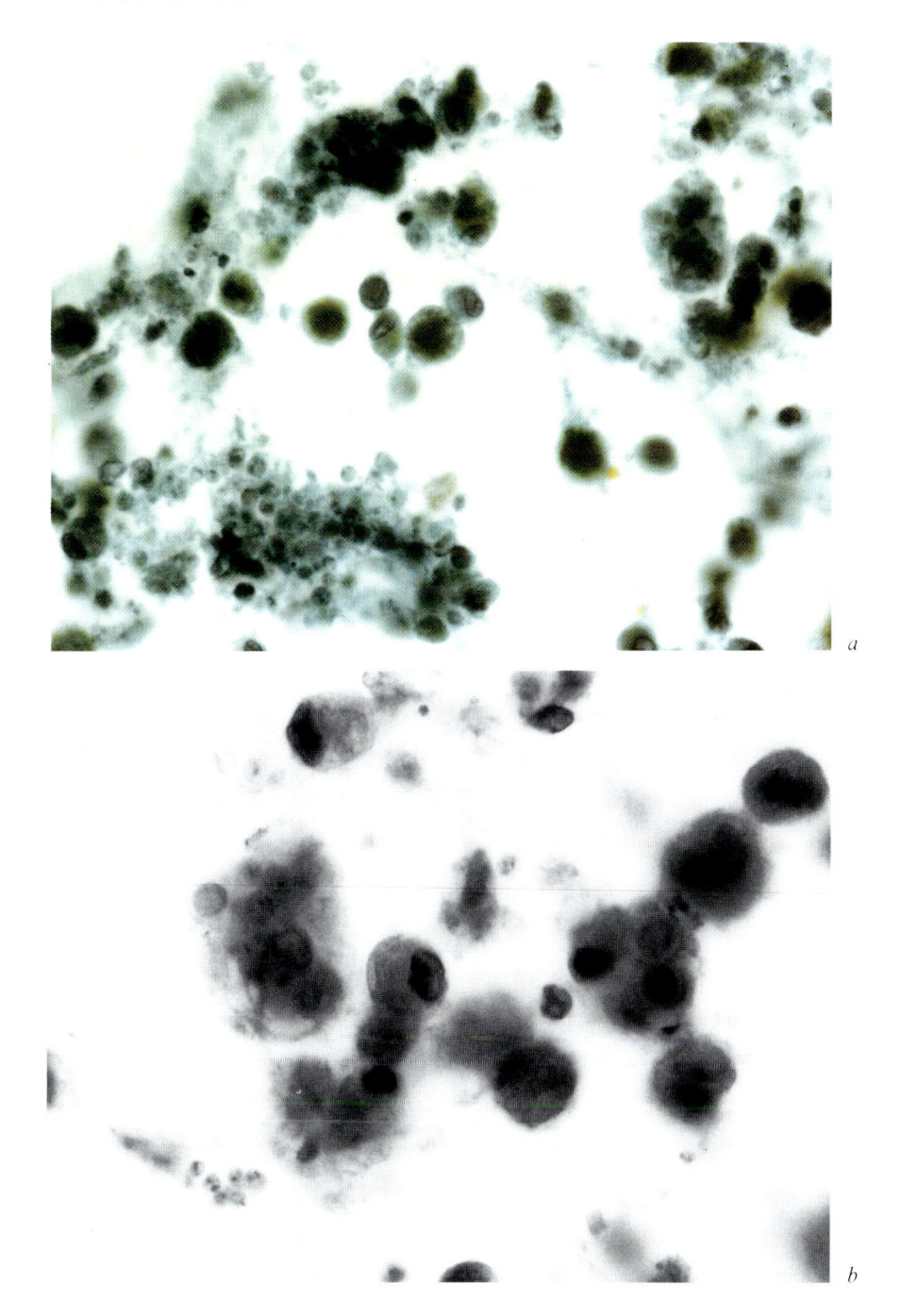

Infectious Diseases

yeast forms bud in a characteristic broad-based fashion, distinguishing them from cryptococcus, with its thin, tapering attachment.

The source of the fungus is not clearly defined, but endemic areas include south, south-central, and Great Lakes areas of the United States, and parts of Canada; scattered cases are reported from Africa and South America.

The lung is the primary target of Blastomycosis, with young to middle-aged adults affected with greater frequency than the other age groups. Participation in outdoor activities appears to be a risk factor for contracting this disease. Clinical syndrome includes an acute pneumonia of abrupt onset with high fever, chills, and cough; patchy infiltrates characterize the chest X-ray. The self-limited form of the disease allows most patients to recover without therapy. A few cases of asymptomatic acute pneumonia have been reported in local epidemics. Unfortunately, in a few patients a progressive form may follow the acute episode, which results in bilateral pulmonary involvement and occasional distant organ infection. Mortality is high in spite of antifungal treatment. A chronic form may involve the lung or other sites, especially the skin, even after recovery from acute pneumonia [121, p. 271].

The microscopic pattern of the pneumonia passes from an acute inflammatory stage to a histiocytic response with granuloma formation. Necrotizing granulomas are constructed of a central zone of necrotic neutrophils without true caseation. Special stains are not needed to visualize the single or budding globes, 8–15 µm in diameter, with thick walls containing either a clear cytoplasmic mass, or varying numbers of granules (fig. 30). Shrinkage of the cytoplasmic mass may produce a halo between the cell wall and mass. All of these features are characteristic, but the most diagnostic is that of the broad-based bud [109]. The organisms may be found either extracellularly within the necrotic granulomas, or within the cytoplasm of macrophages (fig. 31).

The cytologic examination of a bronchopulmonary specimen will reflect the variable inflammatory pattern. Polymorphonuclear leukocytes

---

Fig. 29. Cryptococcosis (BAL): This organism (arrows) can be found both within the cytoplasm of macrophages and free-floating. The size is approximately that of a macrophage nucleus, and the characteristic capsule is best seen when the organism is contained within a macrophage. Because of its thickness, a birefringent center is frequently noted, and should not be confused as mounting medium artifact. Papanicolaou. $a = \times 360$; $b = \times 900$.

Infectious Diseases

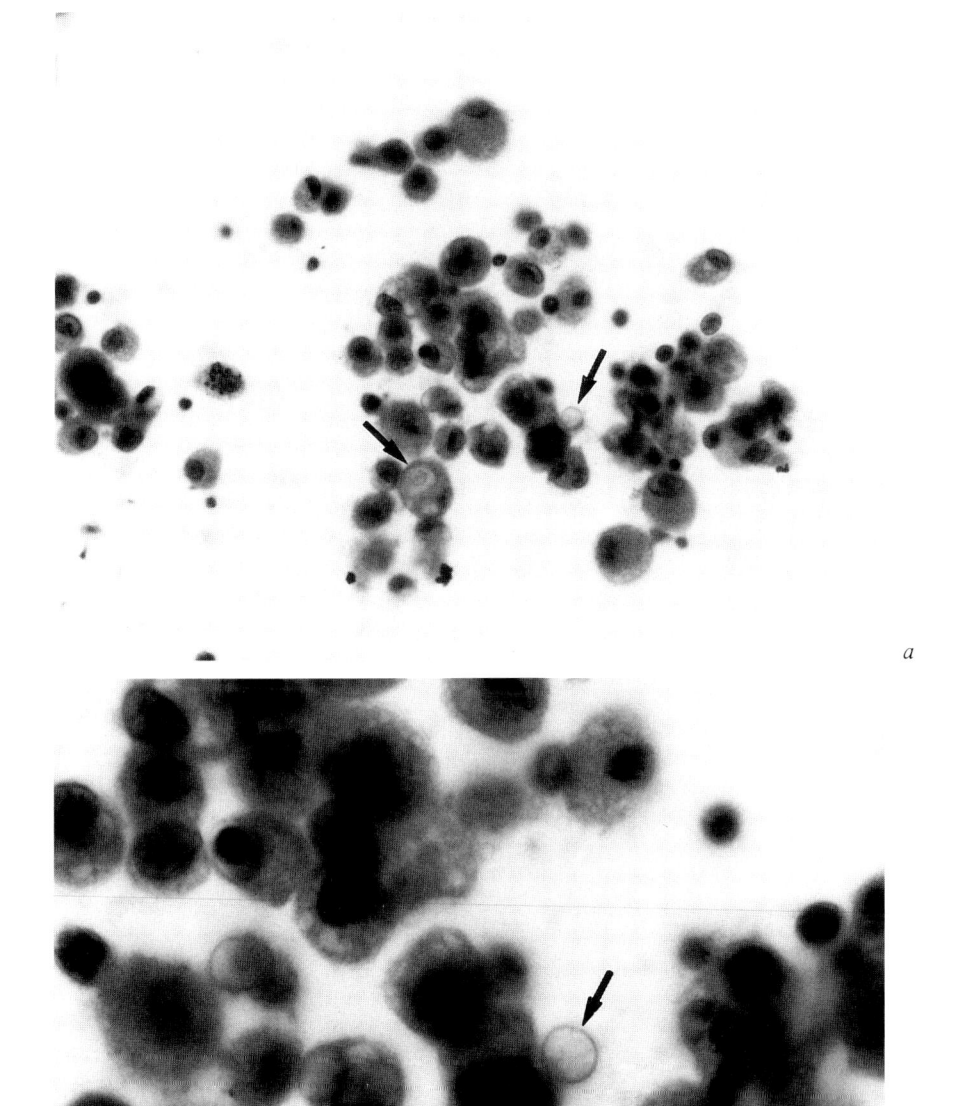

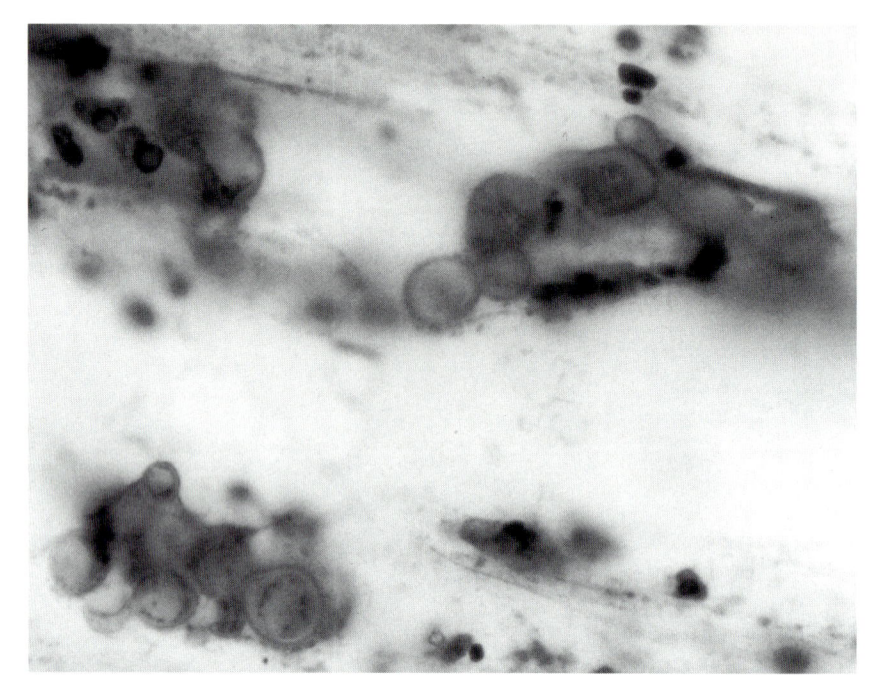

Fig. 30. Blastomycosis (sputum): A hallmark of this organism is the broad-based bud, sometimes forming a chain of organisms. Case courtesy of Dr. William W. Johnston, Duke University Medical Center. Papanicolaou. × 850.

may accompany or alternate with multinucleated giant cells in which the budding yeasts may be found. Organisms have been recovered in pleural effusions. Nothing specific about the inflammatory pattern will provide the diagnosis without the organism [111; 115, p. 104].

Invasive Fungal Pneumonias

Fungi which cause a pneumonia pattern rather than granulomatous disease are outlined in table 3 [121, p. 223]. In the past, such diagnoses were not the target for cytologic interpretation, as these organisms were not recovered from exfoliated or brushed specimens. Transbronchial biopsy in some instances would retrieve diagnostic material. However, with the advent of FNA and enhanced radiologic imaging techniques, needles can be directed to suspected areas in the lung parenchyma and material aspi-

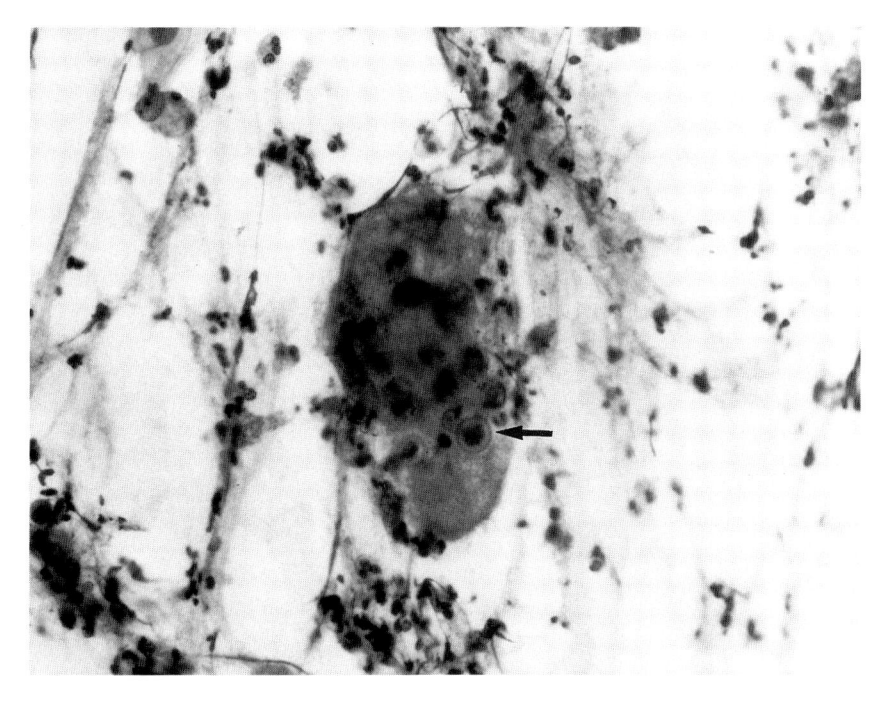

Fig. 31. Blastomycosis (sputum): Elsewhere in the same specimen as figure 30 can be found multinucleated histiocytes containing the thick-walled organisms (arrow). Case courtesy of Dr. William W. Johnston, Duke University Medical Center. Papanicolaou. × 340.

Table 3. Fungal pneumonias: contrasting histologic features [121]

	Aspergillosis	Mucormycosis	Candidiasis	Torulopsis
Organism morphology				
Hyphae	thin (3–5 µm), septate	wide (10–15 µm), nonseptate	–	–
Branching	dichotomous, 45°	haphazard, 90°	–	–
Budding yeast	–	–	+	+
Pseudohyphae	–	–	+	–
Tissue reaction				
Vascular invasion, infarction	+	+	–	–
Acute inflammation, abscesses	–	–	+	+

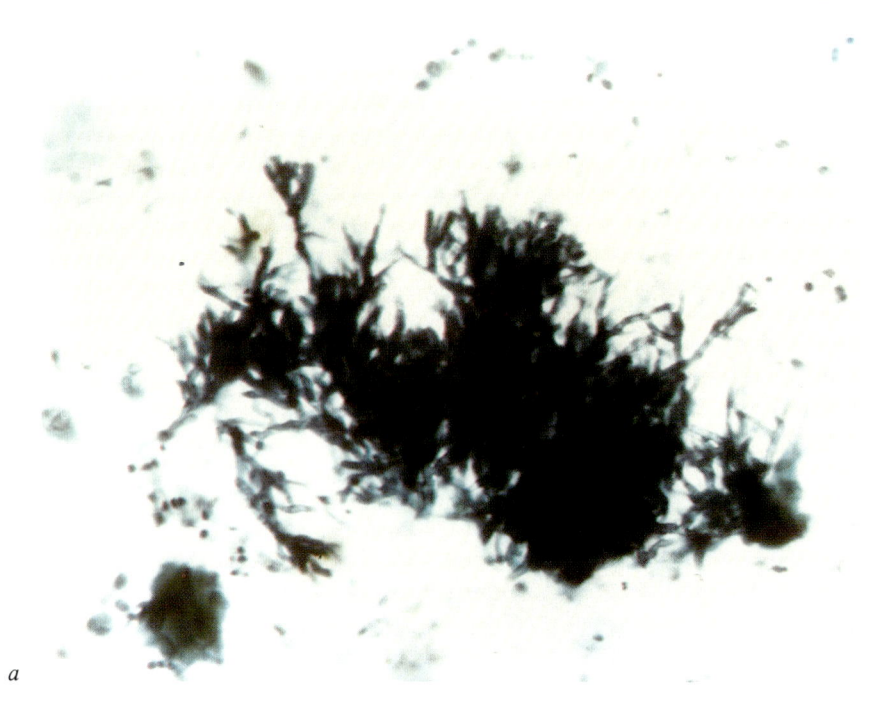

Fig. 32. Aspergillosis (bronchial wash = *a*; FNA = *b, c*): This organism usually is not obtained in exfoliated material as it grows tenaciously into tissue. FNA is an effective way of obtaining diagnostic material, both for morphology and culture. Note the broad hyphae with 45 degree angle branching. The accompanying inflammation is predominantly acute. Vascular invasion with hemorrhage and infarction is common with this organism. *a* = ×170, Papanicolaou. *b* = ×360; *c* = ×850, HE.

rated not only for microbiologic identification, but also for cytologic analysis. These organisms do not need special stains for identification, but show up very well using the routine Papanicolaou stain. Their morphology is sufficiently characteristic to tentatively identify the organism, so that therapy can be started even before definitive culture results are available. This is especially critical in the immunocompromised patient with a life-threatening infection.

Aspergillosis

Aspergillus is a saprophytic organism which occurs as an invading pathogen almost exclusively in patients who are in some way immunocompromised. Acute leukemia patients are particularly prone to this infection.

b

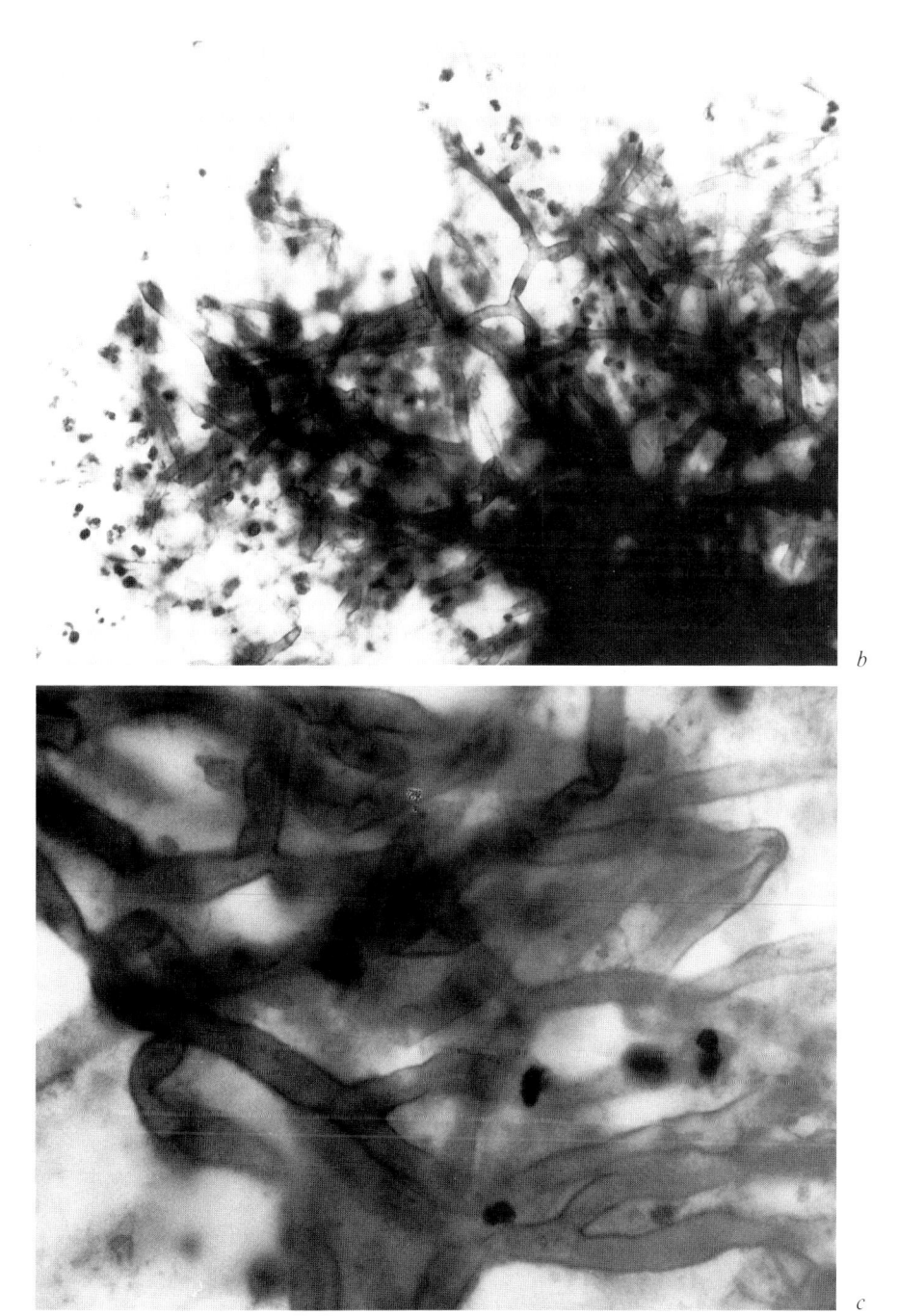

c

Rare cases of invasive Aspergillus in otherwise normal individuals have been reported [121, p. 223].

The clinical course of pulmonary aspergillosis follows the inhalation of air-borne spores which produces a pneumonia, provoking fever, cough, chest pain, and occasional hemoptysis. Chest X-ray findings include patchy infiltrates progressing to dense consolidation. Sputum cultures are frequently negative which makes an antemortem diagnosis difficult. Even with positive culture results, the implication of Aspergillus as a causative agent is difficult since the fungus is a frequent saprophyte. Open biopsy, transbronchial biopsy, and transbronchial and transthoracic FNA are the most reliable means of identifying the organism as pathogenic. Because of the debilitated condition of most infected patients, the prognosis is poor unless very early diagnosis is made and aggressive amphotericin therapy is begun.

The tissue pattern is that of a hemorrhagic infarct with only scattered inflammatory cells. In order to be defined as an invasive process, fungal hyphae should be identified invading blood vessel walls and permeating alveolar septa. Fungi can behave as arterial thrombi when they occlude the lumens. Another pattern is that of a necrotizing bronchopneumonia. A striking gross pattern, a 'target lesion', is formed by a central yellow-grey zone rimmed with a dark periphery. This lesion may be the precursor of the hemorrhagic infarct, caused by vascular invasion. The fungus probably invades the parenchyma through the bronchial walls.

The morphology of the organism is that of a long, thin, septate mycelium, approximately 4 μm in diameter with 45 degree branching (fig. 32). Mycelia frequently run almost parallel to each other, radiating from a central point. Mycelial growth is usually not associated with conidiophores, so that they may be misinterpreted as phycomycosis. The distinguishing feature is that the latter are not septate.

Aside from recognizing the organism as an invasive pathogen, this fungus, with others, can produce dysplastic squamous cells which may be misinterpreted as squamous carcinoma. This is particularly the case when

---

Fig. 33. Aspergillosis, calcium oxalate crystals (sputum): In exfoliated material, not the organism but its product, calcium oxalate, can often be found. Although recognizable only with polarized light, the debris and footprint of the mineral can be recognized in Papanicolaou stained material (*a*). Polarized light is an excellent way of illustrating the calcium oxalate crystals (*b*). Once again, note the acute inflammatory response rather than chronic as in most fungal diseases. Papanicolaou. $a = \times 170$; $b = \times 850$. Case courtesy of Margaret Farley, University of Texas Health Center at Tyler.

Infectious Diseases 61

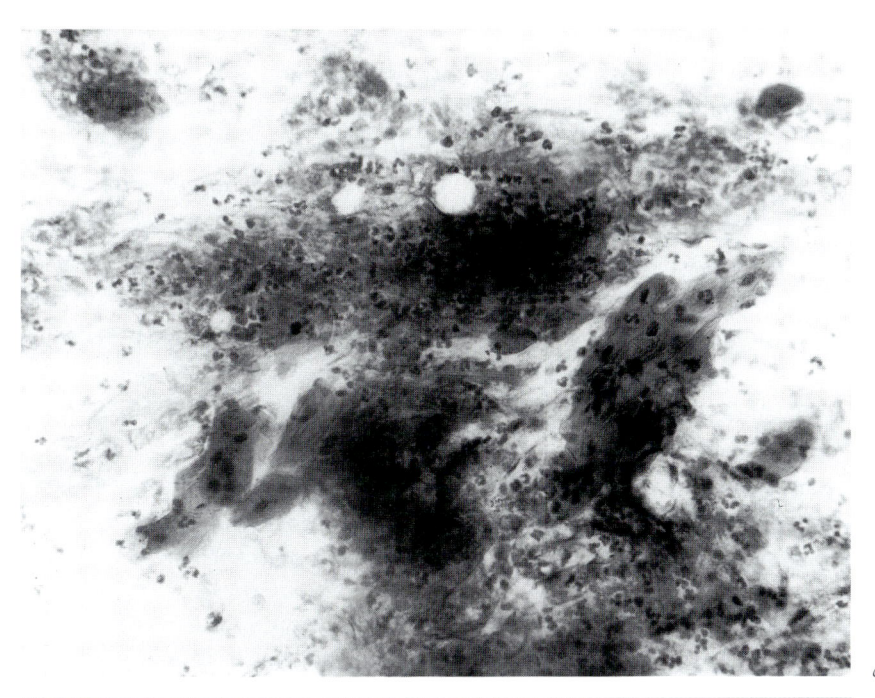

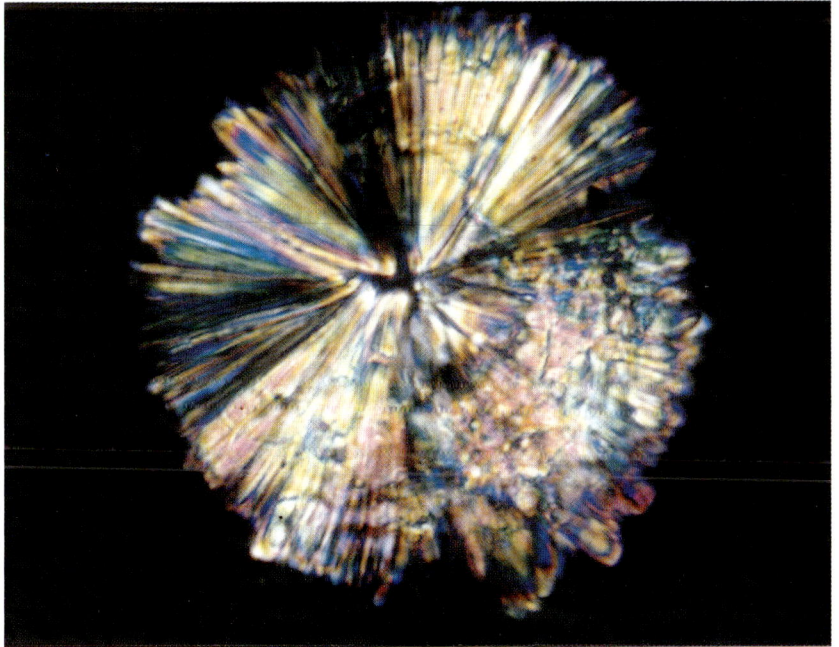

a

b

a cavity develops in a mycetoma (fig. 26). Calcium oxylate crystals can also be seen in large accumulations in association with the hyphae [115, p. 126; 258], and have been retrieved in sputum. These crystals polarize, providing immediate identification. Their presence in a sputum indicates that an Aspergillus infection exists even if the organism is not in the sample [64] (fig. 33). However, other infections, e.g. TB, can accumulate calcium crystals within diseased tissues which can be expectorated [258].

Mucormycosis (Phycomycosis)

The term phycomycosis applies to an acute mycotic infection in which extensive inflammation and vascular thrombi are caused by invasion of vessel walls and lumina by a long list of mycoses including Absidia, Mucor, Rhizopus and Basidiobolus. Once again, underlying debilitating diseases, including diabetes mellitus, the lymphoproliferative diseases, and immunocompromised conditions predispose to these infections. Steroid therapy in otherwise healthy individuals also has been a predisposing factor. The disease pattern consists of fever, chest pain, and possible massive hemoptysis. Chest X-rays reveal patchy pulmonary infiltrates. The organisms are difficult to prove by culture, including direct cultures of lung tissue.

The histologic pattern features extensive parenchymal and vascular invasion by the organism with subsequent hemorrhagic infarcts and scanty cellular infiltrates. These organisms are wider than Aspergillus, 10–15 μm wide, and are ribbon-like; 90 degree branching differentiates these from the 45 degree branches of Aspergillus. Mucormycosis has not been identified in cytologic material at UCLA in the past 15 years.

Fungi Variably Producing Disease

A variety of fungi can be found in respiratory samples; they are usually contaminants, but occasionally are of pathogenic significance. What formerly were saprophytes have now become opportunistic infectious organisms. Therefore, the presence of fungi can no longer be ignored or mini-

---

Fig. 34. Candida (sputum): Usually a contaminant of the upper respiratory tract, especially the mouth, Candida can be seen in immunocompromised persons. The small spores, occasionally budding, provide a Candida diagnosis, although culture is essential to define subspecies of that group. Papanicolaou. $a = \times 360$; $b = \times 850$.

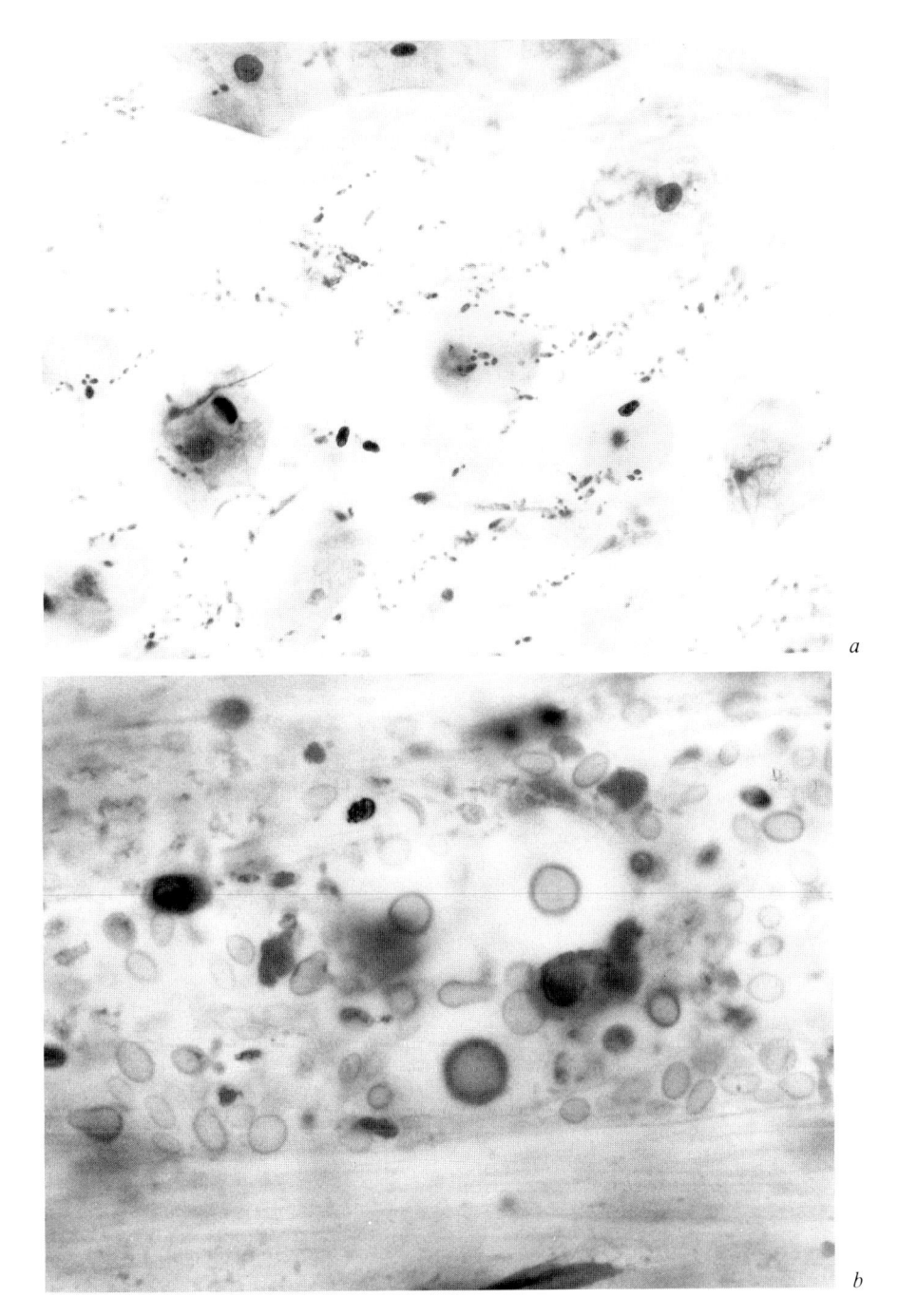

Infectious Diseases

a

b

mized in a respiratory sample. The determination, however, of whether or not a fungal organism is responsible for disease in the patient is left to the clinical judgment of the attending physicians. Definite confirmation of the type of organism is also not the responsibility of the cytology laboratory, but that of the microbiology personnel. However, as reliant on special stains as many pathologists are, experience has shown that the routine Papanicolaou stain is capable of detailing the characteristics of the mycoses sufficiently to obviate the need for special stains. As in any other disease process, if the observer does not consider the possibility, the pathology may not be recognized. Knowledge of infectious diseases endemic to or likely to be brought into the area is important when dealing with probably infectious material.

Candidiasis

Candida species are frequently saprophytic inhabitants of the oral cavity and skin, and occasionally of the respiratory tree. Since Candida located in the mouth can contaminate lower respiratory tract specimens, it must be carefully evaluated as the responsible agent for existing lung disease. The only way of definitely identifying the organism as pathogenic is to locate it within the tissue. In such instances, *Candida albicans* or *Candida tropicalis* is the offending organism. Such infections are usually within immunocompromised patients and will present as a multisystem disease. Significant pulmonary disease, however, is rare [121, p. 228]. The cytologic appearance of Candida species is that of long pseudohyphae with budding yeasts (fig. 34), sometimes found in morulae form.

Actinomycosis

Actinomyces is usually a contaminant of lower respiratory tract specimens, being dragged down by the bronchoscope, as a pickup from the tonsillar area. In order to implicate this organism as a pathogen, tissue sections must be obtained to display its invasion into lung tissue [137].

The clinical setting of actinomycosis is a soft tissue infection, but the lungs can also be involved in about one-fourth of the cases. This is not a disease of immunocompromised patients, although emphysema, bronchitis, and bronchiectasis are usually underlying diseases. The clinical course is that of an acute pneumonia with fever, cough, and a chest X-ray pattern of an infiltrate. The usual causative agent is *Actinomyces israelii,* which is a fastidious anaerobic organism, very difficult to culture, which results in numerous false negative cultures.

Infectious Diseases

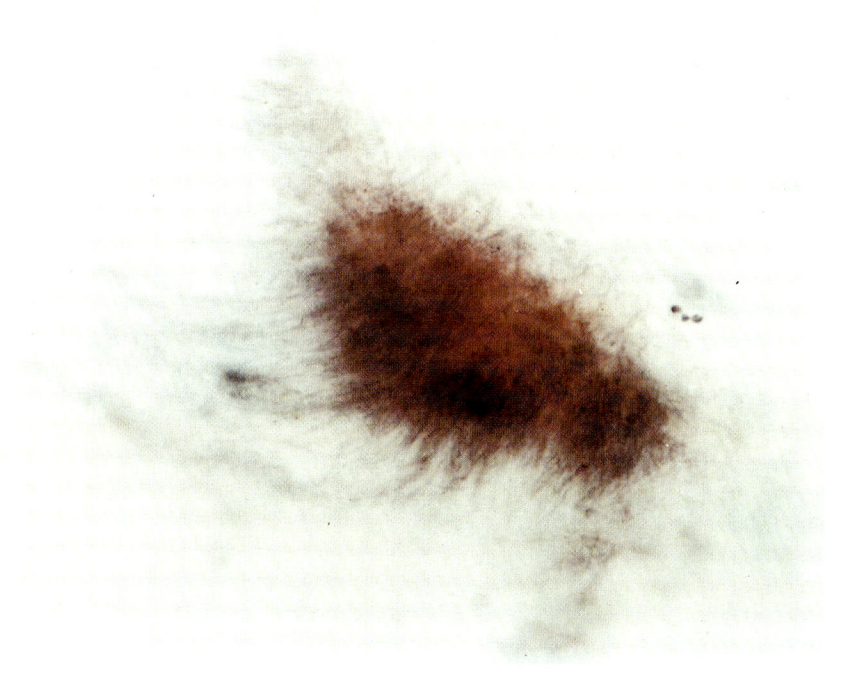

Fig. 35. Actinomyces (bronchial brush): Frequently contaminating a bronchoscopy specimen, this organism should be recognized as nonpathogenic in most instances. Radiating filaments may or may not arise from a central 'sulfur granule'. Such groups should not be mistaken for bacteria-coated fungal hyphae. Papanicolaou. $\times 340$.

The cytology of Actinomyces species is that of a cluster of organisms, with the rod-like filaments radiating from the center in a spoke-like fashion (fig. 35). The central granules, so-called sulfur granules, are not readily recovered in cytologic material. Once again, association with a pathologic condition cannot be made based on the presence in a cytologic sample from the respiratory tract.

Nocardiosis

Nocardia, an organism similar to Actinomyces, produces a disease pattern similar to Actinomyces when the latter is infectious. Nocardia will infect patients with underlying diseases, and produce clinical symptoms which vary from mild chest complaints to acute toxic illness. The chest X-ray pattern ranges from a solitary nodule to widespread infiltrates which

Cytopathology of Pulmonary Disease

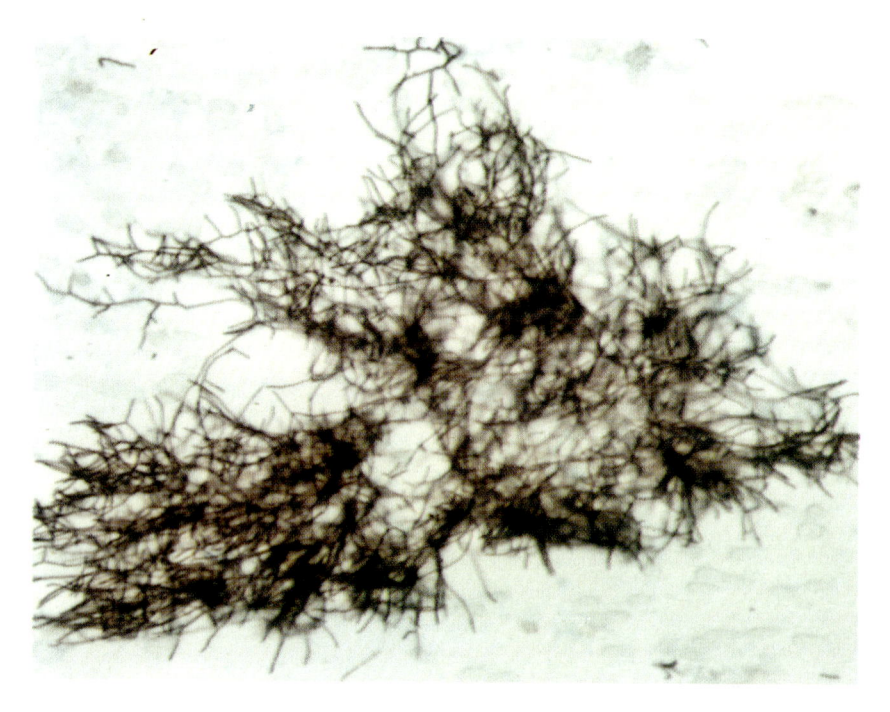

Fig. 36. Nocardia (FNA): These thin but distinct hyphae are arranged in a characteristic right-angle branch, which when superimposed on each other, create a 'Chinese figure' picture. Silver stain. × 170.

are sometimes cavitary. Dissemination via the blood stream is common, especially to the central nervous system. The organism is readily treated by sulfa.

The diagnosis cannot be made by sputum culture in the majority of the cases. Lung biopsy or fine needle aspiration is necessary to obtain material for diagnosis. A necrotizing acute pneumonia with abscess formation is the common picture. Poorly-formed granulomas, predominantly of histiocytes, may surround the necrotic areas. A GMST (Grocott's methenamine silver technique) stain will clearly visualize the organisms. They are also weakly acid-fast and appear as gram-positive with Brown-Hopps or Brown-Brenn. The organism appears as long, branching, filamentous rods, assuming 'Chinese character' configurations, and measuring 0.5–1.0 µm in diameter (fig. 36). Granules such as seen in Actinomyces are not usually present with Nocardia colonies.

Pneumocystis

'*Pneumocystis carinii* was first recognized as a cause of serious lung disease in institutionalized malnourished infants in Europe during World War II; mortality was 50%. Although this neonatal illness is now rare in Europe, it is still seen in some underdeveloped parts of the world' [121, p. 241].

This quote from a recent text on lung disease attests to the rapidly changing status of certain infectious agents. The copyright of 1982 reflects a prepublication date which precedes the era of AIDS-related diseases, in which pneumocystis pneumonia has played a major lethal role. Katzenstein does describe the occurrence of this metazoan infection in 'apparently healthy drug abusers and homosexual men', which has been strongly borne out by the epidemiologic analyses of the AIDS populations [148].

The clinical picture is a pneumonia which occurs invariably in immunocompromised individuals. The onset is either acute or subacute with a dry cough, fever, dyspnea and progression to respiratory failure if treatment is not begun early in the disease. Chest X-ray findings include bilateral interstitial infiltrates radiating from hila to the peripheral alveoli, although occasional localized infiltrates have been reported.

Recovery of the organisms in sputa is rare [147]. Brushings and washings occasionally are productive [109], but the most diagnostic study is the bronchoalveolar lavage. Prior to the use of this technique, open lung biopsy was the most highly diagnostic method, with transthoracic percutaneous needle and transbronchial biopsy being adequate but less successful than the open biopsy. In our institution, BAL has essentially replaced the open lung biopsy for diagnosis of pneumocystis [174]. Equally impressive results have been reported by others [66, 85, 180, 210] (table 4).

The frothy honeycomb 'exudate' within the alveolar spaces, seen on HE sections, is recapitulated in cytologic samples by a rusty brown 'exudate' (fig. 8, 37). This exudate is really closely-packed organisms (fig. 38), which can be clearly revealed by GMST (fig. 39) or Giemsa stain, or by fluorescent emission of Papanicolaou stained material [147]. These small, cup-shaped organisms measure 1–2 µm and are the intracystic forms of the sporozoites [191].

The foamy exudate in the HE sections (fig. 40) requires a GMST stain, but the cytologic specimen stained by Papanicolaou stain is highly diagnostic, and does not require special stains. Weber et al. [272] found that 17 out of 36 cases or 47% did not have the typical intra-alveolar exudate. Katzenstein [121, p. 242] describes the predominant histologic feature as similar

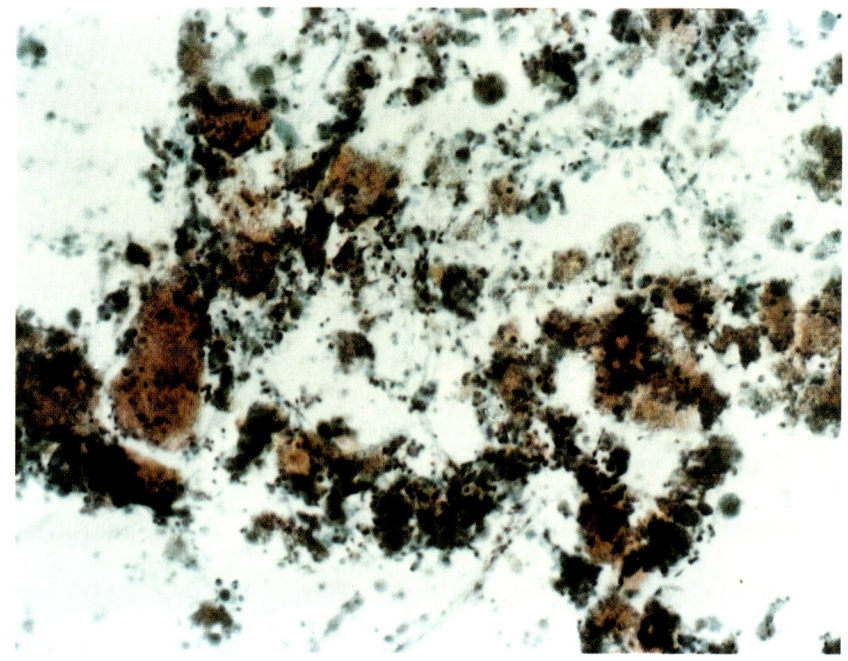

37a

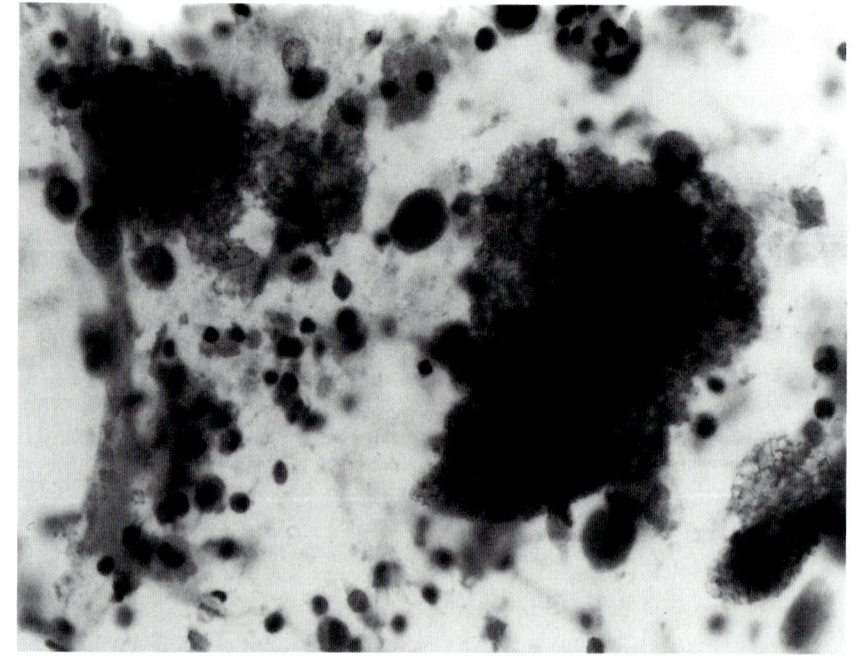

37b

Infectious Diseases 69

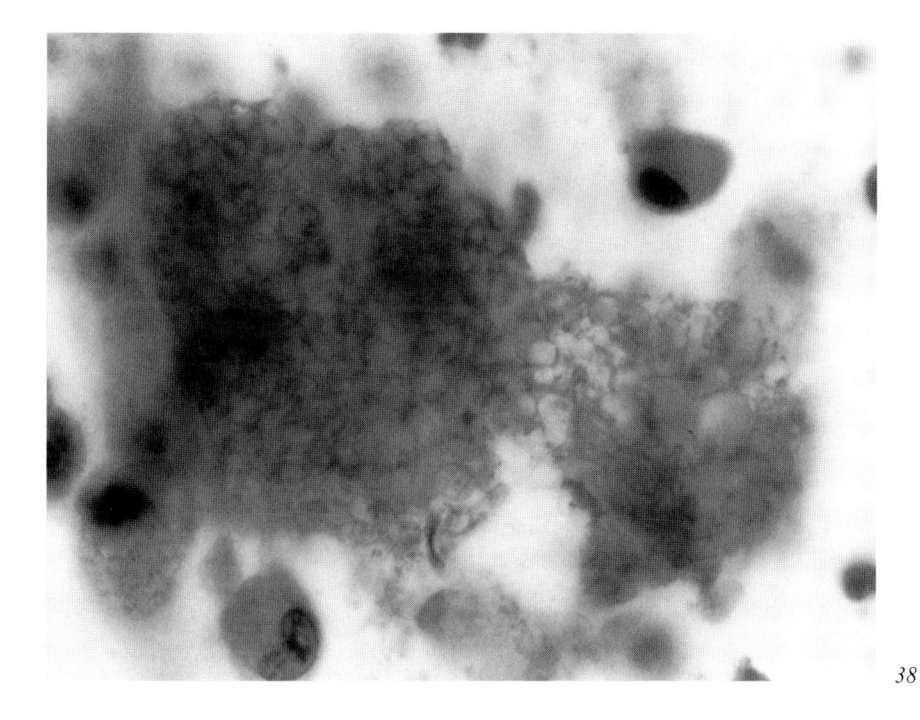

38

Fig. 37. Pneumocystis (BAL): Diagnostic material of this opportunistic infection can be readily obtained with lavage. The large groups of tightly packed organisms present as rusty brown sponges. Although silver stain is still considered the standard of practice, Papanicolaou stained material such as this is considered indisputable. Papanicolaou. *a* = × 34; *b* = × 340.

Fig. 38. Pneumocystis (BAL): Higher power of figure 37 shows the outlines of the organisms. This is not truly an 'exudate', but a colony of organisms. Compare the size of each 'hole' with nearby macrophages. Papanicolaou. × 850.

Fig. 39. Pneumocystis (*a* = FNA, *b*, *c* = BAL): *a* contains pneumocystis organisms stained by traditional silver stain. Note the bipolar shape, but the density of the organisms prohibits true appreciation of the morphology. *b* is stained with a modified silver stain (see 'Appendix'), which provides a transparency to the organisms, allowing the observer to appreciate the concavity or cup-shaped configuration. *a*, *b* = silver stain; *c* = Papanicolaou. × 900.

Fig. 40. Pneumocystis (transbronchial biopsy): The 'foamy exudate' corresponds to the organisms obtained from the alveoli in a BAL. Compare the diagnostic cytologic specimen with the tissue section which is suggestive, but not definitive without special stains. HE. × 340.

Cytopathology of Pulmonary Disease 70

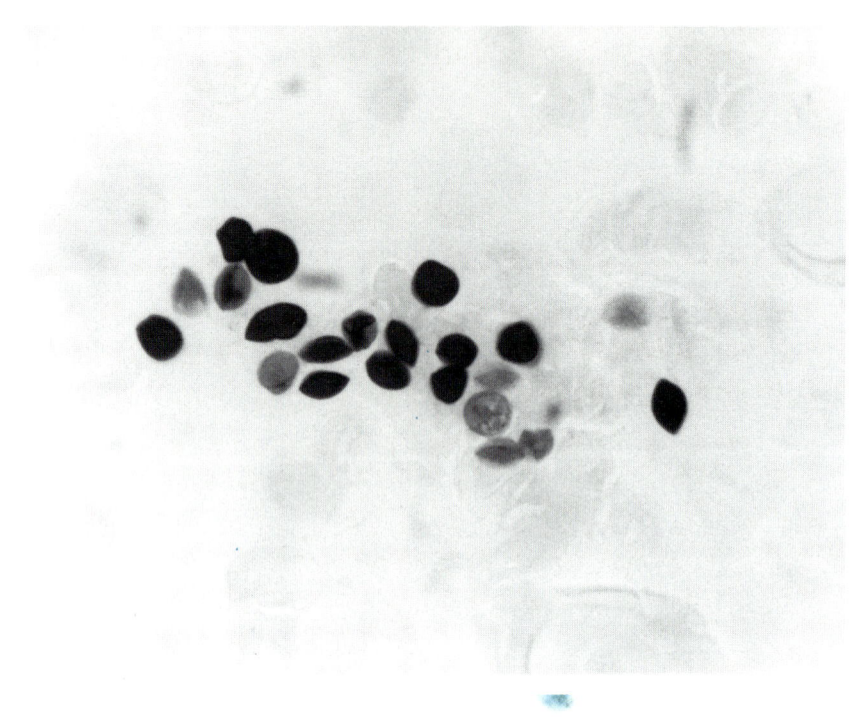

39a

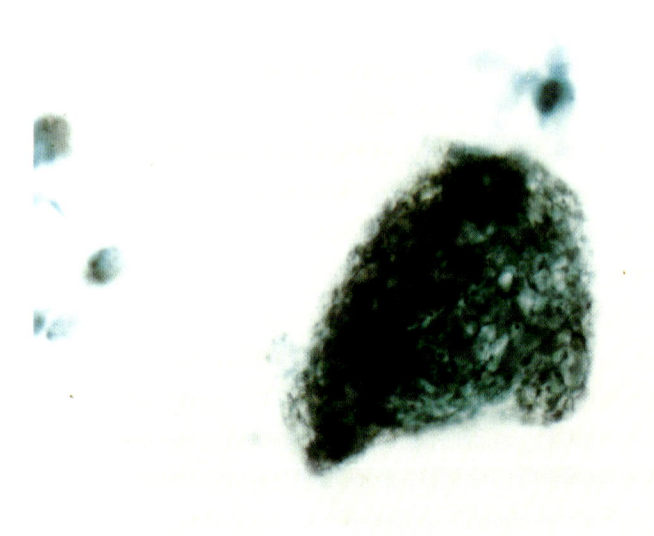

39b

(For legend see p. 69.)

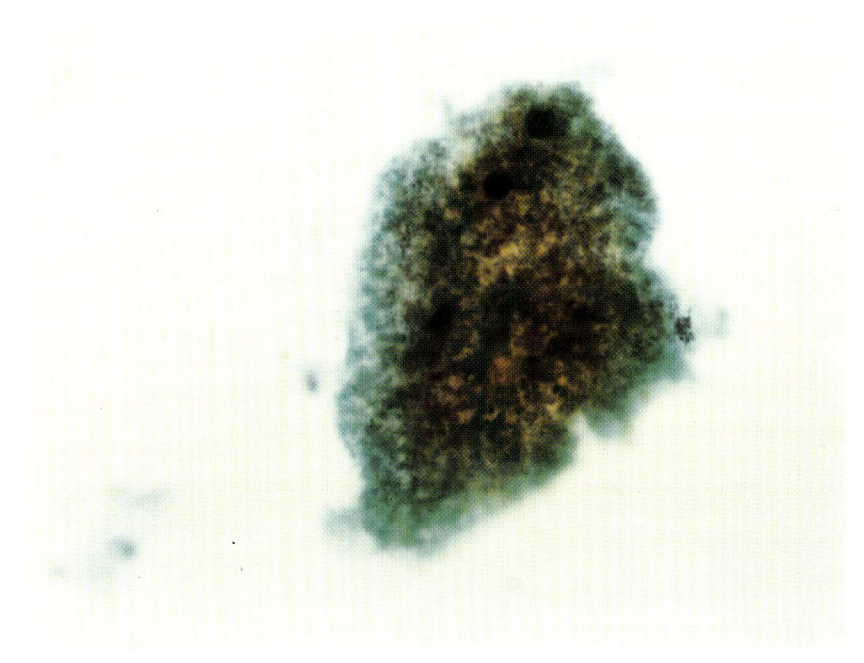

Infectious Diseases

39c

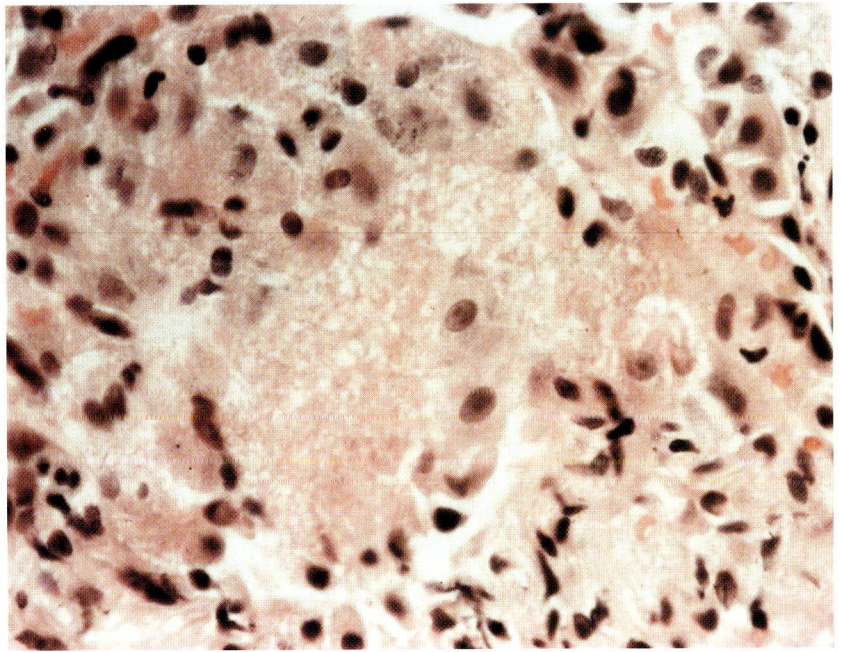

40

(For legend see p. 69.)

Table 4. Bronchoscopy studies showing the yield of *Pneumocystis carinii* [174] (percent values)

Author	BAL	TBB	BR	BW
Pitchenik		90	53	79
Garay	71	98		
Ognibene	89	35		
Broaddus	89	93		
Stover	85	88	41	41
Orenstein	94	73.3	26.7	44.4
Nieberg	100			
Meduri	100 (bilateral)			
Wagner	96	74	12	37
Flick	100	95		
Coleman		79	39	55

TBB = Transbronchial biopsy; BR = bronchial brush; BW = bronchial wash.

to diffuse alveolar damage, an especially prominent finding when the froth is scanty. Hyaline membranes, interstitial pneumonia with a preponderance of plasma cells ('interstitial plasma cell pneumonia') and alveolar lining cell hyperplasia can be noted as well as intra-alveolar hemorrhage and proteinaceous exudates. Rare reactions include granulomas, giant cells, interstitial fibrosis, and calcification. In immunocompromised patients, an absence of inflammatory reaction is common, attesting to the inability of the patients to respond to infectious organisms.

Viral Infections

The significance of viral infection in the lung has become more critical in recent years due to the increasing numbers of immunocompromised patients, and their increased susceptibility to infectious diseases, including the viruses. In the well patient, a pulmonary viral infection is usually self-limited, returning the patient to his previously healthy state. A few patients, especially children, will succumb to an especially virulent strain of virus, or an overwhelming infection. Until very recently, there has been no definitive antiviral therapy, and supportive measures have been the best that medical science could provide for such patients [71].

Infectious Diseases

Table 5. Viral pneumonias: light and electron microscopic features [121]

Virus	Ultrastructure	Inclusions nuclear	Inclusions cytoplasmic	Cellular alteration	Histopathologic features
Cytomegalovirus	100–200 nm, round core double membrane	+	+	cytomegaly	interstitial pneumonia; DAD
Herpes simplex / Varicella-zoster	150–200 nm, round core double membrane	+	–	–	DAD; necrosis
Measles	15–20 nm, tubular filaments	+	+	multi-nucleation	interstitial pneumonia; DAD
Adenovirus	60–90 nm, icosahedral, crystalline array	+	–	smudge cells	necrotizing bronchiolitis; DAD

DAD = Diffuse alveolar damage.

With the demands placed upon infectious disease clinicians to affect a cure in this now large population of immunocompromised patients, diligent search for specific antiviral therapeutic agents has been launched, with some degree of success. As with any other disease process, once a cure has been discovered, specific identification of the infectious agent becomes mandatory to match the diagnosis with the cure. Just because hallmarks of a viral organism are present (table 5), the assumption cannot be made that this virus is indeed causing the pneumonic process. In a normal population, approximately 80% will carry herpes virus and a lesser but significant percentage will carry cytomegalovirus (CMV) within respiratory cells, without actually experiencing a disease.

Therefore, the kind of specimen obtained is critical to accurately sample tissues in question. The recently developed BAL technique has enabled the bronchoscopist to obtain a generous sampling of cellular material of the bronchoalveoli, and thus accurately define the pathology ongoing within the functional component of the lung. This technique has superseded the use of open lung biopsy at UCLA, which definitely benefits these

Cytopathology of Pulmonary Disease 74

already sick patients by not having to undergo major surgery for diagnosis. Needle aspiration via the transbronchial route [215] or the transthoracic [176] route also can obtain diagnostic material of the lung parenchyma without the morbidity of a thoracotomy.

Whatever the route of sampling, the specimens must be handled rapidly to assure that the changes within the cells are quickly fixed so that they accurately represent viral changes and not simply degeneration due to delay in processing. Stains must be fresh and reveal crisp nuclear detail for the same reasons.

The description of the specific viral diseases to follow will emphasize the cytologic findings in the various viral infections. This author recognizes the need for confirmation by viral culture, DNA probes [227], immunocytochemistry, or other specific diagnostic techniques. The changes appreciated in the specimens stained by the Papanicolaou technique can provide a rapid preliminary diagnosis, which will enable the clinicians to begin therapy on an informed basis, before the definitive diagnosis is provided by more sophisticated methods. Avoiding a delay in treatment, albeit currently experimental, may be life-saving to a patient who is threatened by an overwhelming viral infection. Cytologic diagnosis can provide this critical information.

Before the specific cytologic changes of a variety of viruses commonly affecting the respiratory tract are described, nonspecific changes need to be addressed. Cilia with attached cytoplasm, ciliacytophthoria, has long been a recognized consequence of viral attack on a cell. This change is quite nonspecific, but can be especially pronounced in adenovirus infections. It was first described by Papanicolaou [182] in 1956. In addition, nonspecific small, round eosinophilic masses in the cytoplasm can be observed, much like those seen in urothelial cells, presumably of degenerative origin [115, p. 141; 130, p. 580].

The nonspecific changes which present the greatest problem are those of regeneration and repair of the respiratory epithelium. Such atypia may mimic adenocarcinoma or squamous carcinoma, unless the wary observer considers cytologic criteria very carefully. These nonspecifically atypical cells may be found in both sputa and bronchoscopic material and are characterized by enlarged hyperchromatic nuclei and prominent nucleoli. Even when tightly clustered and apparently neoplastic, cilia will confirm their benign nature. The major problem occurs when the cells originate in terminal bronchioles or pulmonary alveoli, are seen in clusters with large irregularly-shaped nuclei, uneven chromatin patterns and large prominent

Infectious Diseases 75

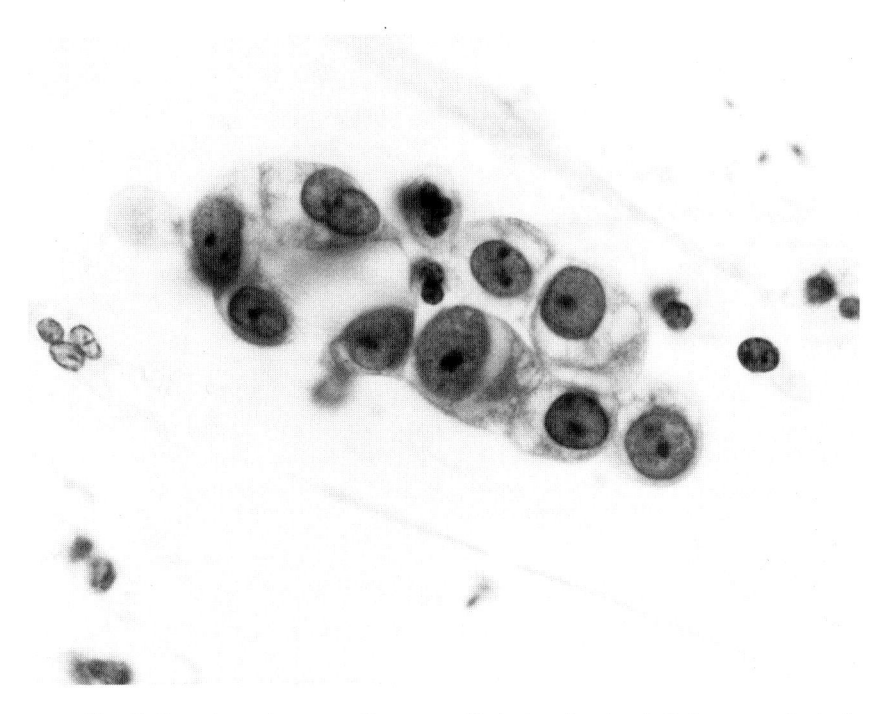

Fig. 41. Reactive columnar cells, unspecified virus (sputum): Columnar cell atypia needs to be distinguished from a well-differentiated adenocarcinoma. Pneumonia is frequently the cause of such benign atypia, and is the most common pitfall in cytologic diagnosis of the respiratory tract. Careful attention to nuclear detail, a history with chest X-ray findings, and follow-up of the patient are all essential ways of avoiding a misdiagnosis. Papanicolaou. × 850.

nucleoli (fig. 41). The lack of cilia is a result of the origin of the cells in nonciliated epithelium. This is the most frequent pitfall for the cytopathologist. Repeat specimens usually assure that an overcall is not made. If the cellular changes are definitely secondary to an infection, the cell changes will disappear as the infection progresses and recedes. If, instead, the changes are secondary to an adenocarcinoma, the atypia will persist, may even become more markedly anaplastic, and will verify the diagnosis of cancer.

Of importance and interest is the altered inflammatory response that many of these patients will manifest, some of them not being able to respond at all. Therefore, little or no inflammatory reaction will be the norm. Diffuse alveolar damage may be the only pattern seen in tissue sections. Careful search for organisms or their hallmarks is therefore an important responsibility of the cytologist even without significant numbers of inflammatory cells. DNA probes are now available to identify infected cells even before any cytopathic effect is evident (see chapter VIII).

Specific Viral Infections

Herpes Virus Type I

The prototype of viral infections infecting cytologic samples is clearly herpes, no doubt because this family of viruses affects the very familiar female genital tract as well as the respiratory tract and numerous other body sites (fig. 42). The clinical picture of patients with pneumonia caused by herpes simplex virus is usually underscored by a debilitating disease or immunosuppression. The parenchymal involvement is bronchocentric with patchy, nodular, or confluent foci of necrosis. Alveolar septa are obliterated, with only their 'ghosts' remaining. Alveolar spaces contain a proteinaceous suspension of necrotic neutrophils and cell debris. Hyaline membranes are equally common. The characteristic intranuclear inclusions will be found in alveolar lining cells (pneumocytes) or alveolar macrophages at the periphery of the necrosis [72]. If necrosis is too extensive, these inclusions will not be identified.

Herpetic tracheobronchitis is a necrotizing lesion seen in most patients with lung lesions but also in patients without. The ulcerated respiratory epithelium is covered by a fibrinopurulent exudate. The intranuclear inclusions can be identified within cells of the intact mucosa (fig. 43) or within submucosal gland epithelium.

Fig. 42. Herpes virus infection (sputum): The same criteria which apply to herpes infection of the female genital tract apply to respiratory tract specimen. Note the ground glass transformation of the nuclei, with margination of the chromatin. Occasional intranuclear inclusions are found in the specimen. The patient was immunocompromised, secondary to chemotherapy for 'oat cell' carcinoma. Diagnostic 'oat cells' were found elsewhere in the specimen. Papanicolaou. × 900.

Fig. 43. Herpes virus (bronchial brushing): The same changes as noted above are found in this specimen of the patient with herpetic tracheal bronchitis. More inclusions are seen, but the disease is essentially the same. This patient was also immunocompromised, suffering from AIDS. Papanicolaou. × 340.

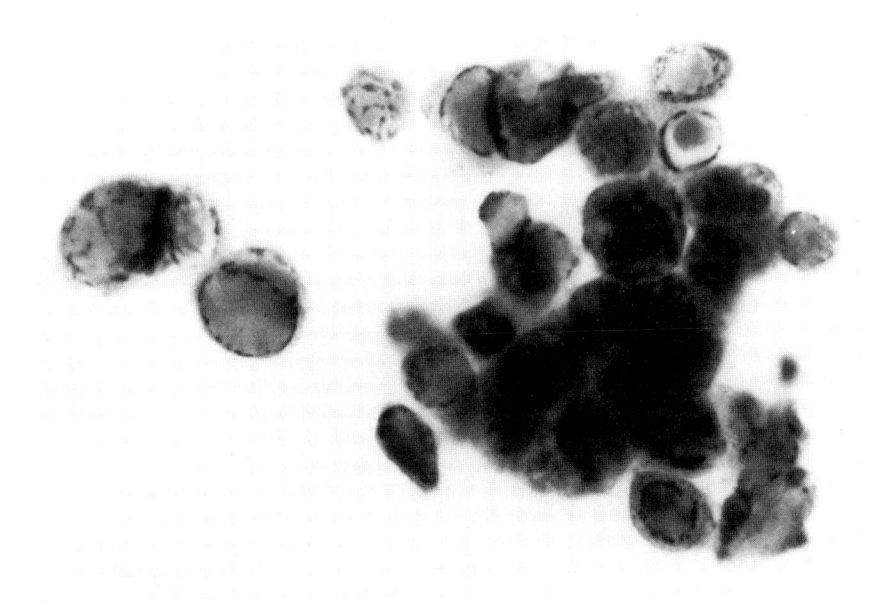

Infectious Diseases

42

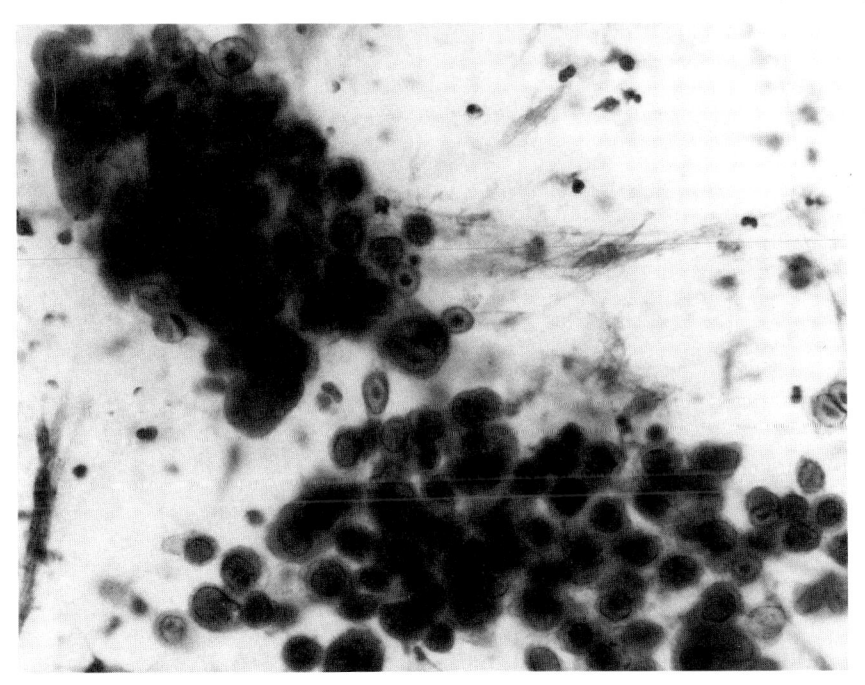

43

Since herpetic tracheobronchitis and esophagitis are not uncommon, a true herpetic pneumonia cannot be inferred from the presence of infected cells in a bronchoscopy or sputum sample. In order to identify herpes as a cause of a pneumonia, the characteristic cellular changes must be observed in samples retrieved directly from the pulmonary alveoli, either by transbronchial or transthoracic needle aspirate. Now, the use of the BAL can retrieve diagnostic specimens from the pulmonary parenchyma [174].

The pathogenesis of both the tracheobronchial and pneumonic forms is probably via a primary tracheobronchial infection which then spreads to the lung parenchyma. Many patients have a previous history of endotracheal intubation, tracheostomy, or burn injury. Damage to the respiratory epithelium is the usual predisposing condition. If there is no tracheobronchitis, the pathway of infection is probably blood borne. Such infections are usually more random than the classic peribronchial distribution.

The classic cytologic lesions can be divided into two types: the groundglass intranuclear inclusion, and the Cowdry type A inclusions which are a round, eosinophilic central body surrounded by a clear halo and then confined by a thickened chromatinic membrane [72] (fig. 44). While characteristic multinucleated giant cells can be seen, they are not so common as in herpetic infections elsewhere in the body. Any or all of these changes may be present simultaneously. Earlier thinking defined the intranuclear inclusion as a later stage or a re-infection manifestation of the disease. However, more recent work has indicated that all stages can be seen in a given sample or over a short period of time in a single infectious period. The cells are not enlarged, which differentiate them from those infected with CMV, and herpetic inclusions are bright red or lavender, not the deeply basophilic inclusion of CMV. Cytoplasmic inclusions, often present in CMV-infected cells, are absent in herpes lesions. Both viruses, however, belong to the same family.

Cytomegalovirus

CMV can be carried by patients who are immunologically intact without any resultant disease. To the immunocompromised patient, however, this infectious agent can be lethal in a large percentage of cases. Bone marrow transplant recipients have a high incidence of CMV pneumonitis, which is the leading cause of death in such patients. The infection may be opportunistic, but most likely is transferred from patient to patient via blood transfusions. The clinical picture is that of fever, dyspnea, and nonproductive cough. The chest films reveal diffuse bilateral infiltrates.

Infectious Diseases 79

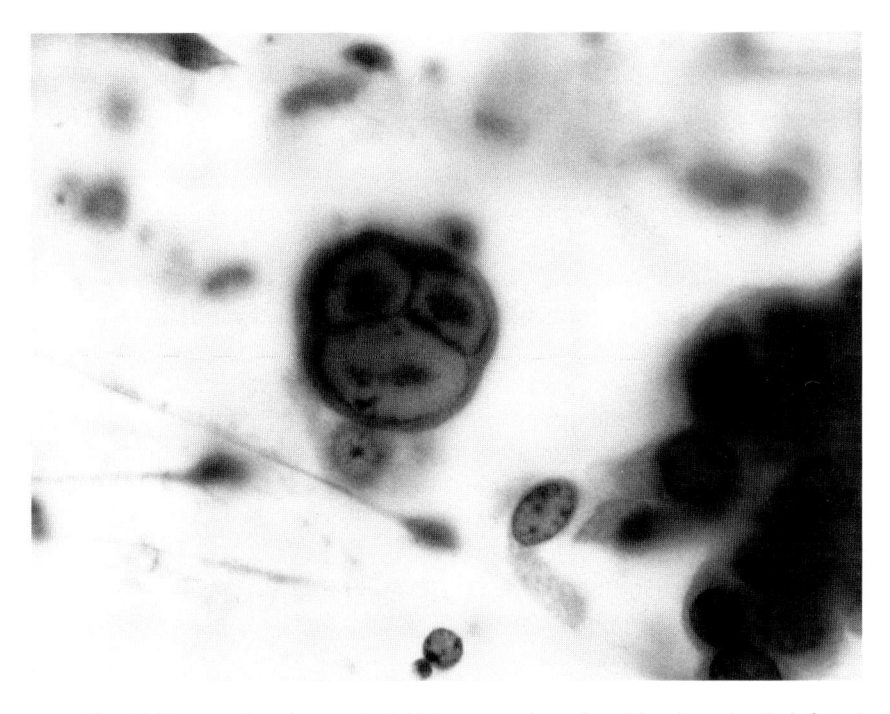

Fig. 44. Herpes virus (sputum): A high power view of multinucleated cells infected with herpes virus. Note the increased size when compared to the nearby columnar epithelial cells. Inclusions are only intranuclear, distinctive from CMV-infected cells which can also contain intracytoplasmic inclusions. The flat-sided nuclear molding is also characteristic of herpes. Papanicolaou stain. × 850.

The histologic pattern is different from herpes pneumonia by the absence of necrosis and the more diffuse pattern. Hyaline membranes, intra-alveolar hemorrhage and proteinaceous exudates are common findings. CMV and pneumocystis carinii often infect the same lung [268].

The diagnostic cell changes include generalized cell enlargement (megalo), and the dramatic large intranuclear basophilic inclusion, surrounded by a well-defined halo and a very distinct chromatinic rim [105] (fig. 45). In contrast to herpes virus infected cells, cells colonized by CMV also frequently have intracytoplasmic inclusions, which are very small spheres (fig. 46), difficult to see unless consciously looked for. These inclusions produce a granular or buckshot appearance to the cytoplasm and can be found in both respiratory epithelial cells and in pneumocytes of the alveoli.

In addition to the changes appreciated on Papanicolaou stained material, the cytoplasmic inclusions can be stained by PAS stain. The staining characteristics of the cytoplasmic inclusions are a reflection of the mucopolysaccharide envelope of the cytoplasmic inclusions that is not present around the intranuclear inclusions. In addition to the respiratory epithelial cells and alveolar lining cells, alveolar macrophages, endothelial cells and interstitial cells are also affected. Rather than wait 7–25 days for viral cultures to yield a diagnosis, the characteristic cell changes are looked for in open lung biopsies, bronchial brushings [6], transbronchial and transthoracic needle aspirates, and now, BALs. CMV probes, using in situ DNA hybridization techniques can be applied to BAL samples to reveal CMV infected cells before the characteristic inclusions are evident [97].

Varicella-Zoster Virus

Varicella virus, of the same family as herpes simplex, indistinguishable from herpes zoster, causes either chicken pox in children or shingles in adults who have had previous varicella-zoster infection. This virus causes pneumonia in approximately 15% of patients with chicken pox, usually adults. Children who are immunocompromised or otherwise debilitated may develop a varicella pneumonia. Adults are not necessarily immunocompromised. The clinical picture is one of a generalized skin involvement. Presenting symptoms include dyspnea, cough and fever. Radiologic pattern is that of a diffuse nodular infiltrate. The mortality can be 10–30%, with the higher figure representing the immunocompromised patient and pregnant women.

If the disease is clinically that of herpes zoster, dissemination will occur in immunocompromised patients, especially in those with underlying malignancies such as Hodgkin's disease. Lung involvement in such patients is very uncommon.

The histology in the lung is that of an acute interstitial pneumonia with hyaline membranes, and proteinaceous exudate within the alveolar

---

Fig. 45. Cytomegalovirus infection (BAL): An unusual multinucleated cell, with characteristic intranuclear inclusions and satellite inclusion. Note the large size of the cell, and the halo rimming the intranuclear inclusion. Papanicolaou. × 900.

Fig. 46. Cytomegalovirus infection (BAL): This undivided double cell contains not only intranuclear inclusions (out of plane of focus), but multiple cytoplasmic inclusions with the appearance of buck-shot. Note the large size of the cells when compared to lymphocytes and red cells. Papanicolaou. × 900.

Infectious Diseases

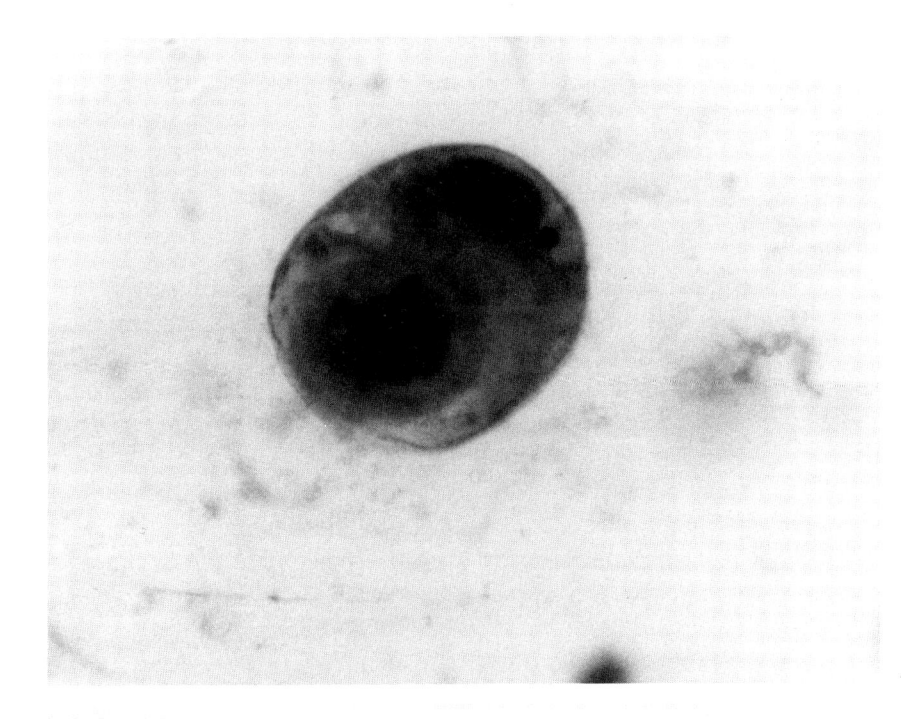

45

46

spaces. A parabronchial distribution has been described, but focal areas of necrosis are the most common picture. The intranuclear inclusions are identical to those of herpes simplex, and are most commonly seen within alveolar lining cells. Healing of this pneumonia has been noted to result in diffuse calcification [121, pp. 212–213].

Measles Virus

Measles pneumonia is extremely rare, and death even more uncommon. However, in immunocompromised children and in rare cases of adults, the disease has a significant impact on the patient. Although skin rashes are usually present, reports of giant cell pneumonia without skin rash have been noted [60] because immunocompromised children may not respond to infection in the common manner.

The histopathology of measles pneumonia is a dramatic scattering of multinucleated giant cells containing eosinophilic intranuclear and intracytoplasmic inclusions. Such inclusions can also be found within endothelial cells and macrophages. These polykaryocytes may contain up to 50 nuclei with abundant eosinophilic cytoplasm and are probably a result of fusion of type II pneumocytes (fig. 47). Accompanying these characteristic histiocytes is an acute interstitial pneumonia with hyaline membranes and intra-alveolar protein. While focal necrosis may occur, it is not a consistent or diagnostic finding, but distinguishes measles pneumonia from the giant cell pneumonia caused by respiratory syncytial virus (see below). Bronchial mucosal hyperplasia with focal squamous metaplasia may also be found [121, pp. 215–216].

Adenovirus

Adenovirus usually does not produce severe disease, but simply the minor flu-like syndrome involving the upper respiratory tract, i.e. the 'common cold'. Pneumonia, although rare, can be fatal in 40% of the patients. These fatalities usually involve children under 1 year, but occasional deaths in previously healthy adults and immunocompromised people have been reported. A sequel to the acute illness may be the development of bronchiolitis obliterans. This can result in prolonged pulmonary impairment with eventual death many months later. Undiagnosed adenovirus infections have been implicated in other forms of chronic lung disease, such as bronchiectasis [121, p. 221].

The histology of pneumonia caused by adenovirus is characterized by destruction of bronchioles and small bronchi. Multiple, eosinophilic in-

Infectious Diseases 83

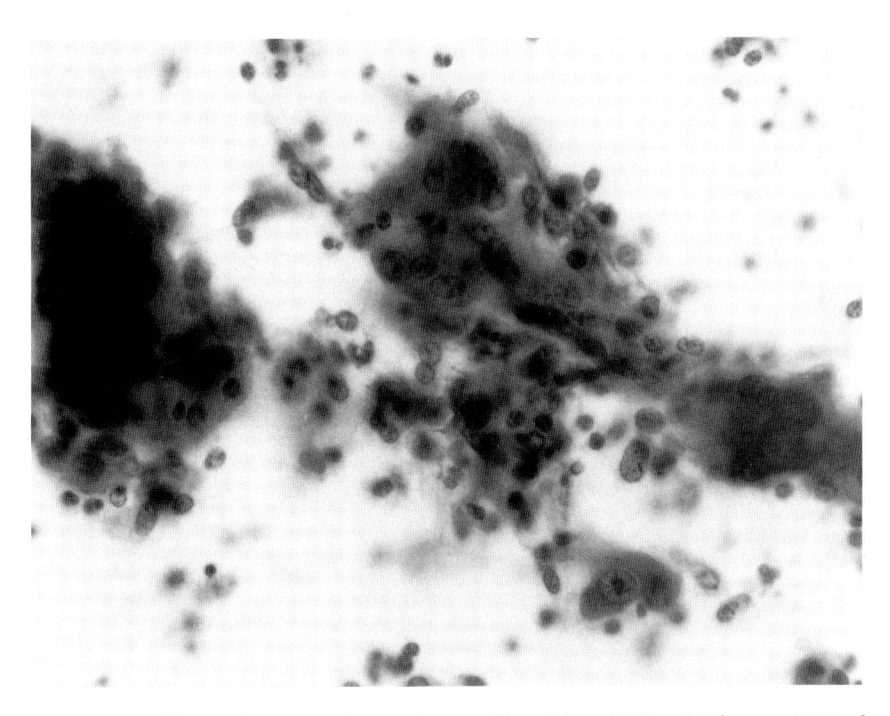

Fig. 47. Giant cell pneumonia (touch prep of lung biopsy): Material from an FNA of a giant cell pneumonia would resemble this material obtained from the touch preparation. Note the multinucleated giant cells and the large epithelioid cells, consistent with type II pneumocytes. Measles and respiratory syncytial virus are the most common viral diseases producing this picture. Papanicolaou. × 340.

tranuclear inclusions, each surrounded by a halo, can be seen in respiratory epithelium, which can be recovered in secretions to be examined cytologically. As the pneumonia progresses the epithelia of bronchi and bronchioles sluff, the lumens become packed with a granular eosinophilic debris resulting in distal airtrapping. Such debris could be expected in BALs or bronchial washings. Accompanying this bronchial damage is an acute interstitial pneumonia with intra-alveolar protein exudate and prominent hyaline membranes.

The intranuclear inclusions are found in the bronchiolar epithelium and alveolar lining cells. Two types can be seen. One is a homogeneous, amphophilic or basophilic mass, almost totally replacing the nucleus. These are termed 'smudge cells', and, due to their enlargement, are very distinct even on low power. The second kind of inclusion is a round, eosinophilic body surrounded by a clear halo which is circumscribed by clumped chromatin. This inclusion is smaller than the Cowdry type A of herpes virus. Ciliacytophthoria is most pronounced with this infection.

Respiratory Syncytial Virus

Respiratory syncytial virus (RSV) may cause a severe bronchiolitis with low mortality except in the immunosuppressed [52], and is a common cause of respiratory infection in the young. The major change in the lung parenchyma is an interstitial pneumonia. Sluffing of the bronchial epithelium and necrotic debris in the lumens are frequent findings.

The cytologic changes include large syncytial cell aggregates, measuring 100 µm or more in diameter. Clear halos surround deeply basophilic inclusion bodies within the cytoplasm of these degenerating cells [121, p. 222; 130, pp. 579–580]. The disease can be similar to measles pneumonia, as both viruses result in giant cell formation. However, RSV more consistently and dramatically produces necrosis.

Influenza Virus

Influenza pneumonia does not have any specific cytologic changes but does produce ciliacytophthoria. Parenchymal changes reflect the picture of diffuse alveolar damage characterized by capillary congestion, interstitial and intra-alveolar edema with hyaline membranes, hemorrhage and inflammation. Necrotizing bronchiolitis and bronchitis can also be complicated by secondary bacterial infections. Bronchiolitis obliterans and interstitial fibrosis may be the end result.

Bacterial Infections

Since bacteria do not produce specific cytologic changes, discussion is limited in a cytology text. Bacteria can be recognized in respiratory tract samples and should be mentioned. However, they are frequently contaminants of the sample during collection [42], so the presence of bacteria does not necessarily imply disease. Acute inflammation is the usual accompaniment to an acute bacterial infection. For an excellent review of pulmonary bacterial infections and their diagnoses, the reader is referred to the article by Bartlett [12].

Infectious Rarities

The pathogenic organisms and their disease processes described above can all be considered common. Case reports occasionally describe exotic diseases caused by unusual organisms. Lung infections caused by *Strongyloides stercoralis* [35, 101, 122, 270] have been the most frequently reported. Isolated case reports describe disease caused by Echinococcus [4], Dirofilariasis [92], Paracoccidioidomycosis [248], and *Paragonimus westermani* [278].

Organisms not producing disease, but described in the respiratory tract include Trichomonads [181], and *Entamoeba gingivalis* [213]; seaweed has been reported to mimic fungus in at least one instance [127].

V. Probable Preneoplastic Lesions and Their Role in Carcinogenesis of Lung Cancer

The only known cell line which develops into carcinoma of the lung and which probably has a precursor stage is the squamous cell. The origin in the respiratory epithelium is controversial. Most pathologists and oncologists equate the development of squamous carcinoma of the lung to that of invasive squamous carcinoma of the uterine cervix because of the microscopically visual similarities. Cigarette smoking is certainly the number one suspect leading to these changes in the lung. The initiators and promoters of cancer in the two sites are probably different, although cigarette smoking is now being considered a risk factor in the development of carcinoma of the cervix [96].

Most theories for the development of squamous carcinoma of the lung begin with transformation of the columnar respiratory epithelium into benign squamous metaplasia, passing through various stages of metaplastic atypia (fig. 48, 49), onto carcinoma in situ (fig. 50), and then to frankly invasive carcinoma [75]. However, several strong voices have cried out against this theory, most particularly Melamed.

In 1963, Melamed et al. [150] reported 12 cases which were cytologically diagnosed as having carcinoma when routine chest X-rays were normal. In the ensuing years, several other articles have been published which claim to have done similar remarkable tasks [69, 91, 164]. In 1977, Melamed et al. [151] presented results of screening 4,000 high risk men,

Fig. 48. Squamous metaplasia with mild atypia (sputum): This mosaic of cells has a consistent nuclear-cytoplasmic ratio, but mild irregularity in chromatin distribution and nuclear shape. This type of metaplasia can be seen in benign pneumonia and bronchiectasis. Papanicolaou. × 900.

Fig. 49. Squamous metaplasia with severe atypia (sputum): The group of cells is not so cohesive nor regular as that seen in figure 48. Nuclear hyperchromasia is more pronounced and nuclear size and shape vary considerably. Such atypia is frequently associated with cancers, although this can be the most severe change present in an individual. Papanicolaou. × 900.

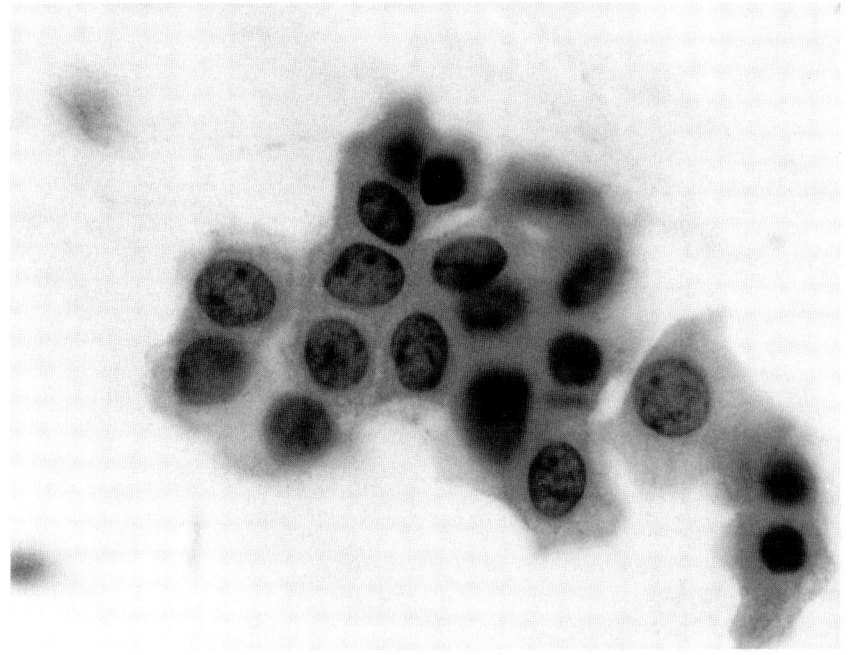

Preneoplastic Lesions and Their Role in Carcinogenesis of Lung Cancer

48

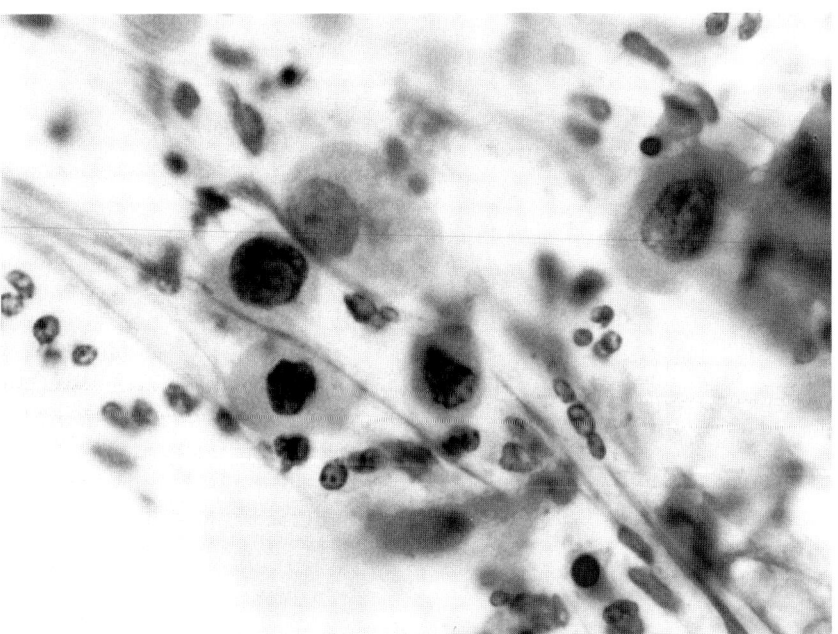

49

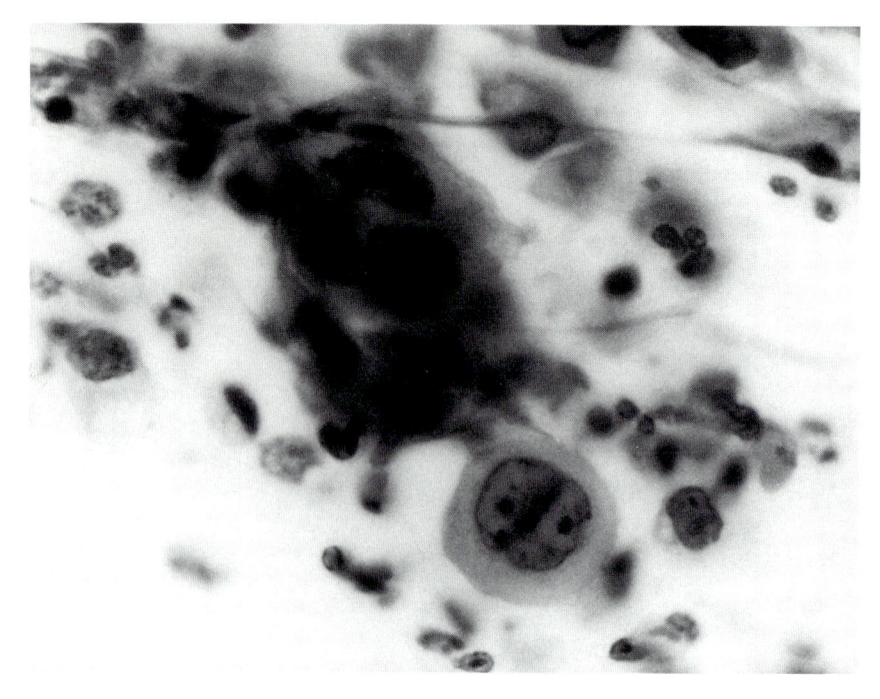

Fig. 50. Carcinoma in situ (sputum): Squamoid cells, with malignant nuclei with cytoplasm evenly distributed around the nucleus indicates a noninvasive tumor. Adjacent to this single large CIS cell is a group of markedly atypical metaplastic cells. Only if cells with aberrant cytoplasmic shapes are seen, should the specimen be identified as diagnostic of invasive carcinoma. Papanicolaou. × 850.

half of the New York City component of the Early Lung Cancer Project. Seven of these 4,000 were diagnosed by cytology as having in situ or insipient invasive epidermoid carcinoma confined to the bronchus. Aside from simply reporting these data, the article speculates on the role of squamous metaplasia and basal cell hyperplasia in carcinogenesis of bronchogenic carcinoma, and opines that squamous metaplasia is probably not a precursor lesion, but that basal cell hyperplasia may be. The authors claim that squamous metaplasia is most common in the lobar bronchus and that early lung cancers primarily involve segmental bronchi. However, basal cell hyperplasia is noted to be a common reaction in segmental as well as lobar bronchi.

Recent experimental evidence supporting the role of atypical squamous metaplasia in carcinogenesis is provided by combined work from the

Karolinska and Tokyo Medical College. Frequent injections of methylcholanthrene into the submucosal areas of beagle dogs resulted in the development of invasive carcinoma in a period of 20 weeks. Careful monitoring of this development saw the cell changes go through stages of mild, moderate and severe metaplastic atypia until carcinoma in situ was reached. Simultaneous measurements of DNA values also saw the transformation of the cell line from diploid through aneuploid values of nuclear DNA [117, 128, 129].

The most comprehensive and long-standing work done on humans has come from the work of Saccomanno who has meticulously catalogued the epithelial cytologic changes in the developmental stages of carcinoma of the human lung [218, 221, 222]. His atlas [217] and other works are worth thorough study. His scheme outlining the cytologic changes from squamous metaplasia to carcinoma is shown in table 6. He has also described reversal or halt of progression of atypical metaplasia using orally ingested 13-cis-retinoic acid [220].

The significance of epithelial atypia is best illustrated by the comprehensive examination of data obtained from the Johns Hopkins Lung Project. Frost et al. [75] analyzed the range of changes seen in sputa examined in 5,226 asymptomatic men screened by cytology and chest X-rays. Table 7 lists the distribution (incidence) and outcome of specimens with the various degrees of atypical cells recovered from these subjects. Such early detection is currently possible only for squamous lesions; in the same study, sputa were useful for detecting only squamous carcinoma. The more peripheral lesions are best detected by other means described elsewhere in this book.

In our daily experience, most metaplasias encountered in sputa and other cytologic specimens are of the mild variety, and usually accompany pneumonia or other inflammatory diseases of the lung, or from urban air pollution [194], aging [192], or other inhalants, e.g. marijuana [55]. However, in Johnston's analysis of respiratory cytology material from his laboratory with inconclusive diagnoses, he found that 60% of moderate to marked atypical metaplasias subsequently were proven to have squamous carcinoma. The remainder of the lesions can regress with cessation of smoking [193]. Therefore, any patient who persists, especially after treatment for inflammatory disease, with atypical metaplasia must be thoroughly worked up for an occult lesion [108, 205]. Even if metaplastic atypia is only an associated change and not a precursor lesion, its presence should be considered significant until proven otherwise.

Table 6. Cytologic criteria for squamous cell metaplasia and epidermoid carcinoma [217]

Regular metaplasia
1. Cells are all about same size
2. Nuclei are same size, with regular nuclear/cytoplasmic ratio
3. Nuclear material is fine and powdery, with rare chromocenter
4. Cytoplasm is usually basophilic
5. Cells usually occur in sheets, but may be single

Metaplasia, mild atypia
1. Cells vary slightly in size
2. Nuclei vary slightly in size, and nuclear/cytoplasmic ratio may vary slightly
3. Nuclear material is still fine and powdery, with rare clusters of nuclear material near the nuclear membrane
4. Cytoplasm may be acidophilic
5. Cells usually occur in sheets, but may be single

Metaplasia, moderate atypia
1. Cells vary moderately in size; some are smaller but most are larger than in mild metaplasia
2. Nuclei vary significantly in size, with moderate variation in nuclear/cytoplasmic ratio
3. Nuclear material is still fine and powdery in most areas, but nuclear masses are abundant, particularly along the membrane
4. Nuclear lobulations, crevices, and nodules are present
5. Cytoplasm may be basophilic, but acidophilia predominates
6. Cells usually occur in sheets, but an increase in singles is found

Metaplasia, marked atypia
1. Cells vary markedly in size, but are generally larger than in moderate atypias
2. Nuclear pleomorphism is marked, and nuclear material is coarse and sometimes clustered about the nuclear membrane; nuclear/cytoplasmic ratio varies, with extremes
3. Nucleoli are present, but are small and may be acidophilic
4. Acidophilic cytoplasm predominates
5. Single cells predominate

Carcinoma in situ
1. Cells vary in size and may be double the size of those in marked metaplasia; single cells are present, but clusters are more common than in invasive carcinoma
2. Nuclear material is coarse and accumulates in large masses, but usually not near the membrane; chromocenters are large and simulate nucleoli, but are not always acidophilic
3. Nuclear/cytoplasmic ratio is decreased in some cells but increased in others, causing obvious nuclear pleomorphism
4. Cannibalism and multinucleation may be present
5. Acidophilic cytoplasm predominates

Table 6 (cont.)

Invasive carcinoma
1. Cells are larger, but may be very pleomorphic and bizarre; they usually are single, but clusters are found
2. Nuclear material is coarse and accumulates in masses unevenly around the nuclear membrane
3. Nucleoli are large and acidophilic
4. Nuclear cytoplasmic ratio is increased in some but decreased in others
5. Cannibalism and multinucleation are common
6. Cytoplasm is acidophilic and basophilic

Table 7. Cytopathology cancer categorization of sputum at initial screen; sputum specimen: mid-day induction, including following 3 mornings mail-in [75]

Initial screen category	n	%	Diagnostic significance: at least this lesion is present, but a more severe one cannot be ruled out
CAN	11	0.2	cancer (in situ, microinvasive, invasive)
MKD	14	0.3	markedly atypical squamous metaplasia (gravely atypical squamous metaplasia; 'suspicious'; marked atypia)
MOD	169	3.2	moderately atypical squamous metaplasia (moderate atypia; moderate metaplasia)
SLI	2,083	39.9	slightly atypical squamous metaplasia (mildly atypical squamous metaplasia; mild atypia; slight metaplasia)
FRI	1,511	28.9	fringe atypical squamous metaplasia (regular metaplasia; 'normal' metaplasia; euplastic metaplasia)
NCE	1,390	26.6	no cancer evidence is present on this specimen
UNS	48	0.9	unsatisfactory specimen
Total	5,226	100.0	

A special situation pertains to bronchial epithelial changes in the neonate [54]. Severely atypical metaplasia (dysplasia) can occur in the newborn following prolonged use (longer than 6 days) of high concentration oxygen fed by intermittent positive pressure respirators. Bronchopulmonary dysplasia as a syndrome is characterized by acute respiratory distress which may completely resolve or can persist with repeated bouts of upper respiratory infections, pneumonia, chronic asthma, and infrequently fatal cor pulmonale.

The cytology reflects the clinical symptoms. Earliest changes in the respiratory epithelial cells are nonspecific and degenerative. After a week or more on oxygen therapy, severely atypical cells are recovered, not necessarily related to the % oxygen concentration inhaled [49].

If abundant keratotic material is obtained from a sputum or a bronchoscopic specimen, then a diagnosis of *tracheobronchial papillomatosis* should be considered. Vacuolated squamous cells are frequently seen in such samples which are easily misinterpreted as well-differentiated squamous carcinoma. The appearance of the gross lesions through the bronchoscope is usually diagnostic [274].

Regardless of the origin of the transformation of respiratory columnar epithelium to 'bronchogenic carcinoma', the most difficult question facing pulmonologists and thoracic surgeons currently is what to do with the occult or in situ carcinoma once it is discovered and verified. Tumors have long been known to incorporate hematoporphyrin derivative into malignant tissue at a higher concentration and for a longer time than normal tissue. The ability to identify early lesions by their UV excited red fluorescence of hematoporphyrin conjugated cells is an inviting concept, especially when visualized through the bronchoscope. Several studies are in progress to not only use hematoporphyrin derivative to localize the tumor to direct brushing and biopsies, but to treat identified areas by laser photoradiation [94, 118].

While there appears to be a morphologic spectrum of change from carcinoid to atypical carcinoid to small cell (oat cell) carcinoma, there is no implication that carcinoid and its atypical counterparts are precursor lesions to small cell undifferentiated carcinoma of the lung. Therefore, the only situation in which premalignant cytologic changes may be appreciated is in the development of squamous carcinoma of the lung [252]. Since this type of lung cancer is still the most common in most series, and has the best prognosis, the diligent search for precursor cells is an important mandate for the cytologist.

VI. Neoplasms of the Lung

General Considerations

Lung cancer has become a major health problem, and is now the number one cancer killer of both men and women in the United States. The causal link with cigarette smoking is now indisputable [8, 40], but an exact scientific basis for the initiation and promotion of lung cancer by tobacco smoke is yet to be proven [104]. Nonetheless, the general opinion of pulmonologists and most other physicians is that the best way to curtail the escalating incidence and death rates of cancer of the lung is for cigarette smoking to cease. The only one of the major primary lung tumors for which this association has not been strongly shown is bronchiolo-alveolar carcinoma.

Not only are the incidence, prevalence, and death rate statistics gory, but the salvage rate is downright dismal. The overall 5-year survival rate for carcinoma of the lung by latest figures is 9%. Squamous carcinoma of the lung still has the most optimistic outlook, 25% 5-year survival rate. Adenocarcinoma and large cell carcinoma patients will have an expected 12% 5-year survival rate, whereas for small cell carcinoma patients, less than 1% of the cases will survive for 5 years. The usual life expectancy, until very recently, for the latter, is less than 1 year. New attempts to accurately stage patients with oat-cell carcinoma, to evaluate resectability, followed by surgical resection has resulted in a few patients surviving more than 2 years.

The occult nature of most early carcinomas of the lung dictates the conditions for poor outcome. Death usually occurs 1 year following clinical evidence of disease [75]. If there were methods for earlier detection in earlier clinical stages of this disease, the salvage rate would most likely be much better [67]. Sputum cytology, utilized for mass population screening, was at one time thought to be the answer [10, 68]. Several large studies were begun, but the results were disappointing (see chapter VII), and the cost to detect an early lesion in a single patient made the total survey cost-ineffective [279]. However, for squamous carcinoma, screening with sputa and chest X-rays appears to be worthwhile; in the Johns Hopkins Lung Project, mortality was reduced by 46.6% in those patients with squamous carcinoma [75]. Identification and screening of individuals at risk to develop lung cancer is now being employed by most physicians [124].

The invention of the fiberoptic bronchoscope has made the collection and diagnosis of respiratory cytologic samples highly reliable [118]. Not only can brushings, washings, and biopsies be obtained through the flexible scope, but fine needle aspirations of both midline and peripheral lung lesions may be performed with precision [119, 120, 145, 178, 179, 215, 219, 265–267]. Accurate staging can be done through the bronchoscope by sampling paratracheal nodes with the fine needle and exploring nonobvious areas of the epithelium with brush and biopsy forceps to determine the presence or absence of in situ lesions. Fluoroscopically controlled transthoracic fine needle aspirates are performed routinely in most major hospitals [27, 138, 235, 285]. For lesions less than 2 cm, FNA provides hope that early lesions will be accurately detected and cure effected [90]. On the horizon, now in the experimental stage, is the employment of hematoporphyrin fluorescence of in situ lesions, directing treatment by laser ablation through the bronchoscope [94, 118]. At the present time, until cigarette smoking is irradicated, and/or until an immunologic preventive is discovered, the accurate workup of a patient suspected of having lung cancer is the best that can be done to increase the quality and length of life of these patients.

The diagnosis of lung lesions is necessarily a team approach. Location of the lesion should determine the initial diagnostic tests (table 8). Some consideration should also be given to the suspected lesion, for certain cell types are more easily obtained by one method of sampling over another [244] (see chapter VII). Bronchoscopists and thoracic radiologists have developed skills to accurately locate and sample lesions, including those of very small dimensions. Once the samples are obtained, they are passed to the cytopathologist and surgical pathologist who are responsible for making a definitive diagnosis from a very minute amount of material. 'At a time when the expectations and demands of our clinical colleagues are increasing, the material on which we must base our diagnosis is vanishing' [161]. This situation dictates extremely careful processing and highly developed diagnostic skills. Intimate cooperation between the cytopathologist and surgical pathologist is a prerequisite to an optimum diagnosis.

Neoplasms of the Lung

This collaboration, coupled with close communication with the clinicians, is essential to guarantee that the diagnosis is a uniform and accurate one. Nothing is more confusing to the clinician than a diagnosis from surgical pathology which disagrees with the cytology findings. Clinicians should be encouraged to challenge the pathologist if their diagnosis does not agree with the clinical intuition. Only by this interchange, unaffected by ego, will the patient receive the best care.

Classification of Lung Tumors

The classification outlined in table 9 is a modification from the current WHO classification of lung tumors [280], which is quite lengthy and unnecessary for the cytopathologist. The first four categories are the most commonly encountered primary lung tumors, but the microscopist must

Table 8. Diagnostic approach to central and peripheral lesions

Central lesions	Peripheral lesions
Chest X-ray (tomograms)	Chest X-ray
Fiberoptic bronchoscopy	Tomograms
Bronchial washings	CT scan
Bronchial brushings	FNA of mass
Transbronchial FNA	Mediastinoscopy
Primary tumor	Biopsy
Paratracheal nodes	FNA
Mediastinoscopy	
Biopsy	
FNA	

Table 9. Classification of cancer of the lung

I.	Squamous carcinoma	VII.	Carcinosarcoma – blastoma
II.	Small cell ('oat cell') carcinoma	VIII.	Sarcoma
III.	Adenocarcinoma	IX.	Malignant lymphoma
IV.	Large cell undifferentiated	X.	Miscellaneous – including melanoma
V.	Carcinoid tumors	XI.	Metastatic
VI.	Bronchial gland tumors		

always anticipate that metastatic disease will be frequently experienced. Most metastatic lesions are carcinomas, especially adenocarcinomas [110, 123], although other entities, such as malignant melanoma, should be considered. The category of large cell carcinoma is infrequently used at UCLA, as we have routinely utilized electron microscopy whenever a cell type is difficult to categorize. Electron microscopy is especially useful to separate true 'oat cell' carcinomas from other small cell neoplasms.

The need to accurately classify lung lesions according to cell type has been a result of the demands of both the radiologist and chemotherapist, who adjust their treatment based on the presumed cell of origin of the tumor [32, 59, 116]. Recently, the inaccuracy of typing lung tumors by light microscopy has been addressed in the literature [89, 113, 152, 209], and now with the use of immunochemical methods, the classification is even more confused [223–225, 261, 262, 264]. Conceivably, the next few years will see a major overhaul of the classification of lung tumors as these more sophisticated diagnostic modalities are tested, their accuracy confirmed, and their significance fully recognized. In our experience, and that of others [152], cellular features in cytologic samples may more accurately categorize a lesion than histologic patterns, the current 'gold standard'!

Perhaps more critical to the good outcome of the patient than cell typing, is the staging of the patient to assess extent of tumor spread. Here again, the diligence of the clinicians and the pathologist to carefully obtain and process specimens for staging is so critical.

The descriptions in this chapter of tissue and cell type are based upon the classic light microscopic criteria. Where there are obvious discrepancies, or chance of confusion, such will be noted. Rare benign lung tumors will be addressed at the end of this chapter.

Squamous (Epidermoid) Carcinoma

Pulmonary squamous carcinoma is the primary lethal cancer in males and the third cancer killer of females. It accounts for 35–50% of lung cancer in males, and 20% in females. This was the first cell type to be linked to cigarette smoking. When metastases do occur, they involve non-regional lymph nodes, adrenals, liver, and kidney, and the contralateral lung. The brain is occasionally involved, but the diagnostic pickup in a spinal fluid is relatively low. Treatment is usually surgical, if the patient is staged as resectable. If not, radiation is the therapy of choice.

The anatomic location of squamous carcinoma is usually subsegmental or in the segmental bronchial junctions, with growth toward the main

Neoplasms of the Lung

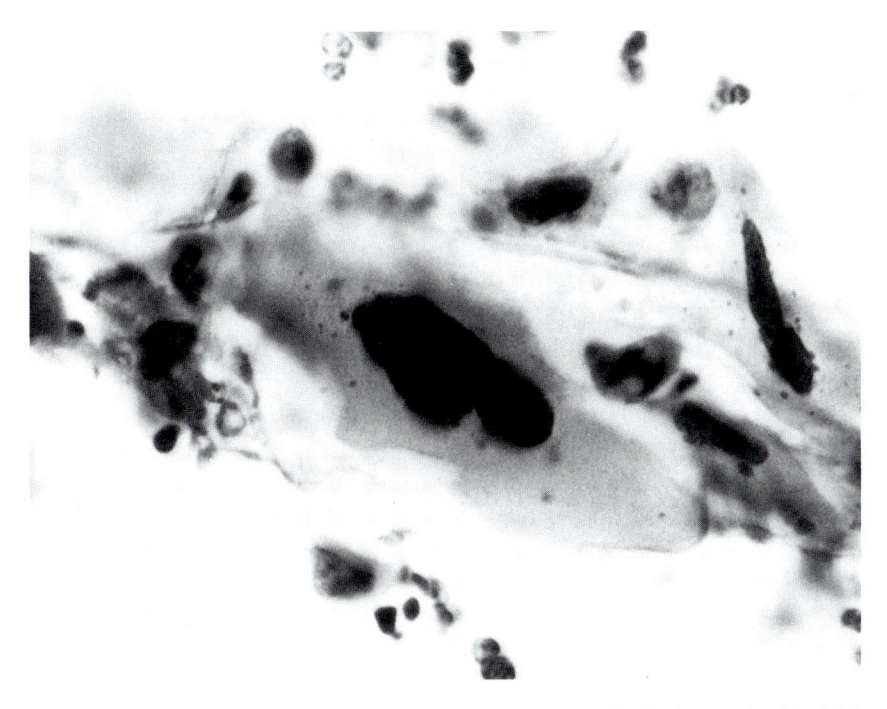

Fig. 51. Squamous carcinoma (sputum): The center cell, the largest in this field, contains multiple hyperchromatic nuclei of unequal size, surrounded by an aberrantly shaped opaque cytoplasm. If photographed in color, the orange of the cytoplasm would be apparent. Accompanying cells display less severe, but significant atypia. Papanicolaou. ×850.

stem bronchus. The tumor locally invades bronchial cartilages, regional lymph nodes, and adjoining lung parenchyma. It is a relatively slowly growing lesion, with metastases occurring late in the course of the disease.

Squamous carcinoma of the lung can be microscopically subdivided into well-differentiated, moderately differentiated, and poorly differentiated. The presence of keratin will automatically classify a squamous carcinoma as well differentiated, even if only a small number of cells exhibit keratin within the cytoplasm. Moderately differentiated tumors maintain squamous cytoplasm, and hyperchromatic nuclei, but do not visually demonstrate keratin. Poorly differentiated tumors, difficult to distinguish from poorly differentiated adenocarcinoma, may require electron microscopy for definition. However, careful attention to nuclear chromatin and cytoplasmic boundaries will help to separate poorly differentiated glandular from squamous lesions. In the former, shared cell borders, often a syncytial arrangement, and delicate nuclear chromatin are the norm. Poorly differentiated squamous lesions have a coarser chromatin in general, and well-defined separate cell boundaries. Nucleoli are more commonly seen and prominent in adenocarcinoma, but their presence or absence is not a critical help in either type of lesion. In instances where electron microscopy is not possible, the term 'bronchogenic' with a suspected cell type is all that may be possible. This writer signs out such cases as follows: 'Poorly differentiated carcinoma, favor squamous (or adeno)carcinoma'.

Cytologic Criteria. Specimens from a patient with classic squamous carcinoma with keratinization will contain cells with large hyperchromatic nuclei, occasionally multinucleated, with a variable nuclear-cytoplasmic ratio (fig. 51). Aberrant cytoplasmic shapes, especially 'tadpoles' (fig. 52) are the hallmark of squamous carcinoma of the lung, and keratinized cytoplasm will categorize the lesion as well differentiated. Occasionally, the lesion will be so well differentiated that anucleate keratin predominates (fig. 53), and no cells with truly malignant criteria are present (fig. 54).

Accompanying the keratinized cells are usually numerous nonkeratinized cells which have similar characteristics, but a very opaque green or

---

Fig. 52. Squamous cell carcinoma (*a* = sputum; *b* = transbronchial FNA): This 'tadpole' (*a*) is the hallmark of squamous cell carcinoma. The nuclear changes are similar to those seen in the large cell in figure 51. Aberrantly shaped cytoplasm confirms its malignancy. Accompanying cells possibly reflect adjacent carcinoma in situ, as cytoplasmic shapes are less irregular. *b* is noteworthy for the abundance of fresh, highly diagnostic material. Papanicolaou. × 850.

Fig. 53. Keratin and necrotic debris (FNA): Opaque cytoplasmic fragments, stained orange, indicate keratin. Nuclear detail is not sufficient to make the diagnosis of malignancy. The accompanying necrosis could be from either a cavitary squamous carcinoma or from the keratinized lining of a tuberculoma or mycetoma. This specimen was from a patient with squamous carcinoma. Papanicolaou. × 340.

Fig. 54. Squamous cell carcinoma (FNA): In contrast to figure 53, these keratinized cells from the same specimen contain nuclei consistent with squamous carcinoma. Great care need be taken to avoid overcalling the contents of a keratinized and necrotic cavity. Papanicolaou. × 340.

Neoplasms of the Lung

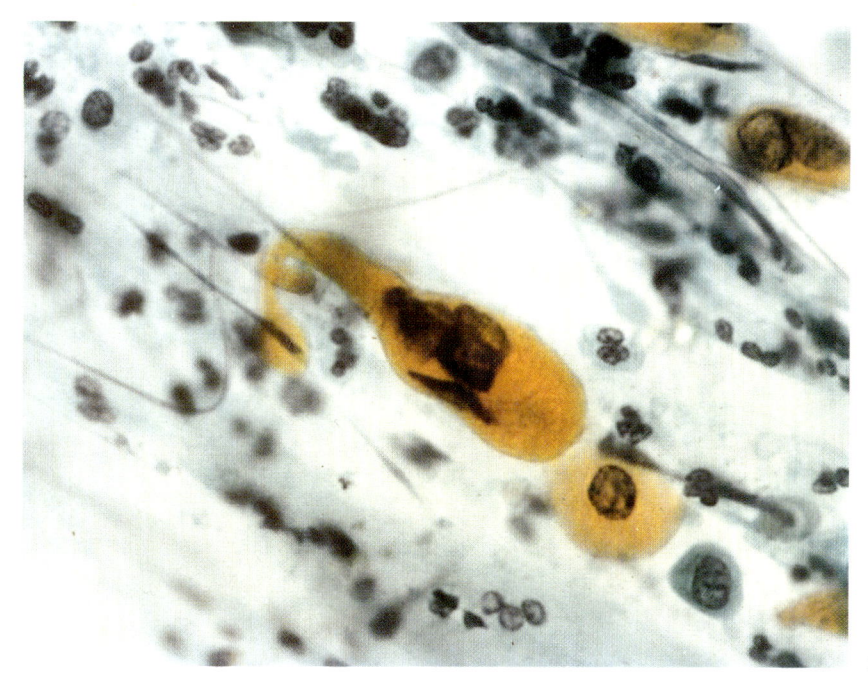

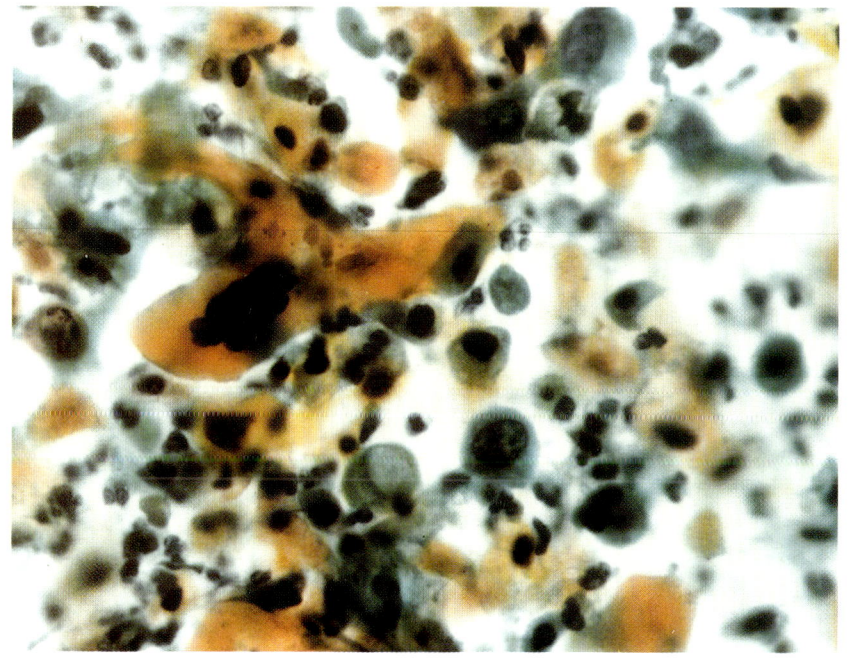

52a

52b

Cytopathology of Pulmonary Disease 100

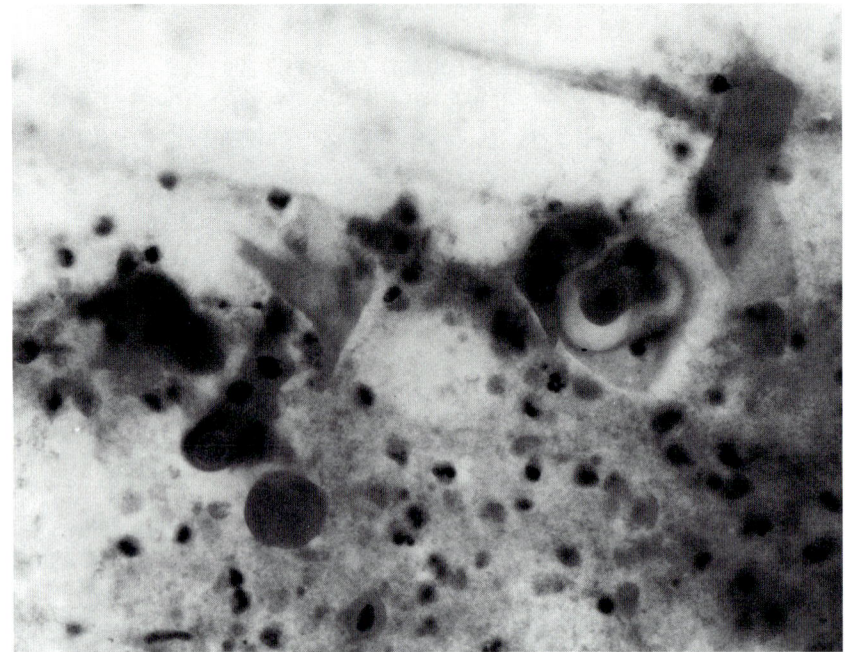

53

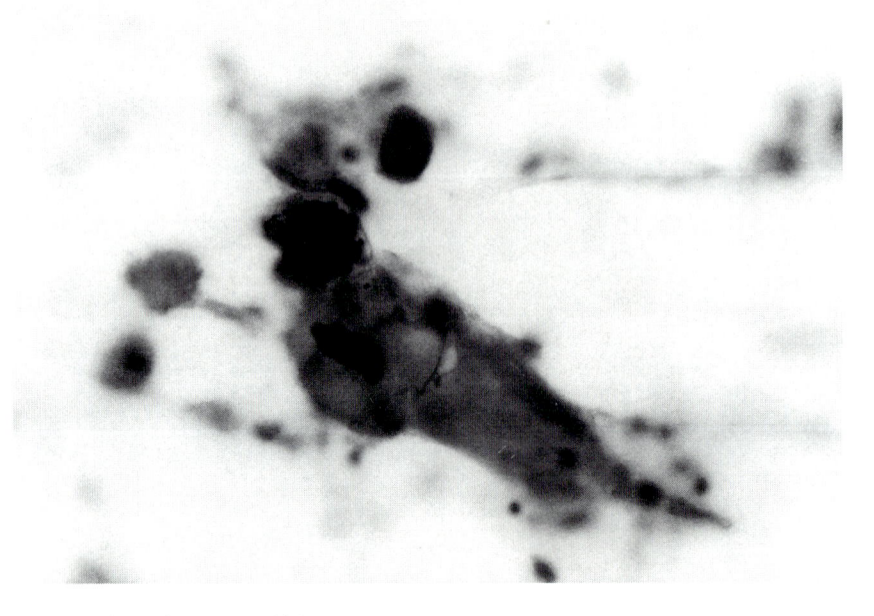

54

(For legends see page 98.)

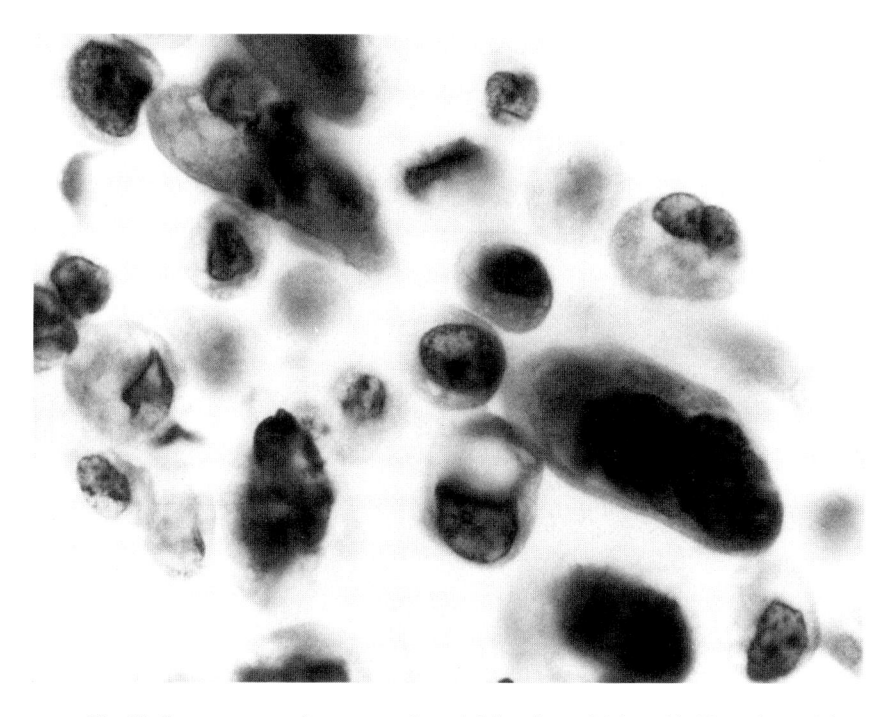

Fig. 55. Squamous carcinoma, nonkeratinizing (bronchial wash): Note the multinucleation, the dark, unevenly distributed chromatin and irregular nuclear membranes. No two cells appear identical, although all are consistent with a nonkeratinizing squamous carcinoma. Occasional vacuoles should not be misconstrued as features of an adenocarcinoma. Such cytoplasmic vacuoles may reflect either persistent mucus production in cells of a transformed respiratory epithelium, or are simply degenerative vacuoles. Papanicolaou. × 900.

blue cytoplasm with endo- and ectoplasm zones (fig. 55). Nucleoli may be a prominent feature but are not a significant criterion. Accompanying the large tumor cells, both keratinized and unkeratinized, are hyperchromatic, often pyknotic nuclei mixed with necrotic tumor debris (diathesis) (fig. 56). Such debris may be the first indication of tumor on the initial cytologic examination, and while not diagnostic, should indicate need for follow-up cytologic specimens [136].

Pitfalls. Major pitfalls of squamous carcinoma include squamous metaplasia, mycetoma, radiation reaction, and chemotherapy (table 10, 11). *Squamous metaplasia* is generally considered a precursor lesion to

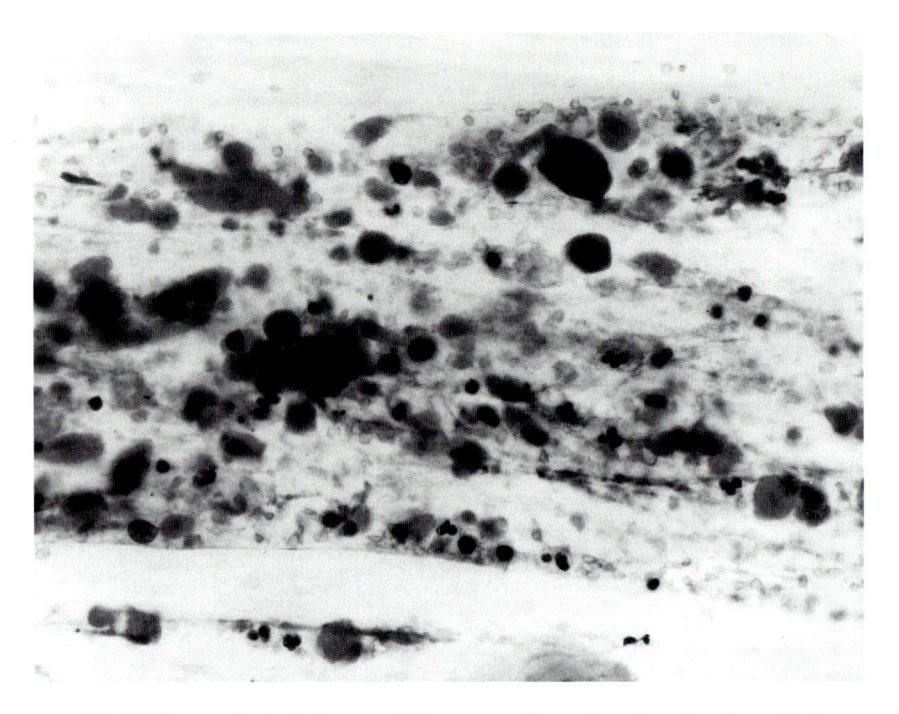

Fig. 56. Tumor diathesis (sputum): Fragments of cytoplasmic and nuclear debris can be found in large streams in sputum and other respiratory specimens in patients with cancers. The marked variation in nuclear fragment size is characteristic of squamous cell carcinoma and should not be interpreted as a small cell carcinoma (fig. 79). Frequently, the cytoplasmic fragments are keratinized, and will suggest the correct diagnosis, which requires malignant cells. Papanicolaou. × 340.

Table 10. Pitfalls of squamous carcinoma

1.	*Squamous metaplasia* = no matter how severe, whether due to underlying malignancy, or repair, must have single malignant cells to make diagnosis of carcinoma; most squamous metaplasia will occur in sheets, i.e. bronchiectasis, pneumonia, etc.
2.	*Mycetoma* = the cavity lining of a fungal infection may undergo extremely bizarre squamous metaplasia
3.	*Radiation reaction* = be especially cautious in postradiation specimens with previous history of tumor
4.	*Busulfan therapy,* other drugs

Table 11. Squamous carcinoma (sc) – cytologic features which distinguish it from similar lesions

	SC	Metaplasia	Repair	Radiation and drug reaction
Cell features				
Cytoplasm				
Border	sharp	sharp	sharp	delicate
Shape	aberrant	uniform	uniform	variable
Quality	opaque	opaque	translucent	often vacuolated
Relation to other cells	separate	separate	separate or syncitium	separate
N/C ratio	variable	intermediate	low	low in large cell
Nucleus				
Border	irregular, variable	smooth	smooth	smooth
Chromatin	coarse clumped	uniform, varies with severity	fine	coarse and clumped
Place in cell	central	central	central	variable
Nucleolus				
Size	usually small	small	large	large
Shape	round/irregular	round	irregular	irregular
Prominence	blends with chromatin	minimal	very	very
Number	single-multiple	single	single-multiple	single-multiple
Pattern of groups	haphazard mosaic, thick sheet	mosaic, flat sheet	attenuated, flat mosaic	relatively normal
Single cells	many	scattered	rare	common
Smear background	diathesis	variably inflamed	variably inflamed	clean

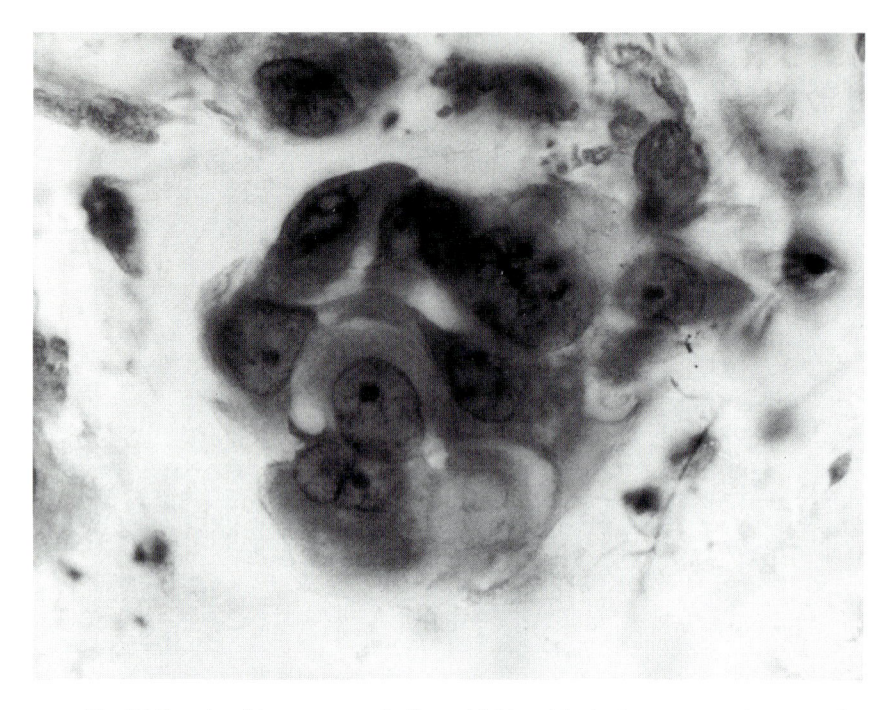

Fig. 57. Repair with severe atypia (bronchial brushing): Opaque cytoplasm, configuration suggestive of a 'pearl', and large irregular nuclei could seduce the observer into a diagnosis of squamous carcinoma. This cell group from the same case as figure 12 has even more severely atypical nuclei, with irregular distribution of chromatin and prominent nucleoli. Most of the cells in the specimen occur in tight clusters. A history of previous bronchoscopy and biopsy within a 2-week period should caution the observer to make a very conservative diagnosis. Papanicolaou. × 850.

squamous carcinoma, just as in the uterine cervix. A spectrum of changes has been identified by several authors [114, 218, 221] and is outlined in table 6. Squamous metaplasia, no matter how severe, must not be overcalled (fig. 57); a 'positive' sample must have single malignant cells to make the diagnosis of carcinoma. An underlying malignancy, repair, bronchiectasis, or pneumonia may be the cause of a metaplasia. If the principle disease is reversible, such as pneumonia, the squamous metaplasia will usually also reverse and disappear in subsequent cytologic specimens following adequate therapy. If the metaplasia persists and worsens, an adjacent tumor should be suspected, including a carcinoma in situ. Such lesions are difficult to locate and accurately diagnose. However, diligent

Neoplasms of the Lung

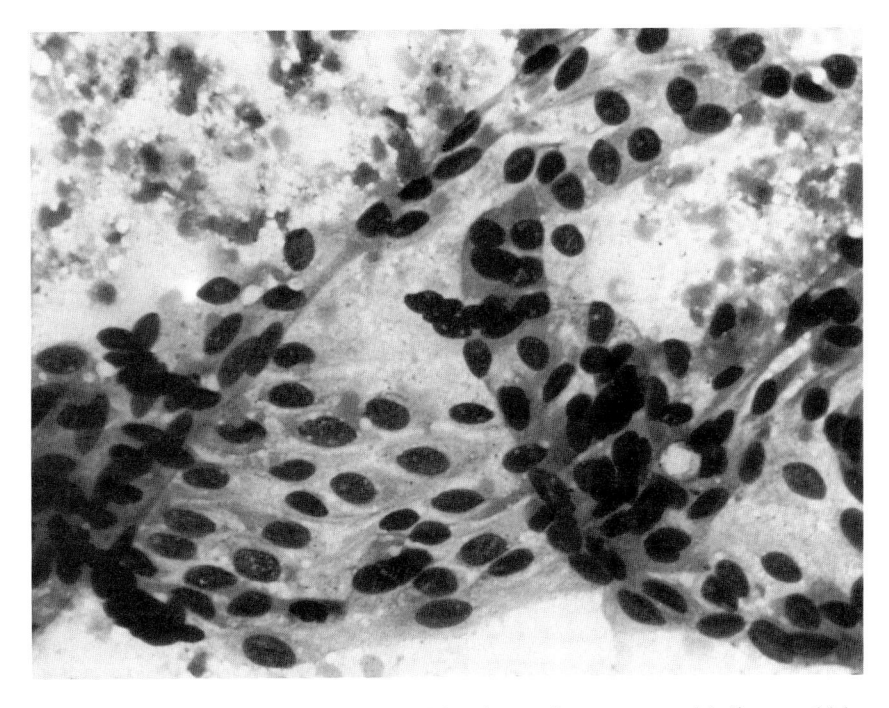

Fig. 58. Repair, mycetoma (FNA): The sheets of squamous epithelium could be interpreted as originating in a squamous carcinoma. Note the regular arrangement and distribution of the nuclei with consistent nuclear-cytoplasmic ratios, even chromatin distribution, and cohesiveness of the groups. Necrosis in the background indicates origin in a cavitary lesion. This sample is from the same case as figure 26, which diagnosis is coccidioidomycosis. Papanicolaou. × 340.

search via the bronchoscope and multiple localized cytologic specimens can be most rewarding to identify the patient with a carcinoma in situ. Current experimental treatment includes hematoporphyrin localization of the epithelial lesion, with laser treatment to irradicate the noninvasive tumor (see chapter V). Carcinoma in situ is usually a multifocal lesion which demands a very thorough examination of the tracheobronchial tree and careful future monitoring.

Mycetomas can be lined by an extremely bizarre squamous metaplasia, which mimics squamous carcinoma (fig. 58). Indeed, squamous carcinoma can be found occurring within the cavity of a fungal or tuberculous infection. Once again, strict criteria of malignancy must be employed to

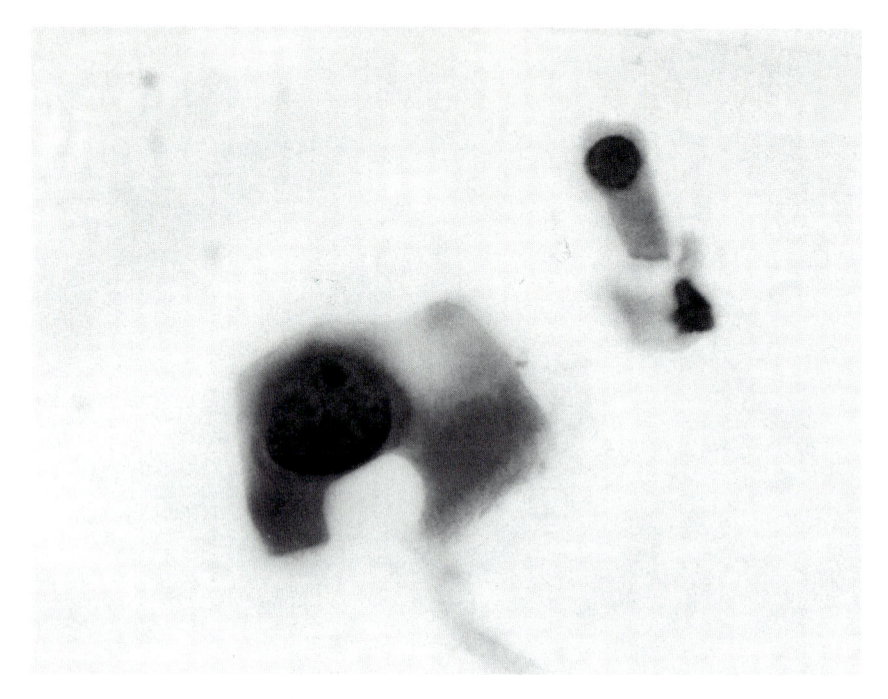

Fig. 59. Radiation atypia (bronchial brush): One year following radiation therapy for squamous carcinoma of the lung, these cells were recovered in a brushing. An abortive attempt at cytoplasmic division and huge nucleus are ominous signs. The presence of cilia places this markedly atypical cell in the benign category. The patient is disease free 5 years later. Papanicolaou. × 900.

avoid over-calling such squamous atypia. Surgical resection of these lesions is usually the treatment of choice.

Radiation reaction causes bizarre cell changes in the lung, identical to those found in the female genital tract, and for that matter, in all other sites of the body. Increased overall cell size, maintenance of nuclear-cytoplasmic ratio, bizarre chromatin patterns and nucleolar shapes, characterize the radiated cell. In the lung, respiratory epithelium usually retains cilia in the majority of well-preserved cells; their presence may assure the microscopist that no matter how bizarre the nuclei appear, the cells are still benign (fig. 59). A biopsy is sometimes needed to confirm the absence of true malignancy.

Chemotherapy can also produce cytologic changes which mimic carcinoma. The original culprit was busulfan, but numerous other chemotherapeutic agents have been documented as producing a cytopathic effect [17] (table 1), a reflection of their intended ability to damage the reproductive portion of the cell. Careful attention to nuclear detail, and comparison with similar known cases is of great help. Clinical history including use of chemotherapy is vital to avoid an uninformed incorrect diagnosis. However, patients undergoing chemotherapy for one malignancy have a greater chance of having a second primary, either from their immunosuppressed state, or because of the chemotherapeutic effect directly on the cell line in question. This is clearly a 'catch 22' situation and demands great skill from the cytopathologist and surgical pathologist to clarify the situation. Watchful waiting and repeat diagnostic samples are frequently necessary before the real answer can be given.

Head and neck squamous carcinomas can shed cells that may contaminate pulmonary specimens. The source of these cells is not always apparent. *Esophageal squamous carcinomas* may erode into the bronchus, or such cells may be regurgitated and be picked up in sputa. Accurate history will warn the pathologist of potential inaccurate interpretation.

Very well or very poorly differentiated squamous carcinomas may present difficulties, the former because the cells exfoliated are so 'differentiated' that they do not look malignant (fig. 53, 54, 60); the latter because the classic features are not obvious (fig. 61).

A fortunately rare tumor, epithelioid sarcoma of soft tissues, has been recovered in a bronchial wash from a patient with pulmonary metastases [1]. Only knowledge of the history would clearly avoid mistaking these cells for primary squamous carcinoma of the lung.

Adenocarcinoma

Adenocarcinoma is found both centrally and peripherally, and presents on X-ray as a bulky mass. Bronchiolo-alveolar carcinoma is usually peripheral and grows in either a nodular or infiltrating pattern. Adenocarcinoma accounts for approximately 30% of lung carcinomas in most series. This is a definite increase over previous years, probably due to the increased incidence of carcinoma of the lung in females, in contrast to the large proportion of squamous carcinomas in men [237]. Adenocarcinoma must always be determined to be either primary in the lung or metastatic from elsewhere. Metastases *from* primary lung tumors can be found in adrenals [155], brain [48], vertebrae, regional lymph nodes and pleura,

Cytopathology of Pulmonary Disease

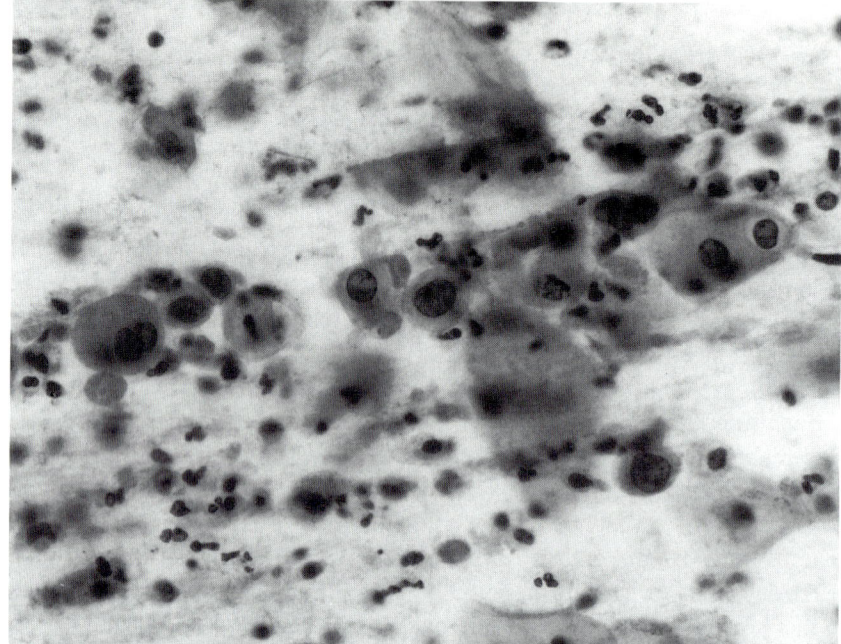

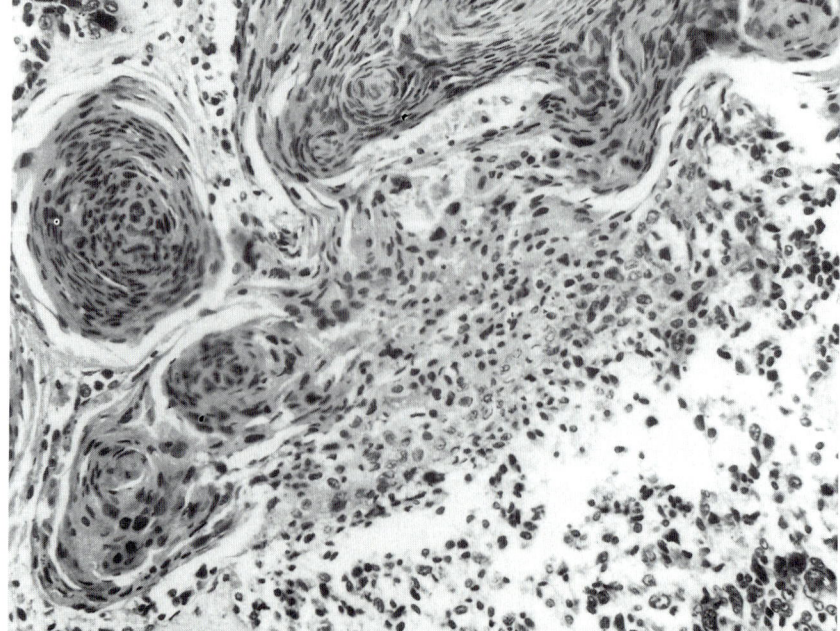

60a

60b

Neoplasms of the Lung

as well as in the contralateral lung. Treatment is usually surgical, if staging indicates a possible cure. The survival rate with surgery is 27% at 5 years. If staging indicates metastatic disease, chemotherapy with or without radiation is performed. The overall 5-year survival rate for adenocarcinoma is 12%.

Adenocarcinoma is subdivided into well, moderately and poorly differentiated types as well as the unique subtype of bronchiolo-alveolar car-

---

Fig. 60. Keratinizing squamous cell carcinoma (*a* = sputum *b* = pneumonectomy): In the very-well-differentiated lesions, pronounced anaplasia of the cells is not always evident because of the maturation of the cells which will exfoliate. Compare the cytomorphology of these 'severely atypical' squamous cells with those in the lumen of the bronchus shown in Fig. *b*. Most of the respiratory epithelium of this major bronchus is replaced by a very well-differentiated keratinizing squamous carcinoma. Note the maturation of the cells, especially those which tend to exfoliate easily, and compare them with those seen in figure *a*. *a* = Papanicolaou. × 340; *b* = HE. × 170.

Fig. 61. Squamous cell carcinoma, poorly differentiated (FNA): The relationship of the cells in this sheet of poorly differentiated epithelium provides the diagnosis of squamous origin. Note the areas indicated by the arrows; such nuclear-to-cytoplasmic molding and well-defined cytoplasmic borders are very characteristic of squamous carcinoma. Papanicolaou. × 340.

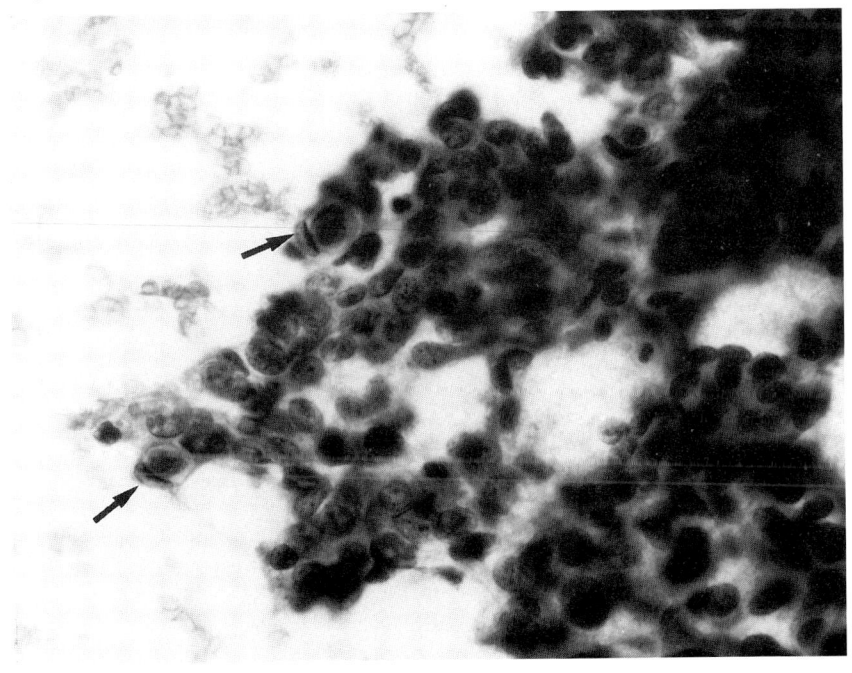

cinoma. The first three types are subcategorized depending upon the amount of mucin production and recapitulation of glandular structures. The poorly differentiated type is often difficult to distinguish from poorly differentiated squamous carcinoma: electron microscopy and mucin stains are often helpful. Bronchiolo-alveolar carcinoma can be divided into type 1 (secretory) and type 2 (nonsecretory), both of which grow along the existing framework of the alveoli [53]. Type 1 is characteristically mucin producing, and clearly an adenocarcinoma. Type 2 has a more hobnail, individual cell appearance as it lines the framework of the alveoli.

Cytologic Criteria. 'Bronchogenic' adenocarcinoma, the most common form, arises from the bronchial lining or the submucosal glandular epithelium. Cells will occur singly (fig. 62) or form a monolayer (fig. 63) or three-dimensional cluster (fig. 64–66) in exfoliated material. Cerebroid nuclei have a finely granular nuclear chromatin. Nucleoli are frequently large and irregular. Cytoplasmic borders are characteristically indistinct, with syncytia being quite obvious in brushings or smears of fine needle aspirates. The degree of cytoplasmic vacuolization is variable, and the diagnosis is not dependent upon the presence of such.

Papillary adenocarcinoma, a rare form, arises from the more proximal bronchial epithelium (fig. 67a) and sheds in clusters and single cells (fig. 67b, 68). Cells are uniformly symmetrical, with finely vacuolated cytoplasm, variable nucleoli and an inconsistent nuclear structure (see fig. 104). Clusters are not usually so three-dimensional as can be found in bronchiolo-alveolar carcinoma (fig. 69a), but both histologic types are difficult to distinguish cytologically. Depending upon the differentiation, cells can be quite pleomorphic and vary considerably in contrast to the relative uniformity of the bronchiolo-alveolar type (fig. 69b). Psammoma bodies, and intranuclear cytoplasmic inclusions [253] have been described in this variant of adenocarcinoma.

Fig. 62. Adenocarcinoma (*a* = bronchial washing; *b* = transbronchial biopsy): Although clusters of malignant glandular cells are usual, dispersed single cells from adenocarcinomas are occasionally seen, and indicate a very high grade lesion. Note the pleomorphism, the remarkably large nuclei, and the prominent nucleoli. Such cells could be mistaken for a lymphoma. The tissue verified the diagnosis of the bronchial washing. Although the pattern is poorly differentiated, a positive mucin stain confirmed the cell type. *a* = Papanicolaou; *b* = HE. × 340.

Neoplasms of the Lung

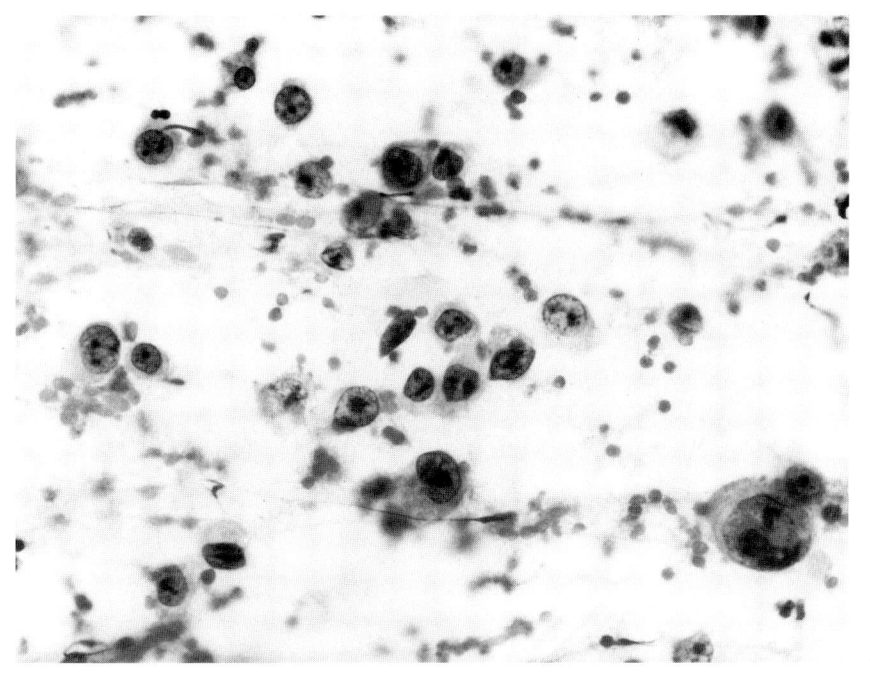

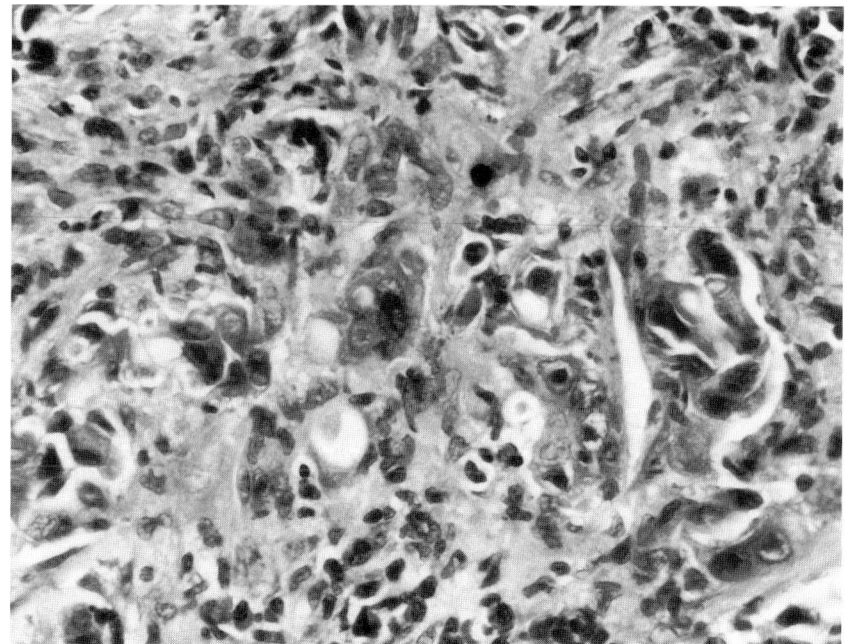

a

b

Cytopathology of Pulmonary Disease

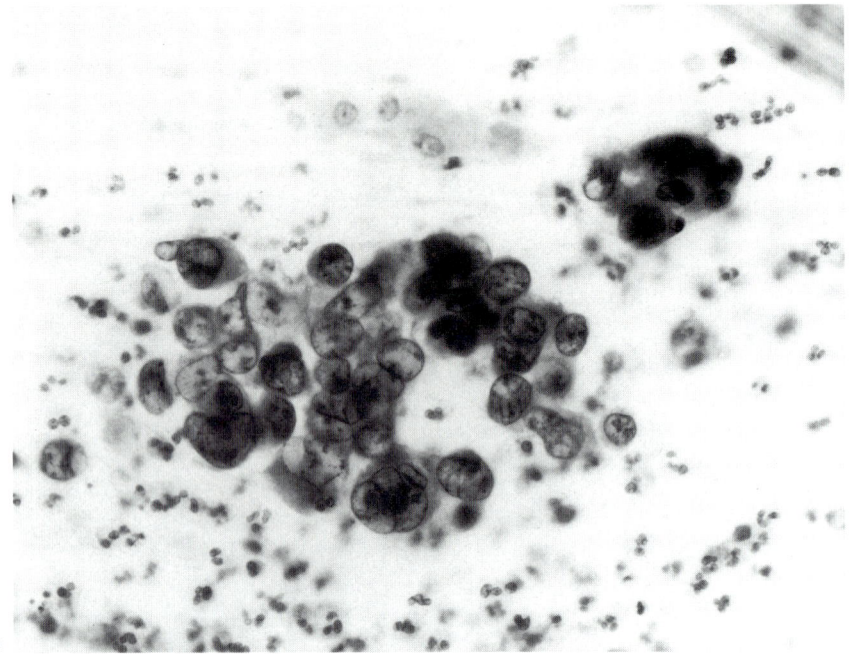

63a

Fig. 63. Adenocarcinoma (*a, b* = sputa; *c* = pneumonectomy): Rather than exfoliating in balls of malignant cells, more high grade lesions tend to occur singly, as in figure 62, or in somewhat dispersed monolayers, as in this case. The higher power view (*b*) reveals the marked pleomorphism and anisonucleosis, unevenly dispersed although fine chromatin, and prominent and irregularly shaped nucleoli. Cell borders are poorly defined, a characteristic of adenocarcinoma. Verification of the cytology in *a* and *b* is obtained by tissue section. Although the growth pattern is moderately differentiated, the individual cells correlate well with those seen in the sputum sample. *a* = × 340; *b* = × 850, Papanicolaou. *c* = × 170, HE.

Fig. 64. Adenocarcinoma (*a* = sputum; *b* = bronchial brush; *c* = pleural fluid; *d* = pneumonectomy): The exfoliating cells aggregate somewhat differently depending upon the sampling method, but the individual cells are quite similar. To assure that metastases in a pleural effusion are from the primary in the lung, and not from a second primary, comparison of all available specimens on the same patient is mandatory. The tissue (*d*) from the lung of the same patient whose samples are illustrated in figure *a–c*, contains both papillary clusters and singly occurring cells, which correlate well with the cytologic samples. *a–c* = Papanicolaou. × 850; d = HE. × 340.

Neoplasms of the Lung

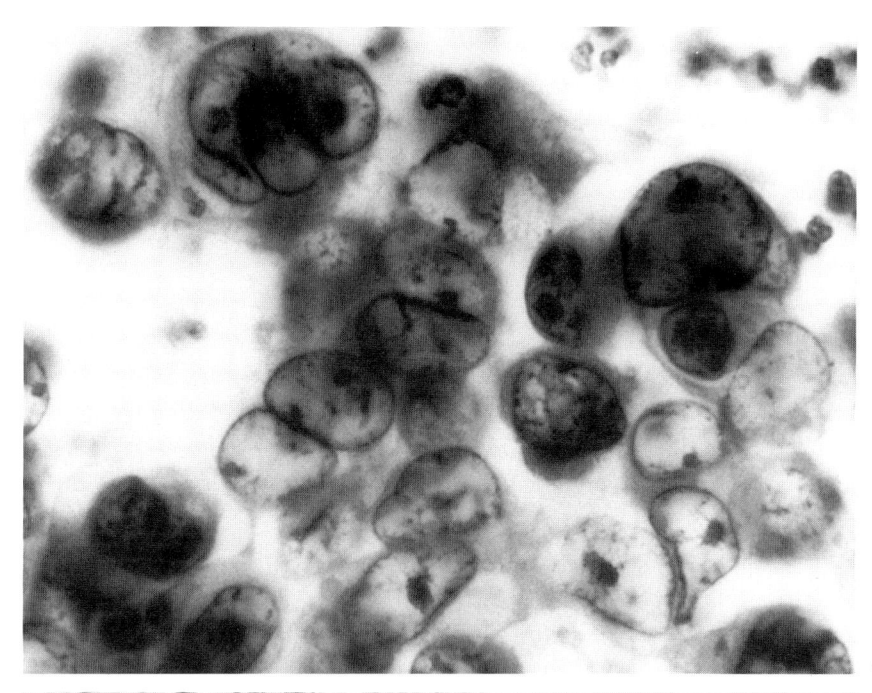

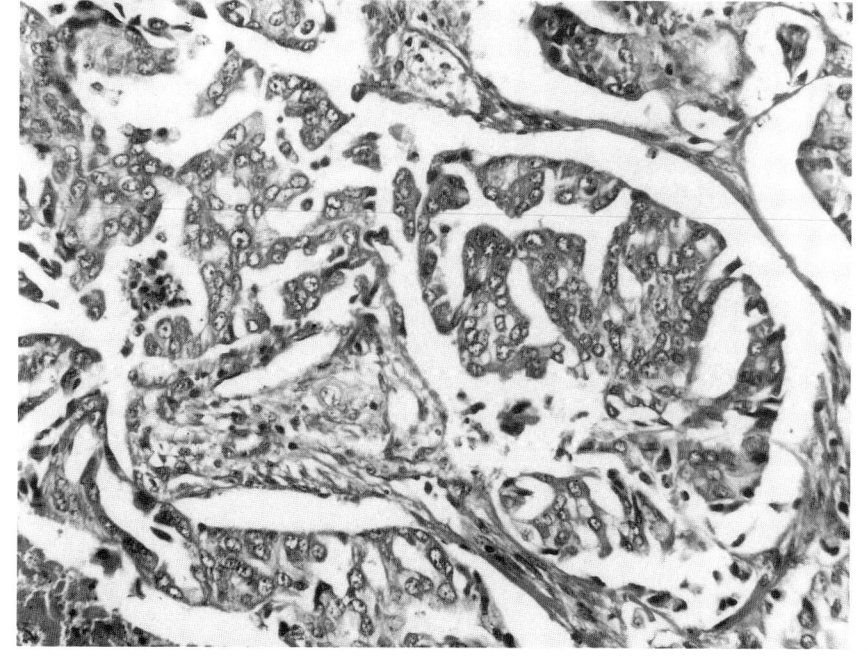

63b

63c

Cytopathology of Pulmonary Disease

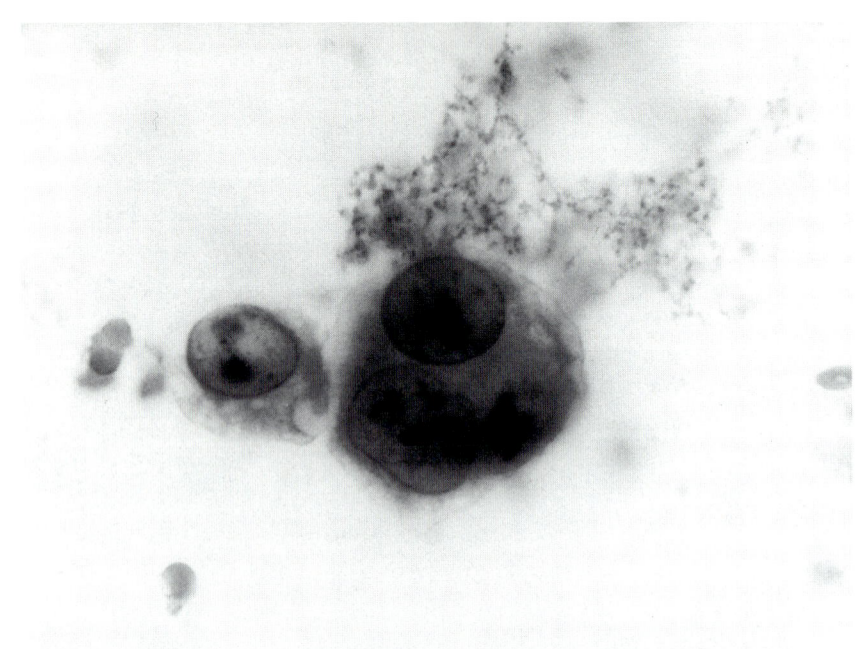

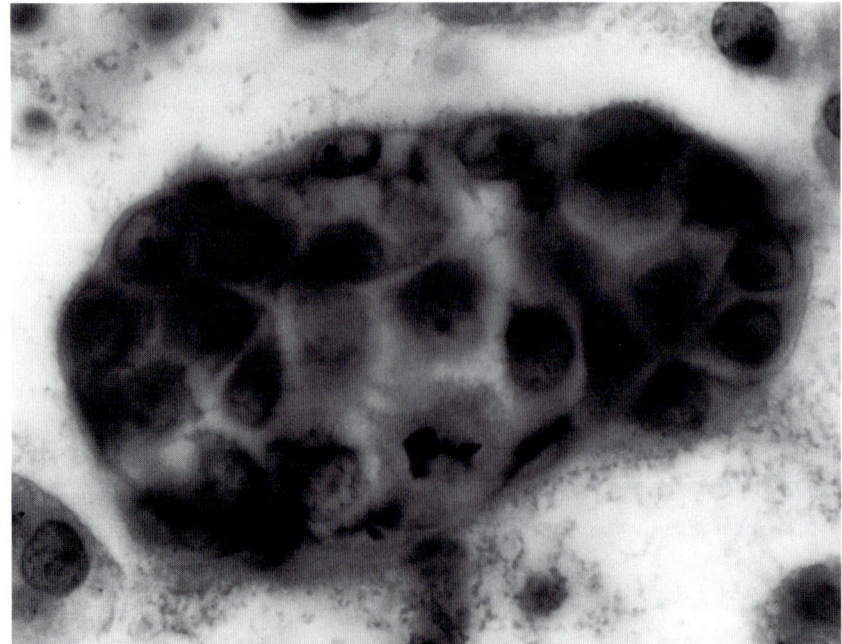

64a

64b

(For legend see page 112.)

Neoplasms of the Lung

64c

64d

(For legend see page 112.)

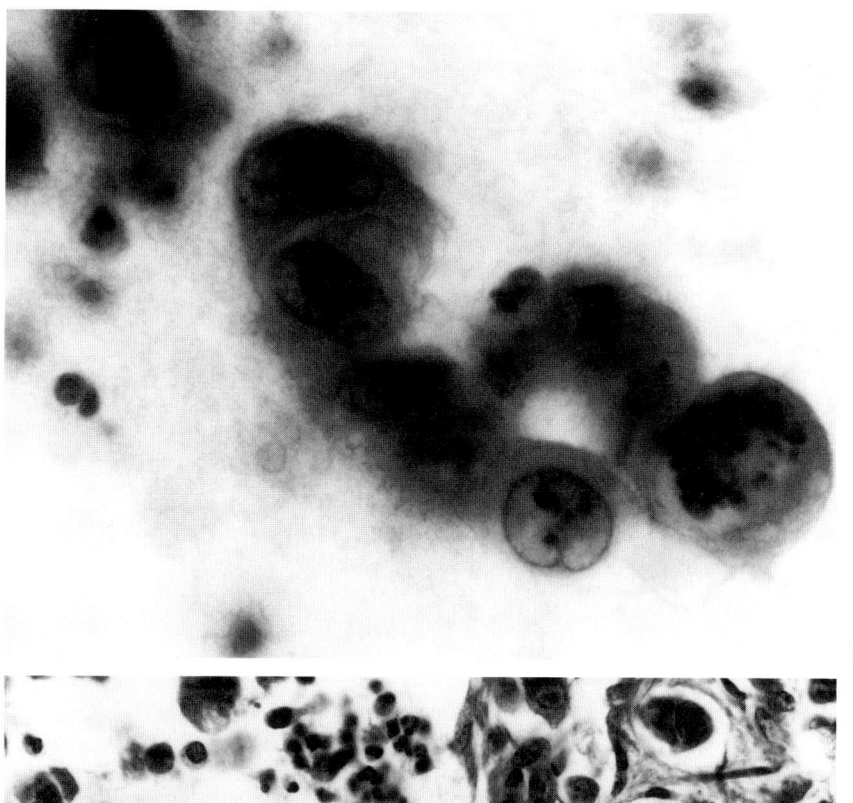

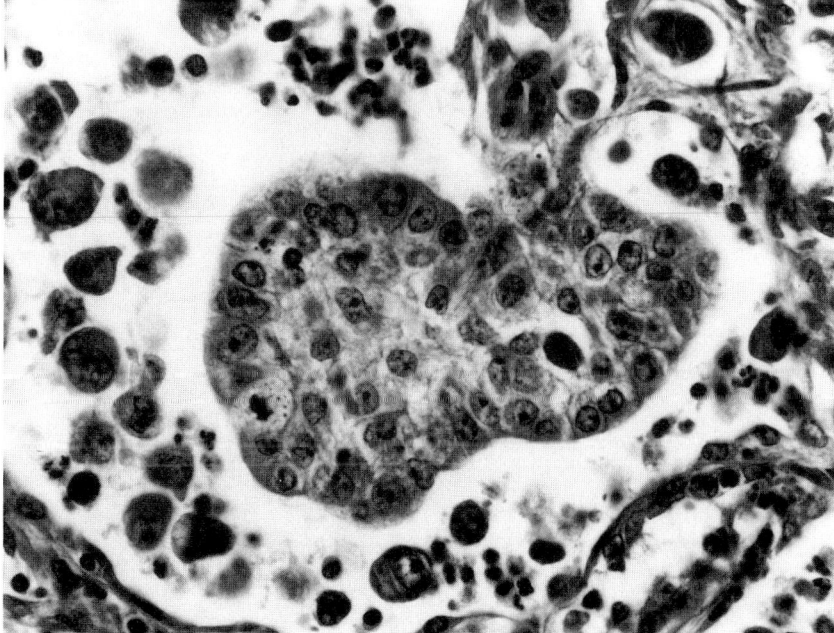

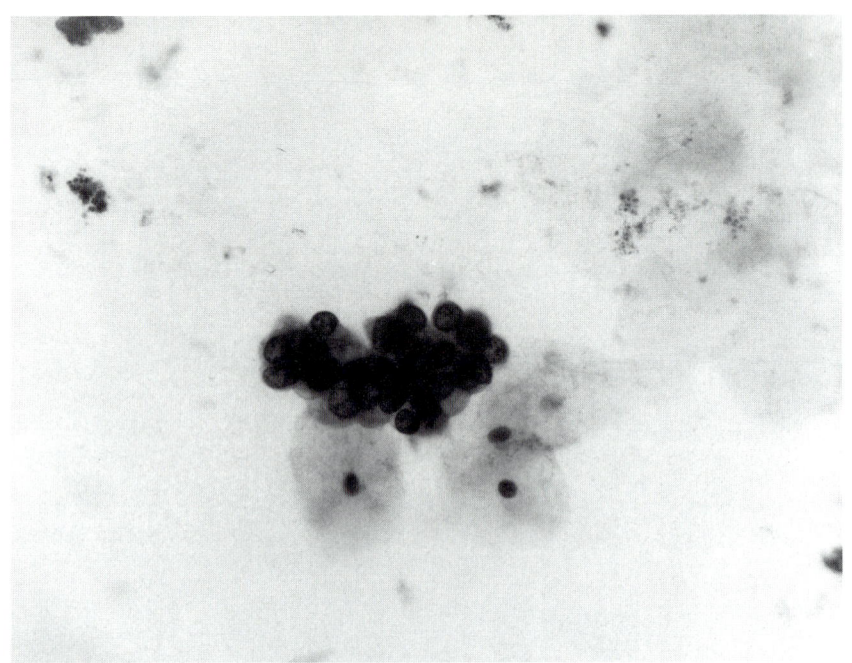

Cytopathology of Pulmonary Disease

65a

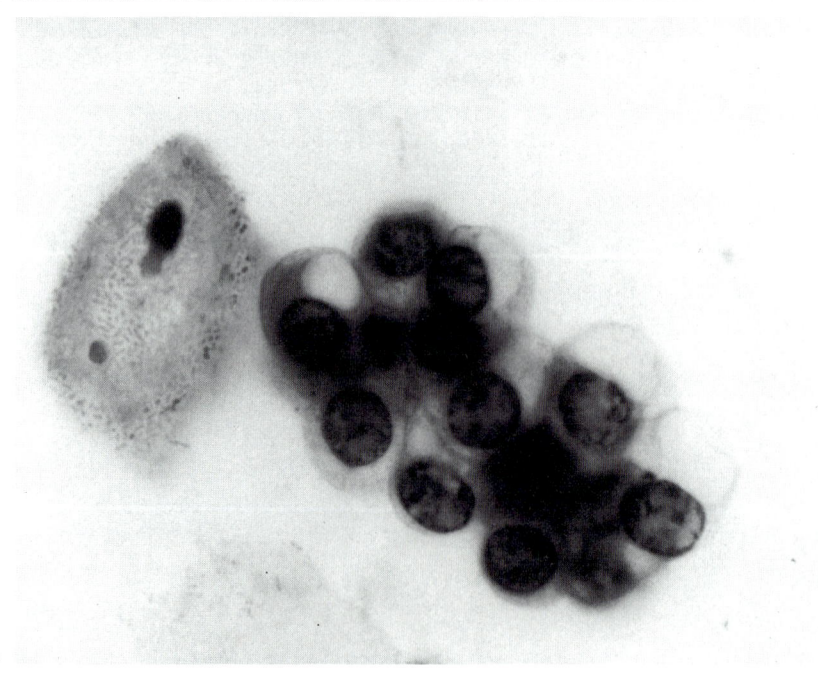

65b

(For legend see page 118.)

Neoplasms of the Lung

65c

65d

(For legend see page 118.)

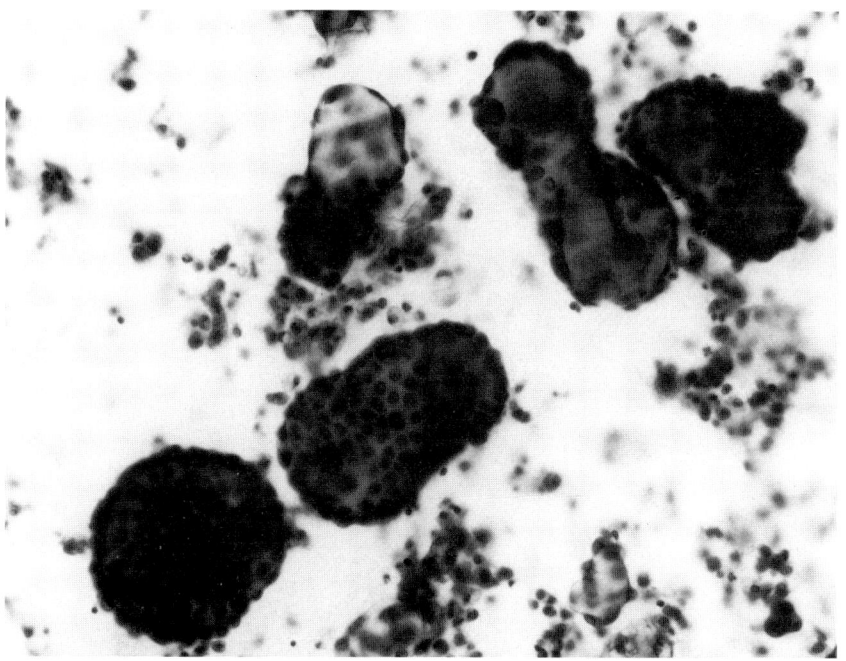

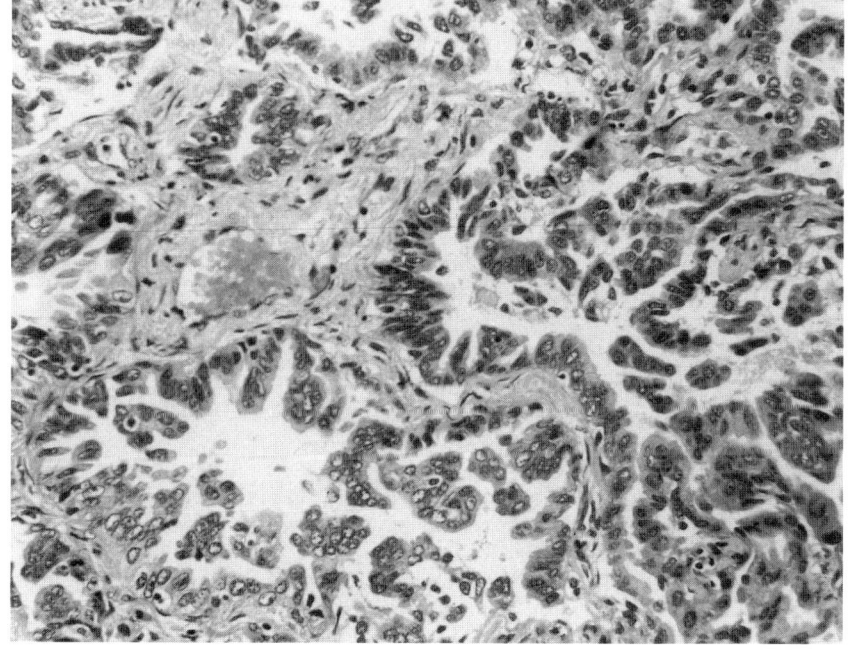

Cytopathology of Pulmonary Disease   118

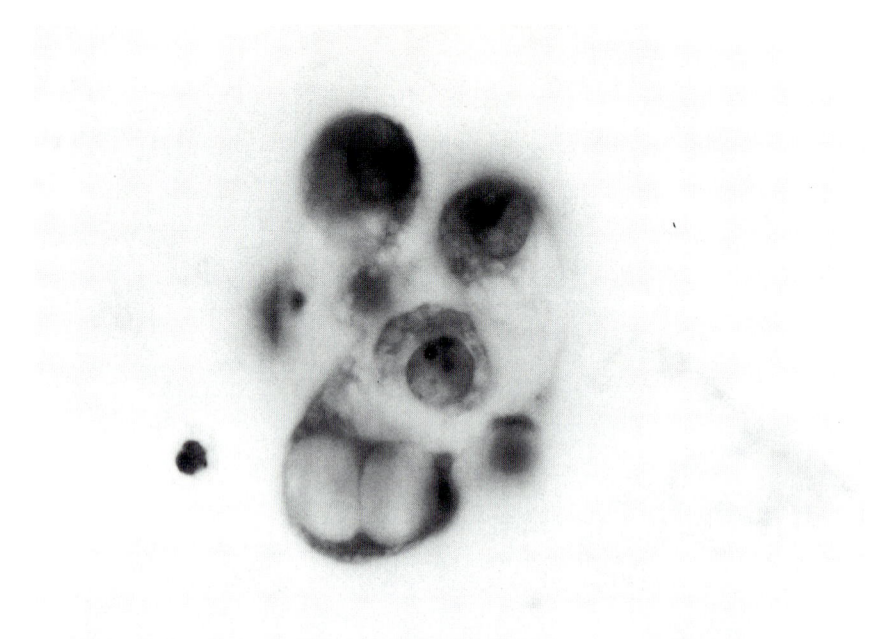

66a

Fig. 65. Adenocarcinoma – bronchiolo-alveolar carcinoma (*a, b* = sputum; *c* = pleural effusion; *d* = pneumonectomy): This group of small cells (*a*) could easily be mistaken for a group of reactive columnar cells. A higher power (*b*) reveals irregularly distributed nuclear chromatin and uneven nuclear membranes. However, extreme caution should be made in diagnosing such cell groups when features are not blatantly malignant. Pleural fluid (*c*) from the patient whose sputum samples are illustrated in figures *a, b* contains the same kind of cells verifying that those cells in the sputum are indeed adenocarcinoma cells. The question of a primary breast cancer must be raised because of the cytomorphology. The patient was worked up for a breast lesion, and the primary was felt to be in the lung. This lung tissue (*d*) verifies the origin of the cells seen in the samples from the same patient in figures *a–c*. *a–c* = Papanicolaou. *a* = × 340, *b* = × 850, *c* = × 170; *d* = HE. × 170.

Fig. 66. Adenocarcinoma (sputum): The three-dimensionality of cell groups from adenocarcinoma is illustrated by the three photographs (fig. a–c) taken at different focal planes through the same group of cells. The importance of focusing through groups stained by the amazingly transparent Papanicolaou stain cannot be overemphasized. Papanicolaou. × 900.

Fig. 67. Adenocarcinoma (*a* = pneumonectomy; *b* = bronchial brushing): The location of the tumor will dictate the cellularity of the cytologic sample. This pneumonectomy section shows the tumor to be intraluminal. *b* displays the yield of cells from such a lesion. When the tumor is located as in *a*, an enormous quantity of diagnostic material can be expected. A transbronchial biopsy, although indicated, is generally not necessary for diagnosis of such a situation. *a* = HE; *b* = Papanicolaou. × 85.

Neoplasms of the Lung 119

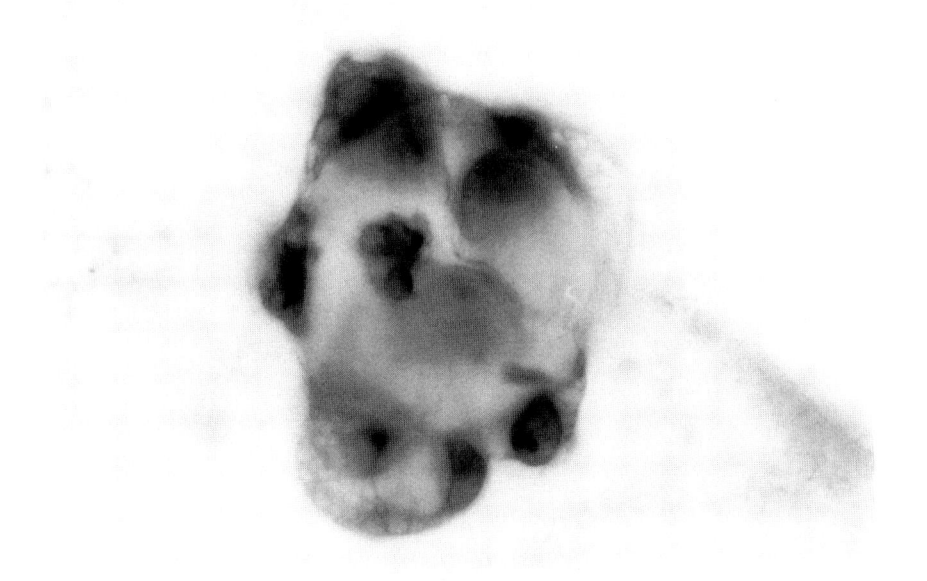

66b

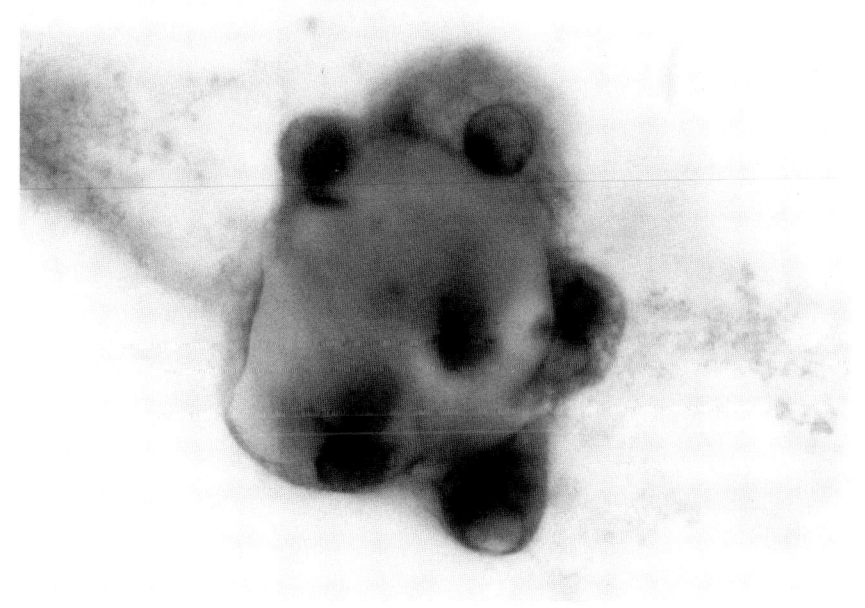

66c

67a

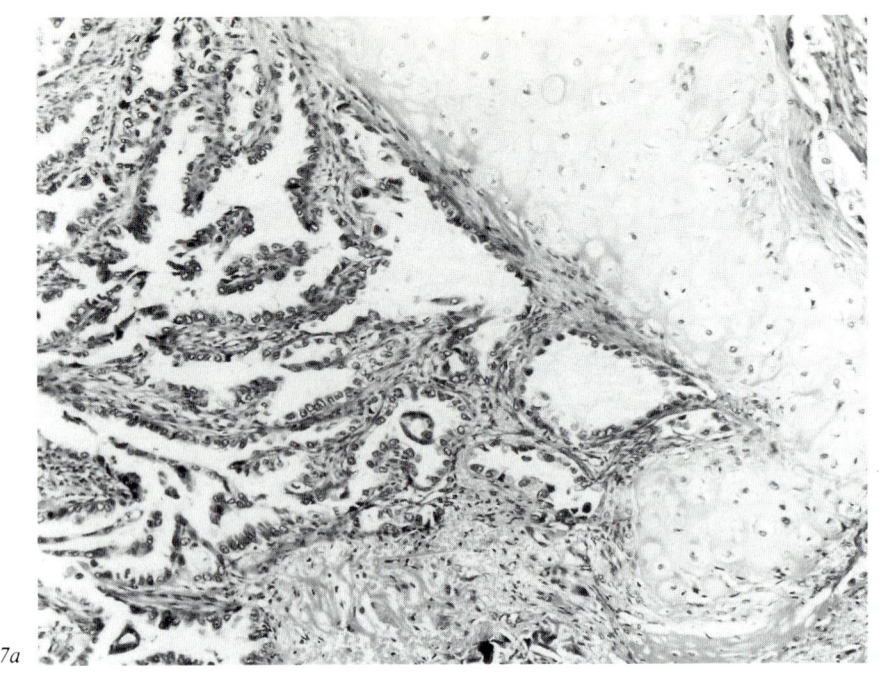

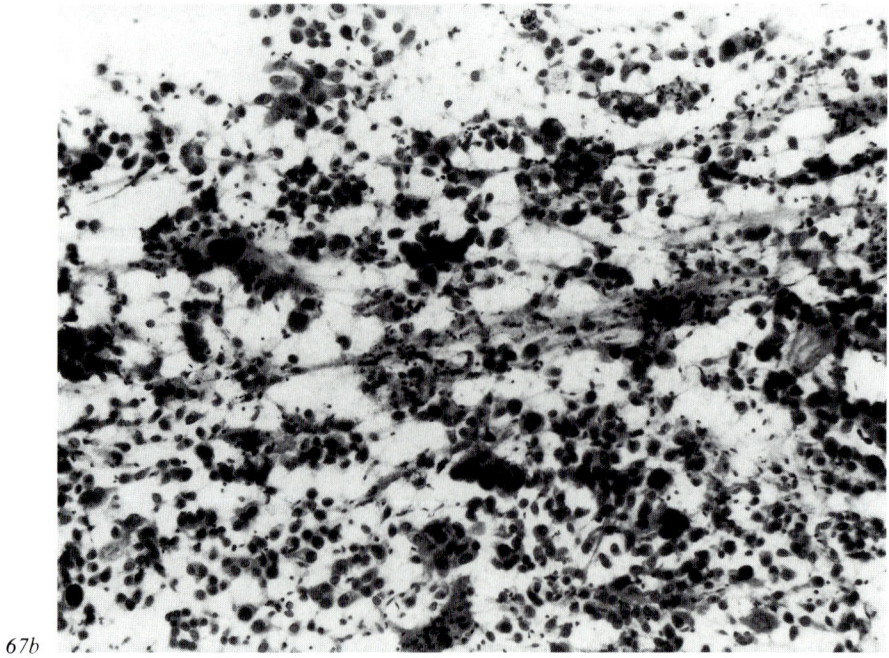

67b

(For legend see page 118.)

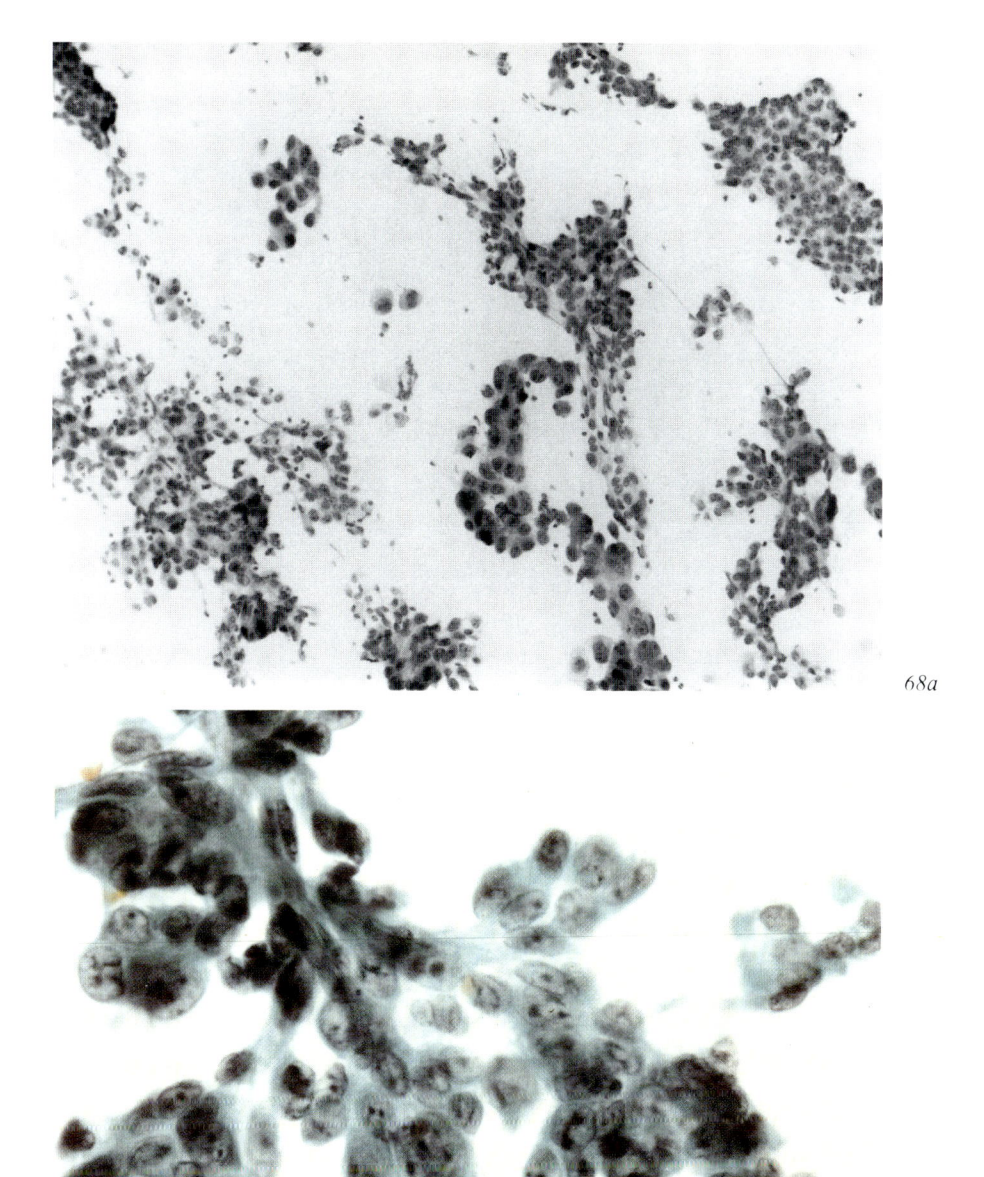

Neoplasms of the Lung

68a

68b

(For legend see page 123.)

Cytopathology of Pulmonary Disease 122

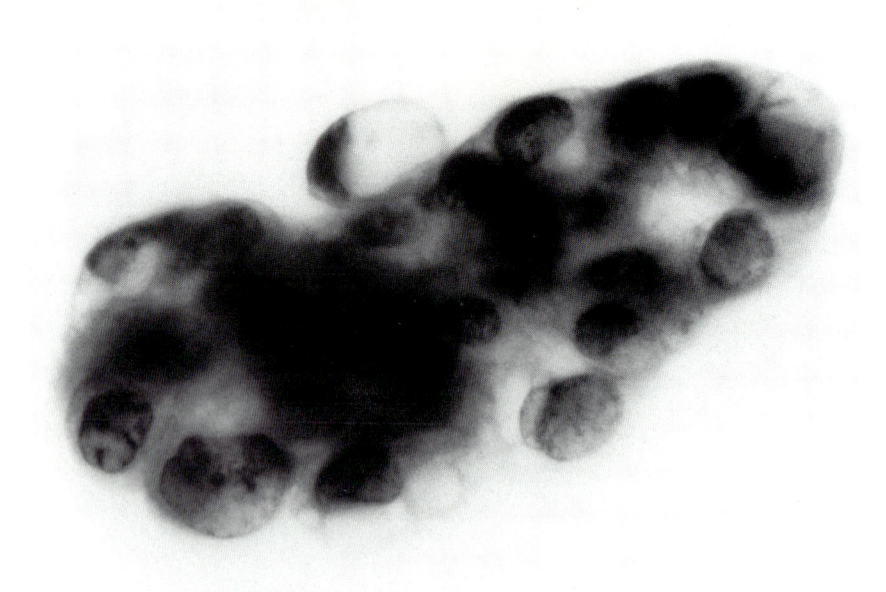

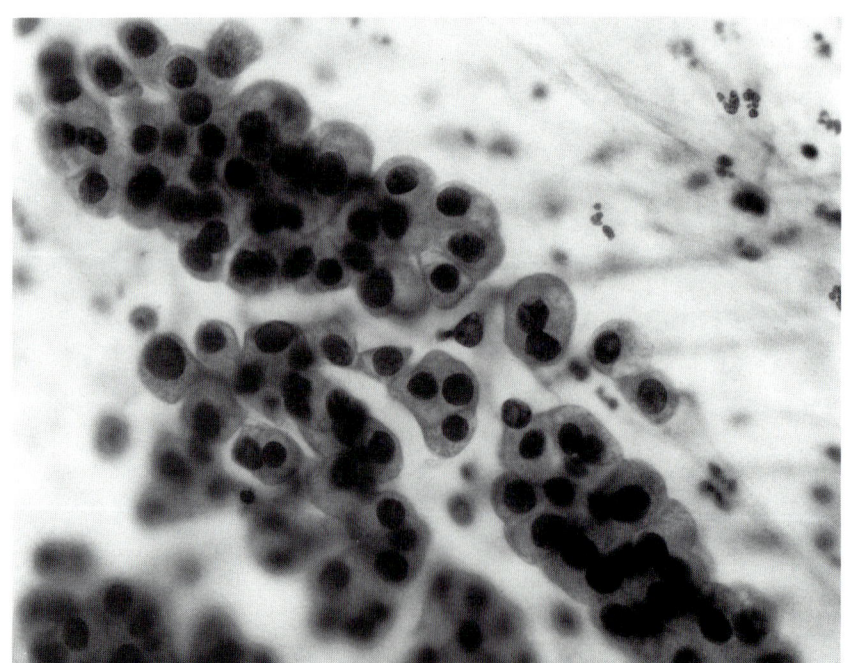

69a

69b

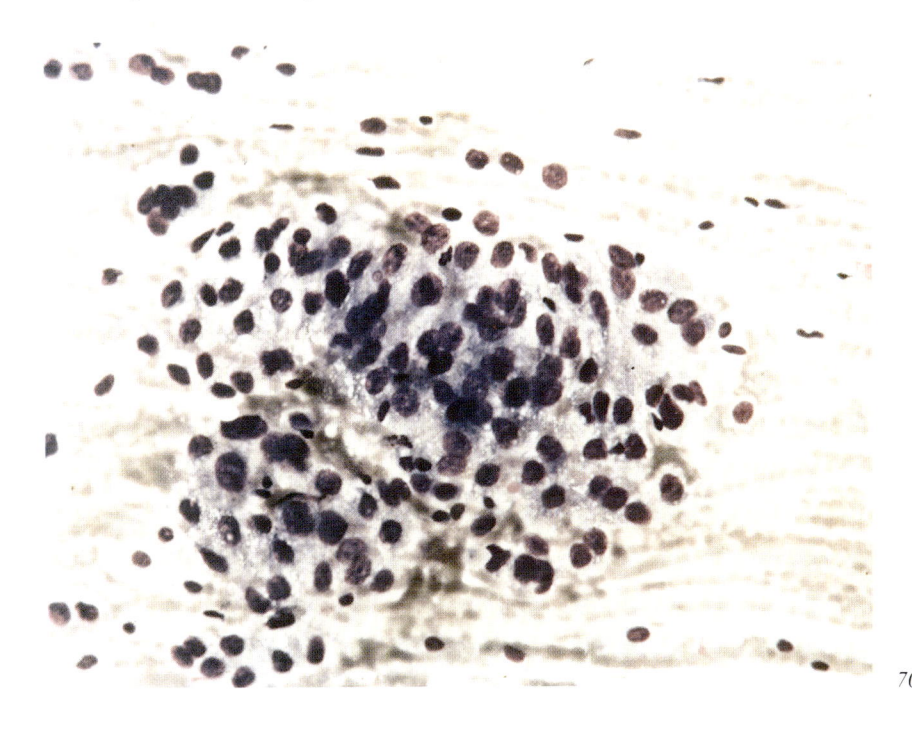

Fig. 68. Moderately differentiated adenocarcinoma (transbronchial FNA): The excellent cellular yield is made possible because of transmural penetration of the bronchial mucosa by the thin needle guided through the bronchoscope. Higher power (*b*) reveals cells having pale nuclei, prominent nucleoli, and indistinct cytoplasmic borders, all characteristic of adenocarcinoma. The papillary configuration of the fragment (*b*) provides a tissue pattern equivalent to a histologic section. Papanicolaou. $a = \times 85$; $b = \times 340$.

Fig. 69. Bronchiolo-alveolar carcinoma (sputum): This lesion is extremely difficult to diagnose because of the variability of cytologic presentation. The group of cells in *a* (a glandular cluster complete with cytoplasmic vacuoles) should be contrasted with the dispersed monolayer of cells seen in *b*. Monolayers of uniform cells could be mistaken for streams of alveolar macrophages. Such streams are often mixtures of tumor cells and alveolar macrophages. The distinction between the two cell populations is often difficult, a characteristic feature of bronchiolo-alveolar carcinoma. Papanicolaou. $a = \times 850$; $b = \times 340$.

Fig. 70. Bronchiolo-alveolar carcinoma (FNA): This transthoracic needle aspirate was obtained from a 2-cm discrete, peripheral mass, under fluoroscopic guidance. The uniformity of the cells is misleading. The gross presentation of the aspirate was mucoid, further adding to the diagnosis. MGG. $\times 340$.

Bronchiolo-alveolar carcinoma probably arises from the Clara cell, and more rarely from the type II pneumocyte [41]. Two cytologic presentations reflect the two distinct histologic patterns. Cells may occur in three-dimensional clusters (fig. 69a); or, groups of strikingly uniform cells are recovered intermixed with abundant histiocytes, which can appear very atypical, making the distinction between histiocytes and tumor cells quite difficult [249] (fig. 69b). Single cells may have a hob-nail appearance, with cytoplasm flaring from an eccentric nucleus [229]. Nuclear size can be uniformly round and when seen in clusters, a lack of molding is striking (fig. 70). Nucleoli are conspicuous but small and uniform. Chromatin pattern is usually powdery, and vacuolization of cytoplasm varies. Abundant mucus is usually evident in the background, and reflects the excessive mucus production [57], a common complaint in patients with this tumor. Roger et al. [206] were able to increase their accuracy of cell typing bronchiolo-alveolar carcinomas as distinct from bronchogenic adenocarcinomas from 52 to 90% using the following criteria: 'bronchiolo-alveolar carcinoma mainly exhibits tight clusters of uniform tumor cells in sputum preparations and more rarely single cancer cells and that the presence of pleomorphism, prominent nucleoli, and numerous single tumor cells

Table 12. Cytomorphologic features of different types of bronchiolo-alveolar carcinoma [249]

	Secretory	Nonsecretory	Poorly differentiated
Cellular arrangement	tightly packed clusters	sheets or loose clusters	discrete or loose clusters
Nuclei			
1. Shape	round or ovoid	round or ovoid	irregular
2. Size (μm)	25–35	25–35	30–60
3. Prominent nucleoli	frequent	infrequent	frequent
4. Multi-nucleation	unusual	occasional	common
Cytoplasm			
1. Abundance	abundant	less abundant	scanty
2. Vacuolation	foamy or vacuolated	not vacuolated	not vacuolated
Cohesion between cells	good	good	poor

Table 13. Pitfalls of adenocarcinoma

1.	Any *reactive* or *pneumonic* process ✓
2.	In order to avoid pitfalls, be certain of radiologic evidence for tumor, continuity of cytologic picture from one specimen to another – if it varies be aware that process is benign and reactive ✓
3.	Differentiation from *metastatic adenocarcinoma* may be impossible; conference with clinicians may clarify the issue

Table 14. Adenocarcinoma – cytologic features which distinguish it from similar lesions

	Adenocarcinoma	Pneumonia	BAC[1]
Cell features			
Cytoplasm			
Border	distinct	indistinct	distinct
Shape	round/oval	round/oval	round
Quality	delicate vacuolated	vacuolated with neutrophils	delicate
Relation to other cells	shared borders	shared borders	distinct/separate
Cilia	absent	usually present	absent
N/C ratio	variable	variable	uniform
Nucleus			
Border	slightly irregular	thin, uniform	smooth
Chromatin	finely/coarsely granular	fine, somewhat granular	usually fine
Place in cell	eccentric	eccentric	central
Nucleolus			
Size	large	small	small
Shape	round/irregular	round	round
Prominence	very	visible	very
Number	usually single	single	single
Pattern of groups	round – three-dimensional	irregular flat	variable: papillary-single cells
Single cells	rare	rare	frequent, with histiocytes
Smear background	dirty	inflamed	clean – much mucus

[1] BAC = Bronchiolo-alveolar carcinoma.

a

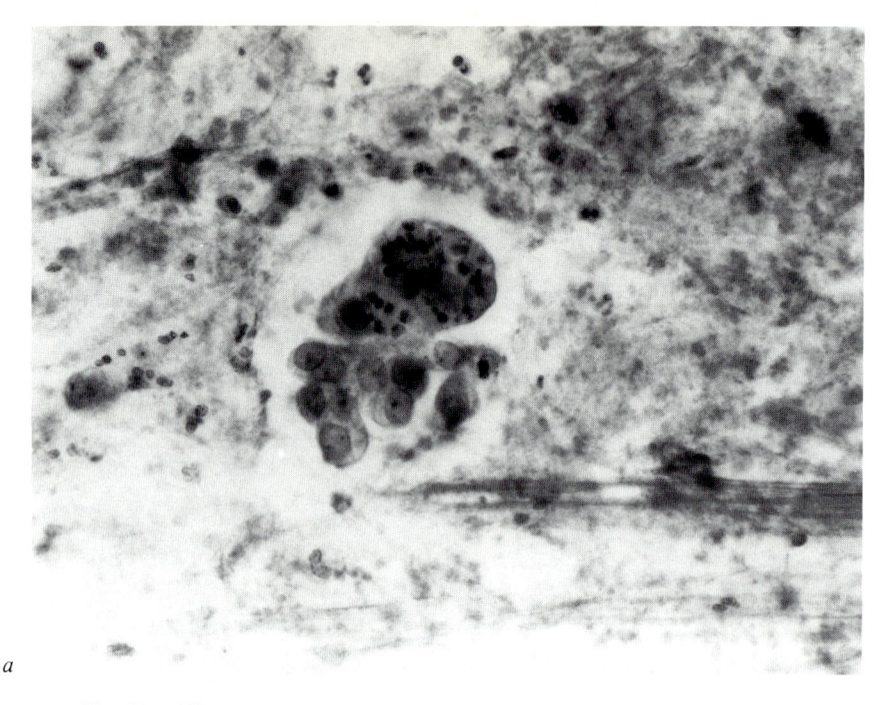

Fig. 71. Diffuse alveolar damage with severe atypia (*a, b* = sputa; *c* = segmental resection): Cells in sputa from this patient were repeatedly diagnosed as adenocarcinoma. In this group (*a, b*), the intracytoplasmic neutrophils provide a clue that this lesion was instead inflammatory. However, the lesion proved lethal after several years of repeated episodes. Etiology was never established. The atypia seen in multiple sputum samples is obvious in the respiratory epithelium of this patient (*c*). Individual nuclear changes are consistent with malignancy, but the overall pattern is that of an inflammatory lesion. *a* = × 340; *b* = × 850, Papanicolaou. *c* = × 340, HE.

favors a diagnosis of bronchogenic adenocarcinoma.' Tao et al. [249] recognized the variety of histologic patterns as reflected in cytologically distinct subtypes (table 12).

Pitfalls. Reactive and pneumonic processes can mimic adenocarcinoma [106, 146] (fig. 71) (table 13, 14). In a prospective study, Bewtra et al. [21] cytologically followed 9 patients with radiologically proven *pulmonary infarction*. Specific cell changes consisted of 'three-dimensional, papillary clusters of reactive bronchiolo-alveolar cells' atypical enough to be mistaken for adenocarcinoma. Aiding in the correct diagnosis are the

Neoplasms of the Lung

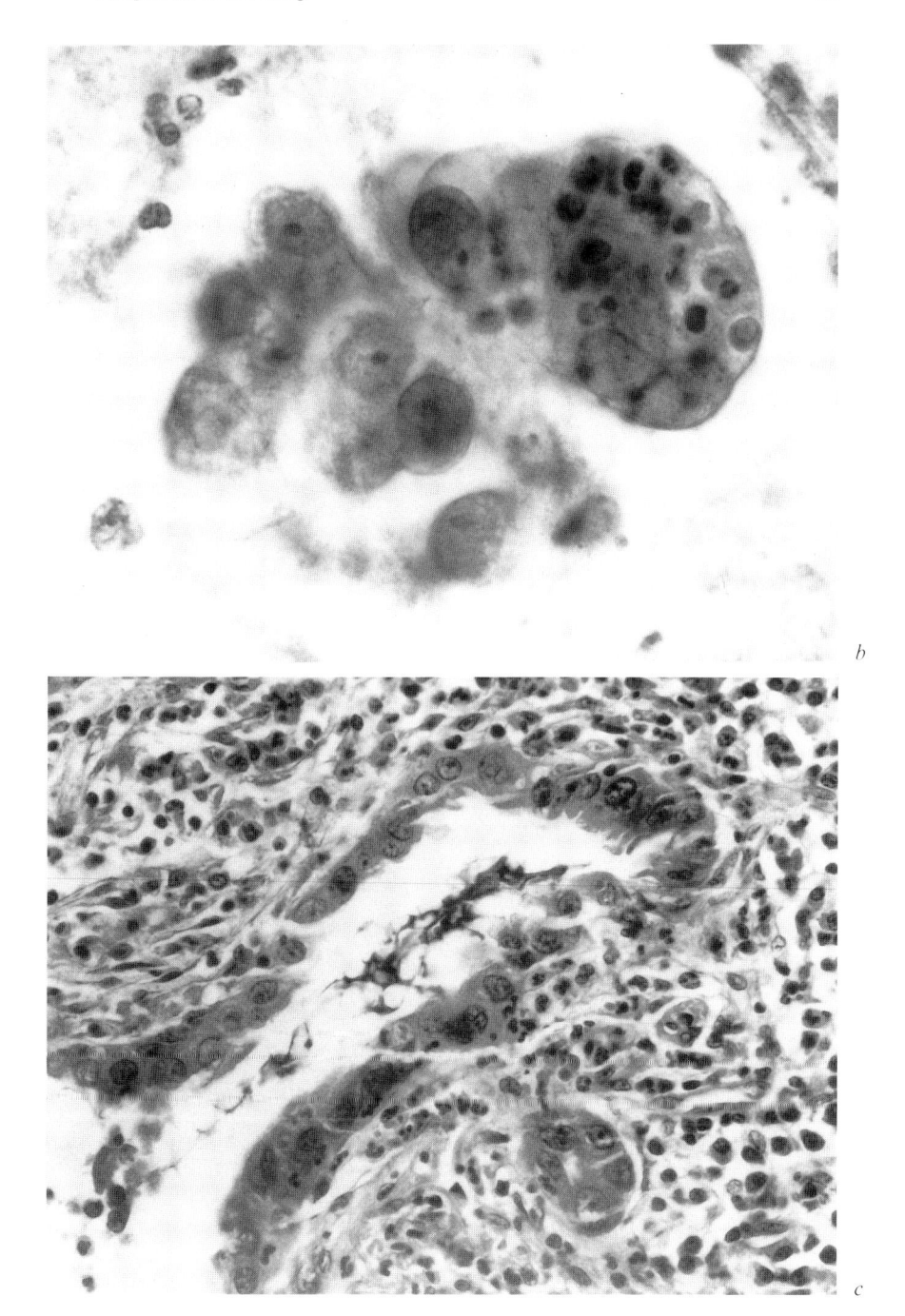

b

c

Cytopathology of Pulmonary Disease 128

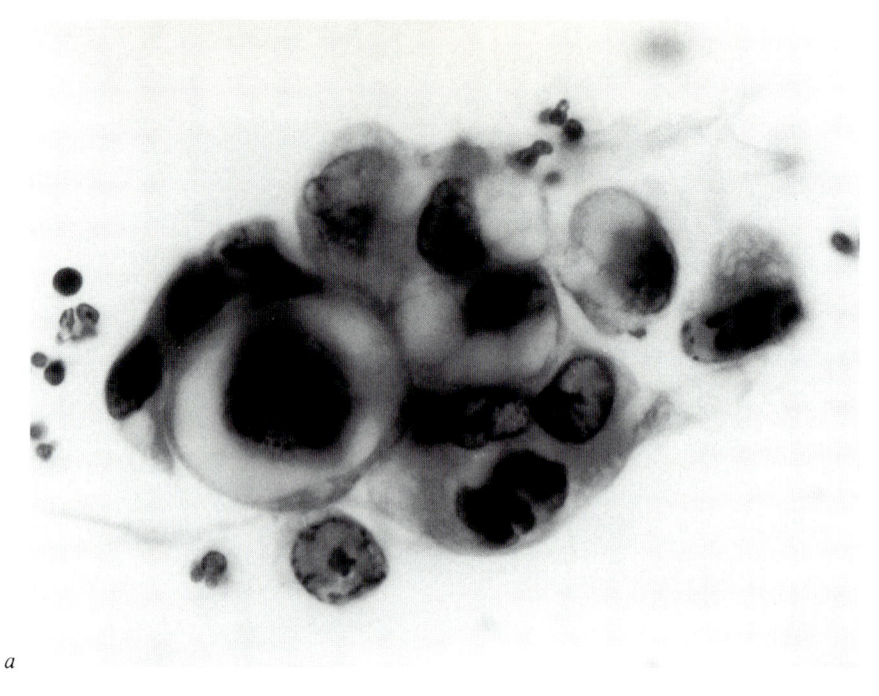

a

Fig. 72. Squamous carcinoma (*a* = sputum; *b* = sputum; *c* = pneumonectomy): The cytoplasmic vacuoles in *a* could persuade the observer that the lesion is of glandular origin. Further inspection of the specimen (*b*) reveals keratinized cytoplasmic fragments, deciding the diagnosis of squamous carcinoma. The tissue (*c*) confirms the diagnosis of squamous carcinoma by virtue of the intraluminal keratin, but also reveals the source of vacuolated cells. This case is a good example of the validity of the term 'bronchogenic'. *a* = × 850; *b* = × 340, Papanicolaou. *c* = × 340, HE.

following factors: the incidence of such atypia is low, 2/9 patients; the atypia is transient and inconstant, occurring typically during the second to third weeks postinfarct.

In order to avoid such pitfalls, radiologic evidence of a tumor should be present, and the cytologic picture should be continuous from one specimen to the other, if not becoming more atypical. Treatment of the lesion by antibiotics will clear the cytologic atypia if the process is inflammatory, but if a neoplasm is present, even in association with a pneumonia, the atypical cells will persist after the pneumonia is cleared.

Misinterpretation of a *squamous 'bronchogenic' carcinoma* may occur when vacuoles are present in the cytoplasm of some squamous tumor cells

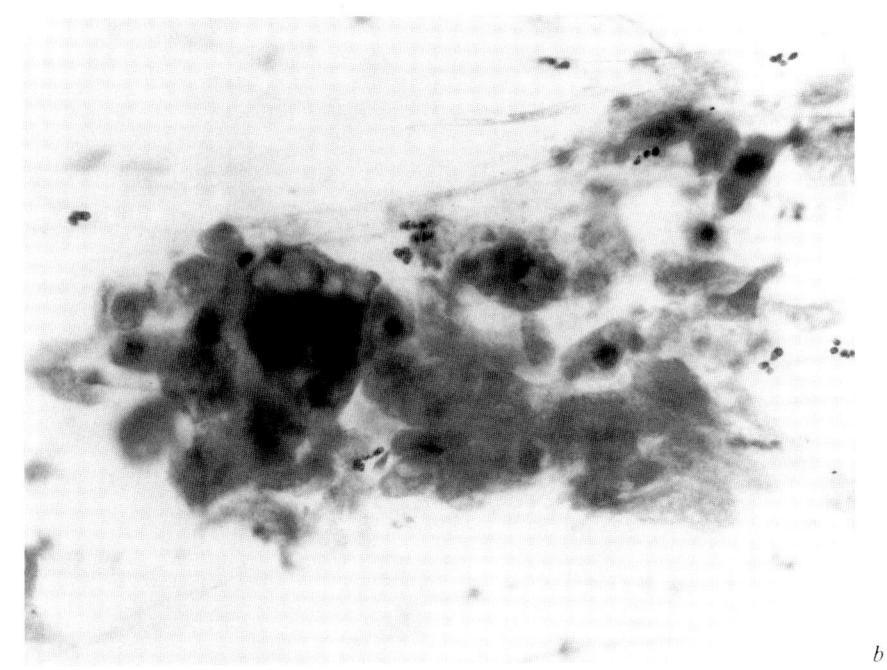

Neoplasms of the Lung

b

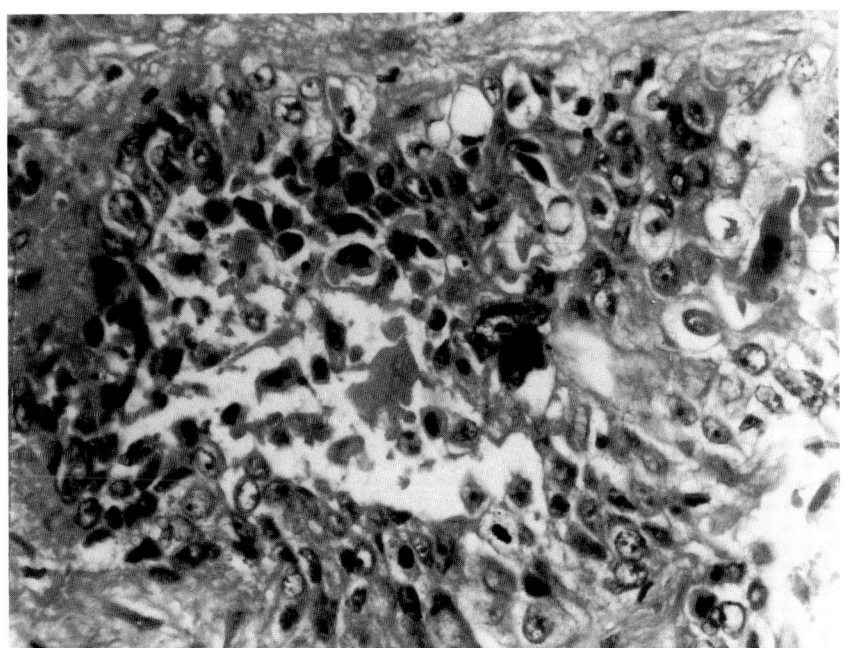

c

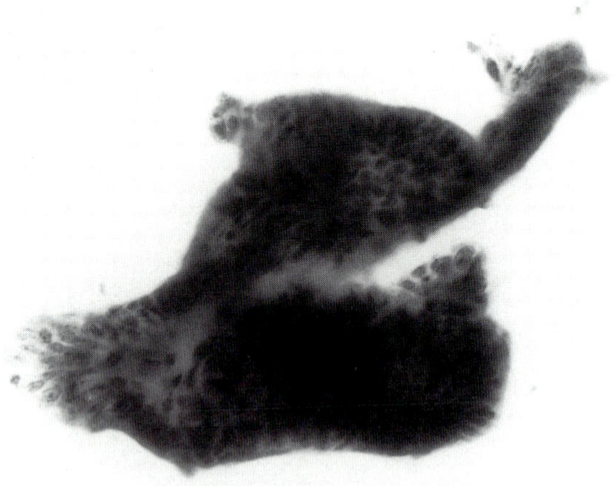

Cytopathology of Pulmonary Disease

a

Fig. 73. Adenocarcinoma of the colon, metastatic to the lung (*a* = sputum; *b* = FNA; *c* = segmental resection): This remarkable tissue fragment (*a*) was spontaneously expectorated and strongly suggests the organ of origin by the very tall, narrow (carrot shape) columnar cells and the sharp luminal borders. The three-dimensionality of this fragment is indicated by the density. A large tumor fragment was aspirated from a lung nodule (*b*). The elongated slender epithelial cells, aligned along the edges of the fragment, recapitulate the histology seen in *c*, so characteristic of colonic carcinoma. Note the debris in the background, indicating necrosis and possible cavitation. Tissue from the same patient as *b*, confirms the origin in a colon primary, even without examination of the primary tumor. The very tall, slender, epithelial cells, polarized perpendicularly to the basement membrane, and with a sharp luminal margin, are all features characteristic of colonic carcinoma. Note the inflammation and necrosis which coincide with those findings in the FNA. *a, b* = Papanicolaou. *a* = × 180, *b* = × 170; *c* = HE. × 170.

(fig. 72a). Careful search of the sample for other criteria of cell type (fig. 72b) will usually clarify the issue. If not, a diagnosis of 'bronchogenic, non-oat cell carcinoma' is usually acceptable to the clinicians to treat the patient. Tissue confirmation is important to educate the cytologist and categorize the tumor (fig. 72c).

b

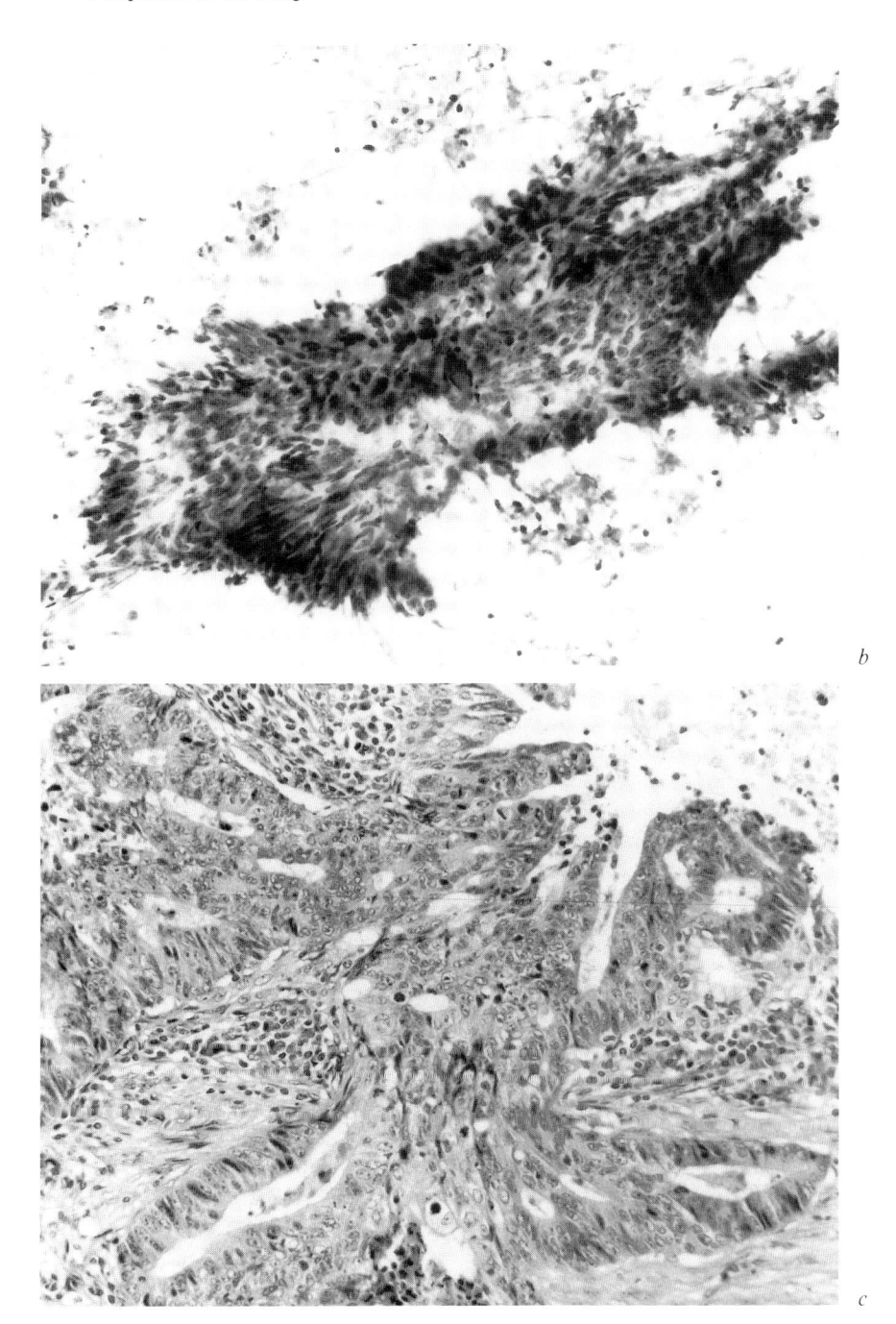

c

A report of an FNA of a *sclerosing hemangioma* describes the similarities and differences of that rare pulmonary lesion compared with bronchiolo-alveolar carcinoma [269].

'Creola bodies' are glandular structures which exfoliate after stimulation of the epithelium in such diseases as asthma or chronic bronchitis [167, 168]. These groups of respiratory epithelium have surface cilia and small uniform nuclei vertically arranged perpendicular to the basement membrane.

Distinction between a *metastatic adenocarcinoma* and a primary adenocarcinoma of the lung is often difficult. Consultation with clinicians to elicit history of a possible distant primary is essential to avoid a wrong diagnosis. The most common adenocarcinomas to travel to the lung are from breast and colon [123]. Certain metastatic carcinomas will mimic the normal histology of the primary site, especially colonic carcinoma which has elongated cells with 'carrot'-shaped nuclei [130, p. 670; 153] (fig. 73). Breast cancer cells (fig. 74, 75) will sometimes appear in morulae or balls, but will also assume a tandem or 'Indian file' arrangement. Highly specific immunochemistry, such as prostate-specific antigen, can also be of help. The primary tumor should be stained in concert with the metastatic sample to make sure that the parent tumor has the same immunologic character as the metastatic lesion. The problem arises when metastases lose their membrane antigens and the primary tumor is still membrane antigen positive. Microscopic comparison with tissue or cytology from the suspected primary site is still the choice method of resolving diagnostic uncertainties (fig. 76–78).

Small Cell 'Oat Cell' Carcinoma

Small cell undifferentiated ('oat cell') carcinoma is located centrally with a tendency toward early spread and invasion of bronchial, hilar, and mediastinal lymph nodes, and soft tissue. The prevalence of this lesion is

---

Fig. 74. Adenocarcinoma of the breast, metastatic to the lung (a = lung; b = sputum): Carcinoma of the breast usually metastasizes to the lung in solid tumor aggregates. When it exfoliates into sputum (b) clusters of neoplastic glandular cells are the rule. Note the smoothness of the outer edge of the group, with the suggestion of cytoplasmic vacuolization and cell separation which could be mistaken for windows. This is the classic pitfall between mesothelial cells and breast carcinoma cells. a = × 360, HE; b = × 900, Papanicolaou.

a

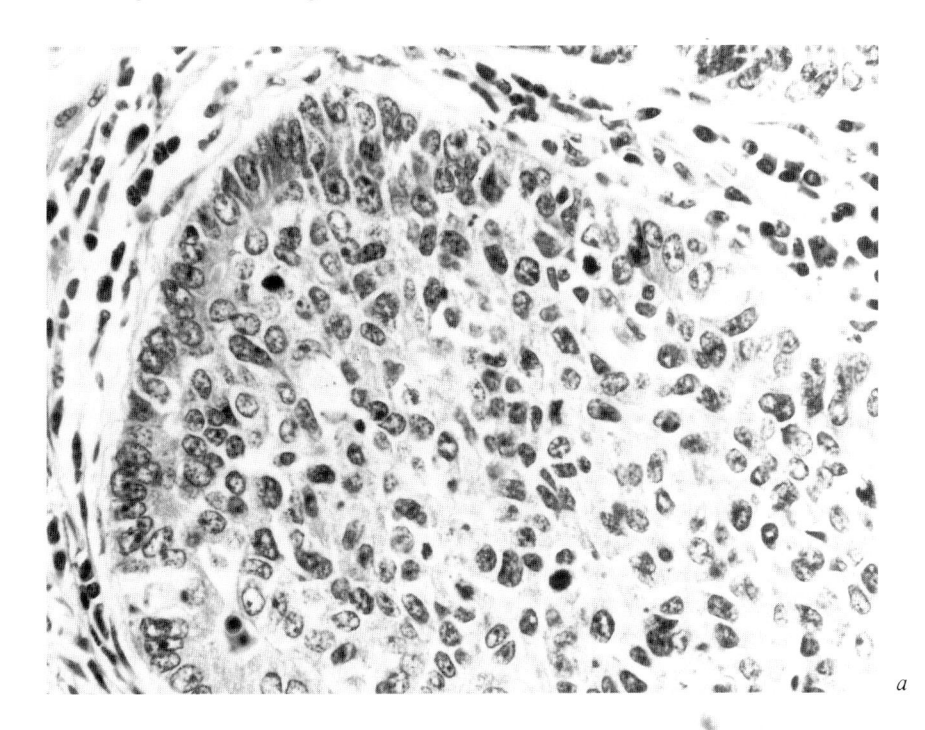

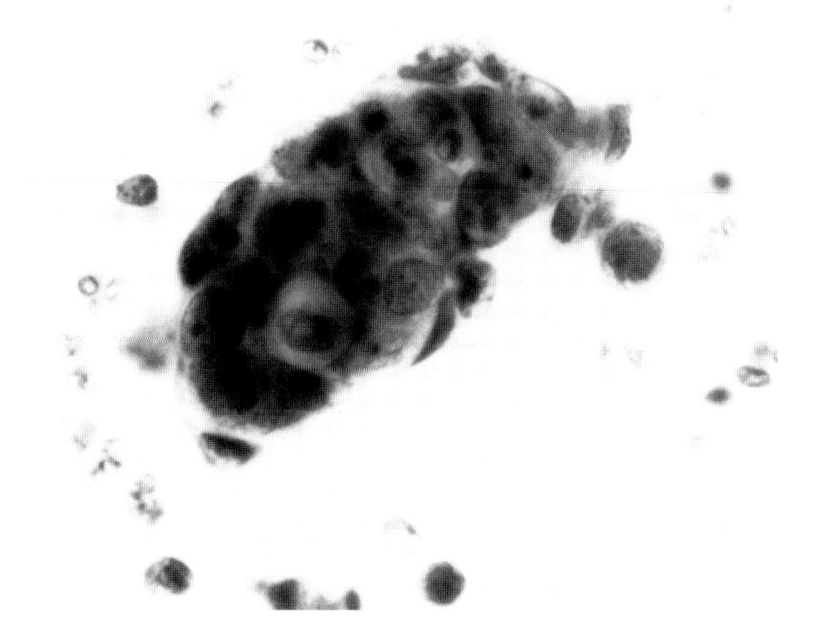

b

Cytopathology of Pulmonary Disease 134

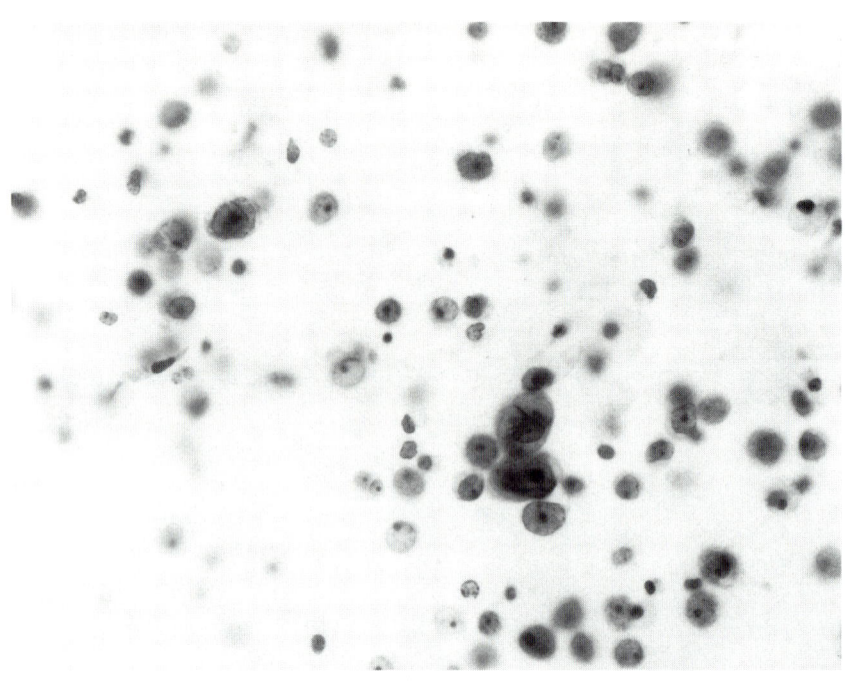

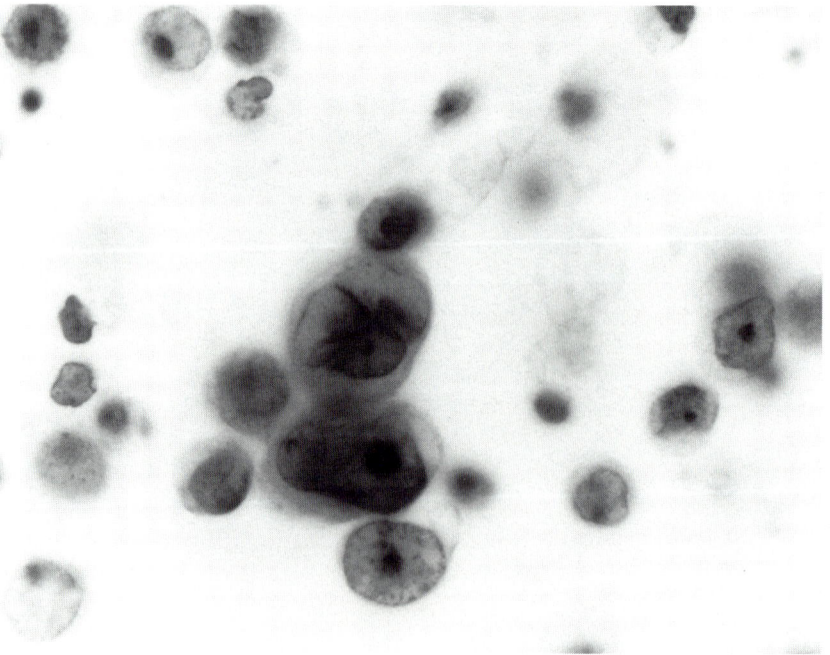

75a

75b

Neoplasms of the Lung 135

75c

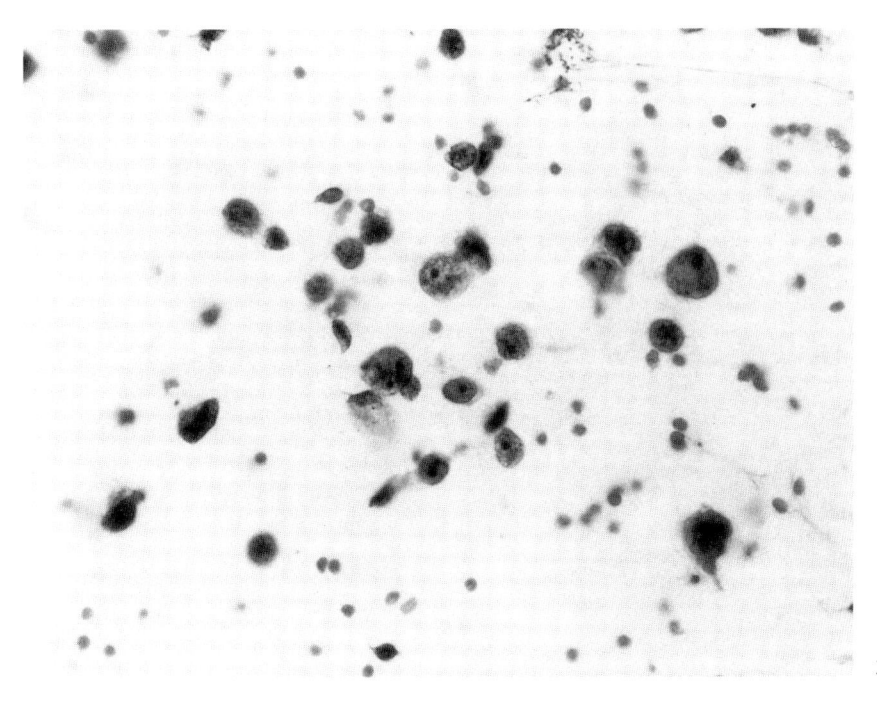

Fig. 75. Adenocarcinoma of the breast, metastatic to the lung and pleural cavity (*a, b* = sputum; *c* = pleural fluid): Compared with figure 74, these cells have exfoliated in both sputum and fluid as individual cells. There is no question as to the malignant nature of these cells, but they are not classically those seen in carcinoma of the breast; in fact, they could be mistaken for a large cell lymphoma (see fig. 89). Papanicolaou. *a* = ×340; *b* = ×900; *c* = ×340.

Fig. 76. Adenocarcinoma of the cervix, metastatic to the lung (*a* = FNA; *b* = cervical biopsy): All adenocarcinomas are not primary in the lung, and in fact, most are metastatic. Also, not all carcinomas of the cervix are squamous. This needle aspiration of a lung nodule was initially thought to be primary until the tissue, shown in *b*, was examined and the similarity between the two appreciated. *a* = ×340, Papanicolaou; *b* = ×180, HE.

Fig. 77. Adenocarcinoma of the pancreas, metastatic to the lung (*a* = FNA; *b* = lung): The pleomorphism of this pancreatic carcinoma can be appreciated when compared with the cluster of more well-differentiated tumor epithelium in the corner of *a*. Comparison with the tissue in *b* reveals the variable pattern of well-differentiated and more pleomorphic areas. *a* = ×340, Papanicolaou; *b* = ×170, HE.

76a

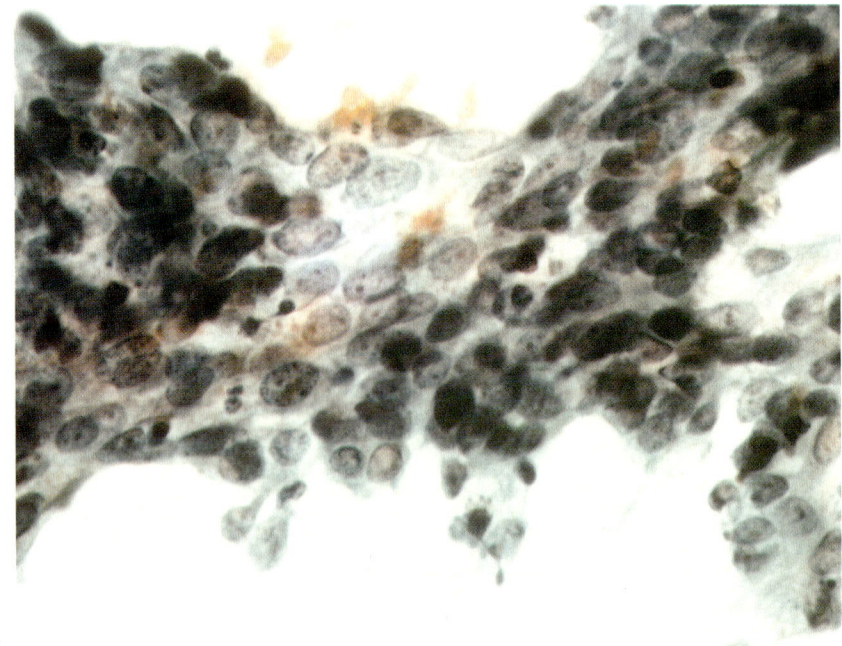

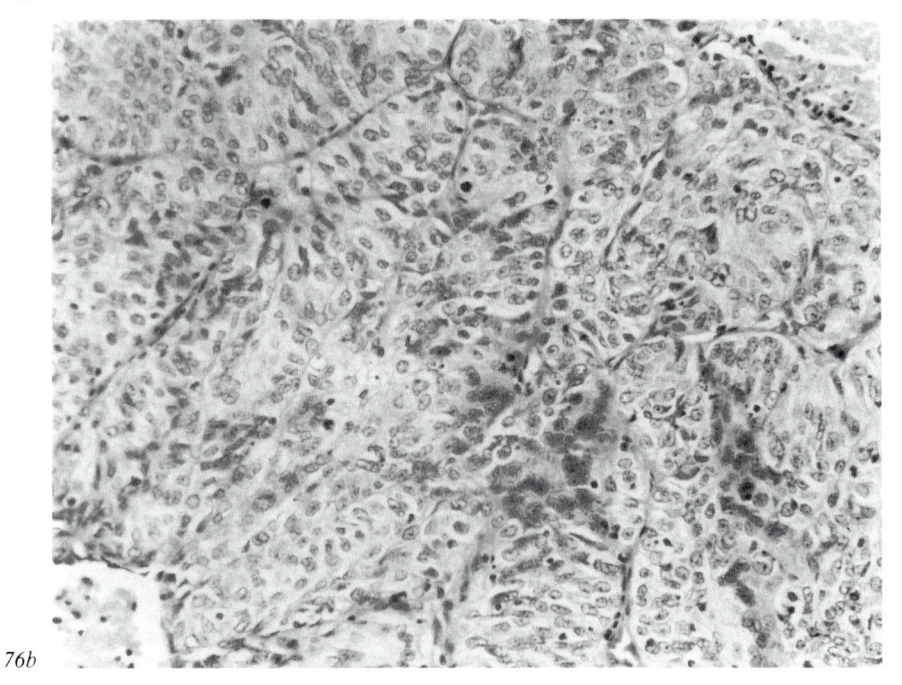

76b

(For legend see page 135.)

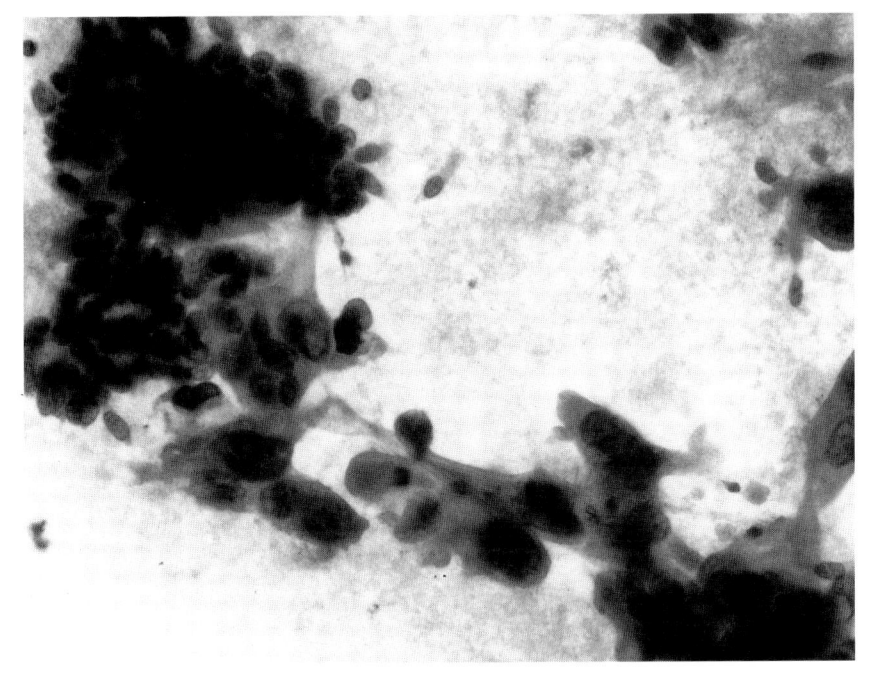

Neoplasms of the Lung

77a

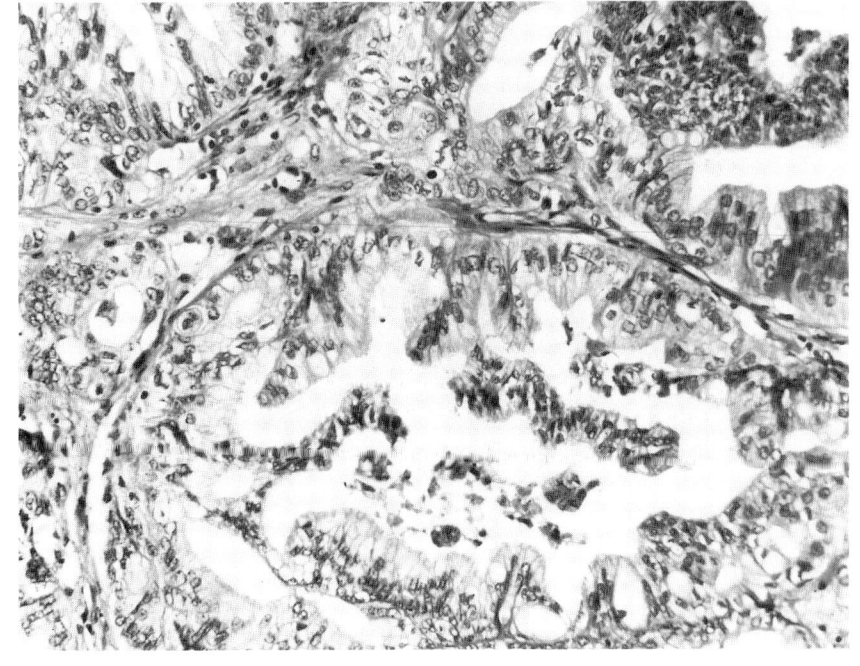

77b

(For legend see p. 135.)

a

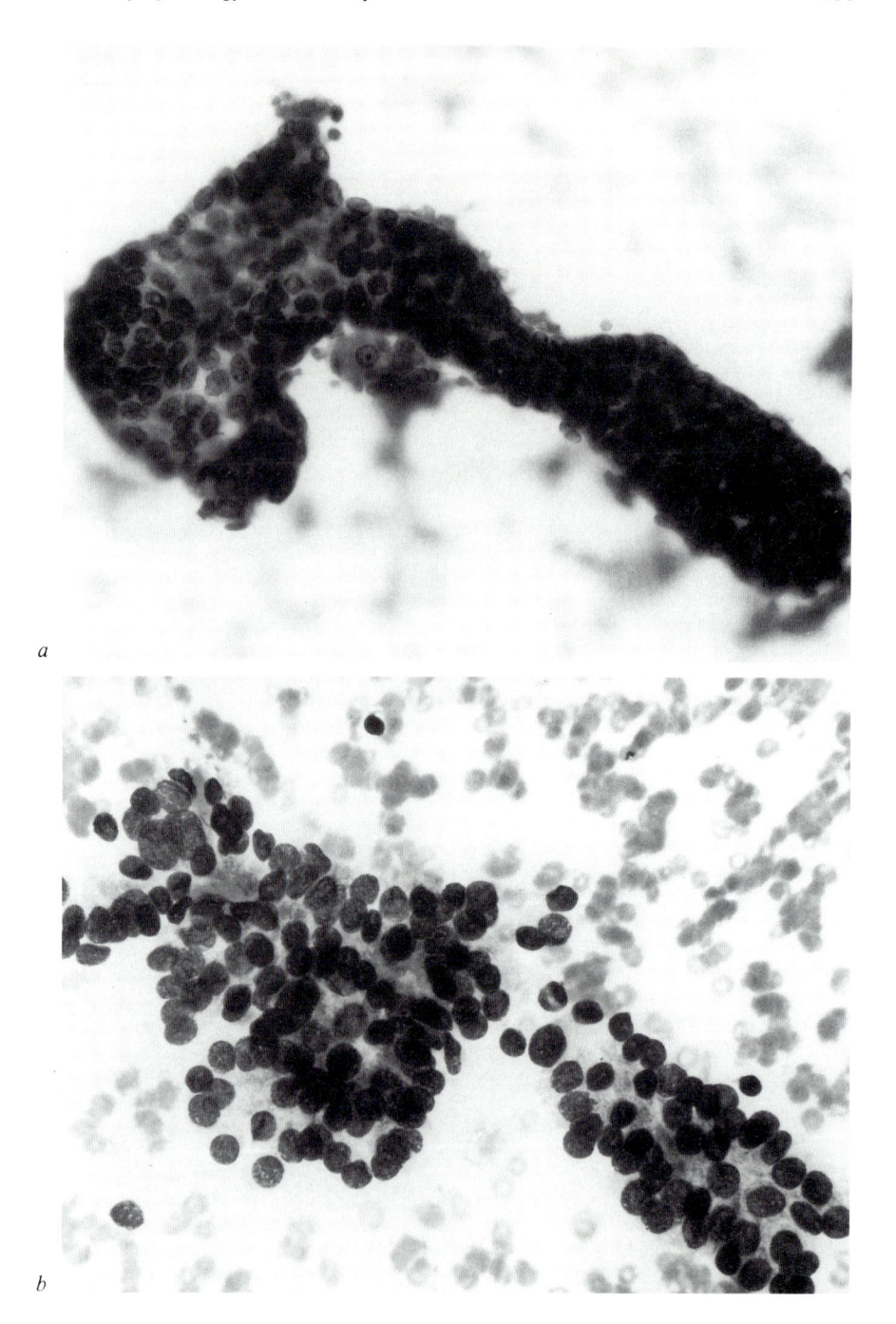

b

Neoplasms of the Lung 139

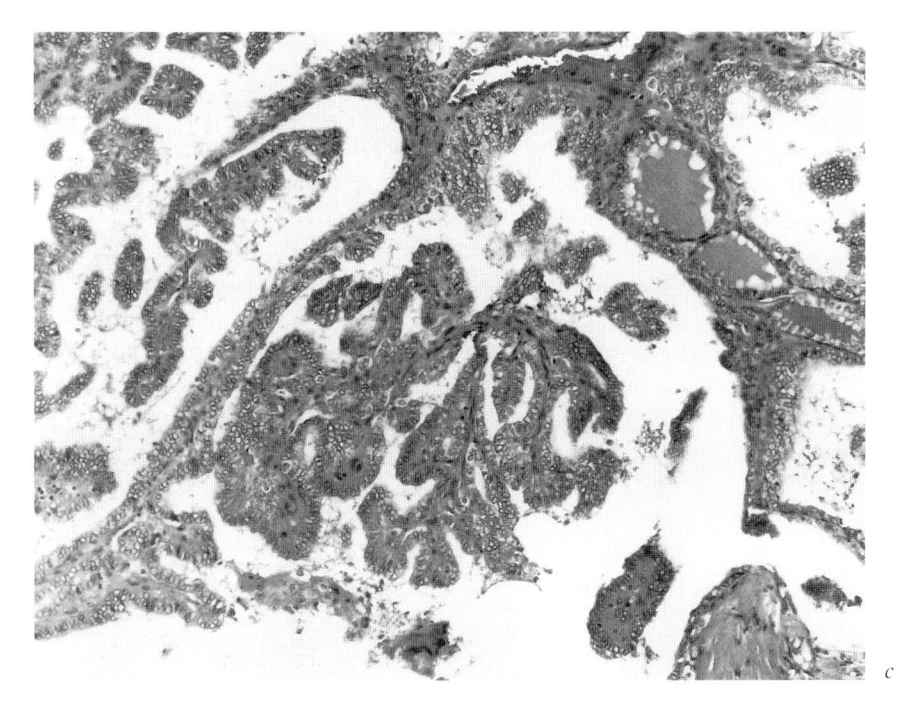

Fig. 78. Papillary carcinoma of the thyroid, metastatic to the lung (*a, b* = FNA; *c* = thyroid): Tissue fragments aspirated from a lung nodule confirmed the diagnosis of origin in the thyroid. Although the cells are uniformly small with regular chromatin, the configuration of the tissue fragments is that of a papillary neoplasm. Careful search for intranuclear cytoplasmic inclusions was futile, and while suggestive of papillary carcinoma of the thyroid, are not necessary for a diagnosis. Note the excellent comparison with the tissue in the original tumor. *a, b* = ×340. *a* = Papanicolaou; *b* = MGG. *c* = ×85, HE.

approximately 25% of all lung cancers with a strong association with cigarette smoking.

This is a multisystem disease [2], with metastatic foci frequently becoming clinically evident before the primary lesion is apparent [18, 98]. Metastases can be found in liver, adrenal, brain, kidney and abdominal lymph nodes. Such biologic behavior accounts for the very poor survival rate, which is currently much less than 1 year. Treatment is traditionally radiation with adjuvant chemotherapy. However, rare cases which are staged to be free of metastatic disease have now survived surgical resection for more than two years; adjuvant chemotherapy is usually employed.

This tumor group is perhaps the most fascinating of all the primary lung tumors. 'Undifferentiated' is a misnomer: these tumor cells are capable of producing a variety of hormones and are thus considered among the amine precursor uptake decarboxylase (APUD) family of cancers [15, 98, 183, 184, 241]. This capability is no doubt responsible for the propensity of 'oat cell' carcinomas to create a paraneoplastic syndrome [165].

The cell of origin is generally accepted to be the Kulchitsky cell [98, 282]. Two cell types, 'lymphocyte-like' and intermediate, can be seen in the same lesion in tissue and cytologic samples, and may represent degrees of maturation of the same cell line. However, Horai et al. [99] and Miyamoto et al. [156] present evidence that the differences in chromatin may correlate with responsiveness to therapy and prognosis. In this author's opinion, the lymphocyte-like cell is probably a degenerating form of the intermediate cell.

Cytologic Criteria. In sputum samples, streams of small hyperchromatic cells, not tightly adherent but closely related to each other, can be highly diagnostic, even in a single specimen (fig. 79). The cell size is slightly larger than a lymphocyte in the 'lymphocyte-like' cell type, and considerably larger with a more open chromatin network in the 'intermediate' cell type [284] (fig. 80). Very scanty, almost indiscernible cytoplasm surrounds a nucleus polygonal in shape. Chromatin is powdery, with very inconspicuous nucleoli, if any can be noted at all. Molding, onion-skinning, and Indian-file, or tandem arrangements, are diagnostic and are maintained in pleural fluids (fig. 80c). Nuclear fragments accompany these tumor cells, and add to the diagnosis. In brushings, these fragile cells are easily attenuated when smeared and assume the elongated pointed form which provides the name 'oat-cell', and corresponds to crush artefact seen in tissue.

Fig. 79. Small cell undifferentiated 'oat cell' carcinoma of the lung (sputum): Streams of associated but disconnected small tumor cells provide definitive diagnosis of this tumor cell type, even if no more than this amount of material is seen in a single sputum. Note the inconspicuous cytoplasm, absence of nucleoli, and smudgy nuclear chromatin. Nuclear molding, and tandem arrangement or 'Indian filing' are additional characteristics of oat cell carcinoma. Compare the cell size with the neutrophils scattered in the background of *a*. Papanicolaou. $a = \times 340$; $b = \times 850$.

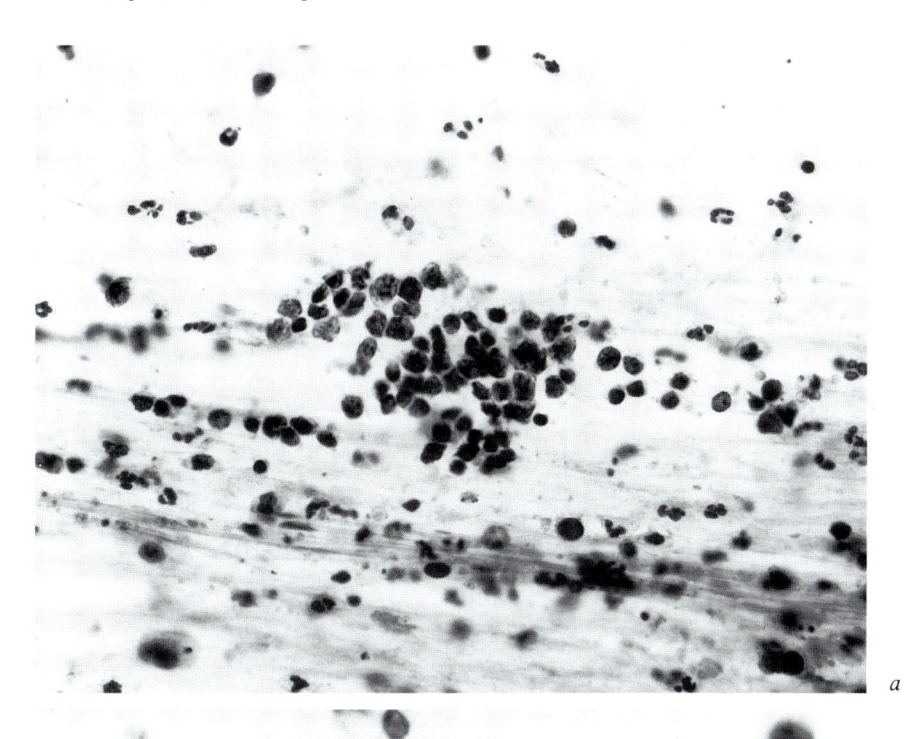

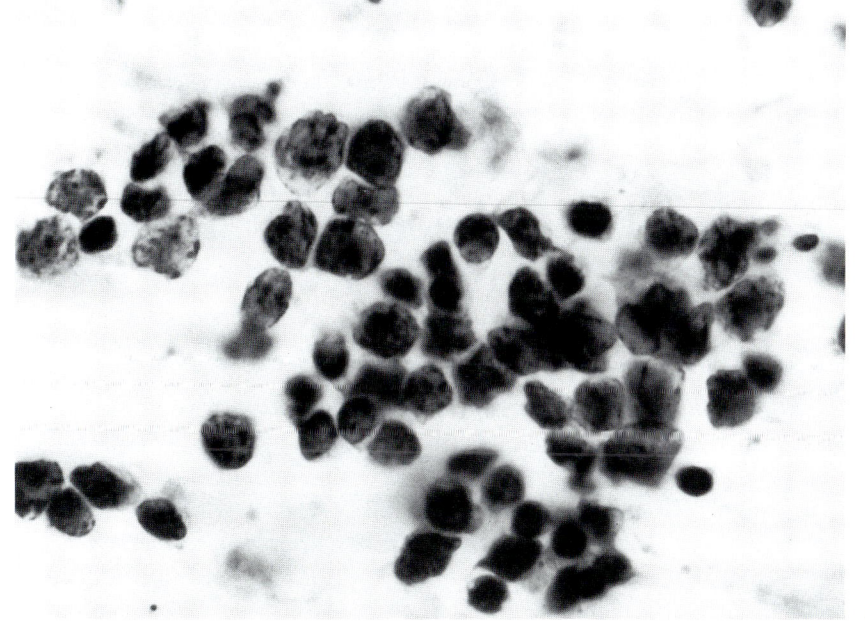

Neoplasms of the Lung

a

b

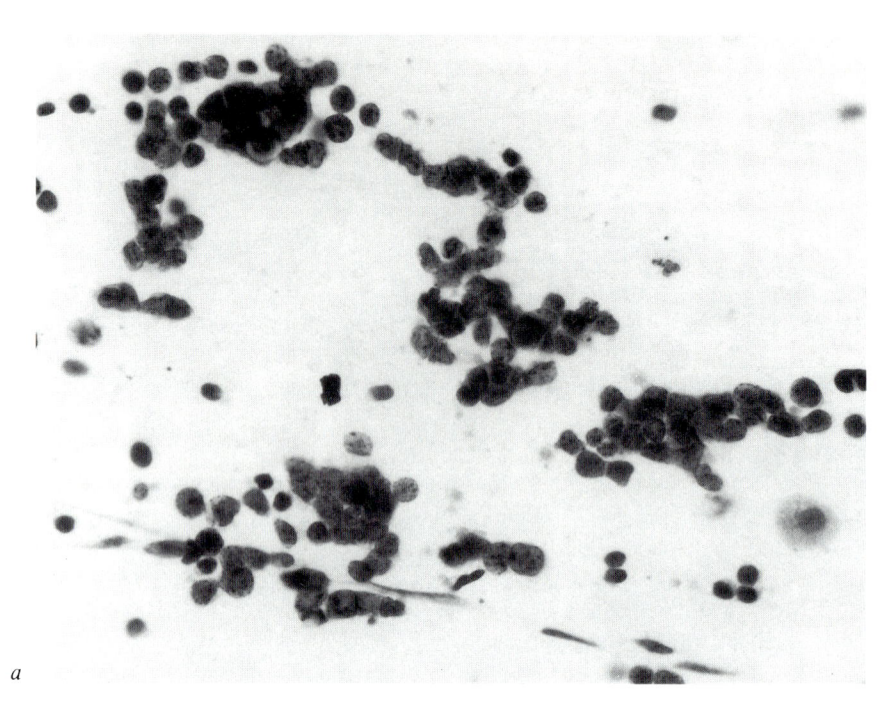

Fig. 80. Small cell undifferentiated 'oat cell' carcinoma of the lung (*a, b* = sputum; *c* = pleural fluid): Compare the size and chromatin distribution of these cells with those in figure 79. In *a* note the pathognomonic features of Indian filing, nuclear molding, salt and pepper chromatin, absence of nucleoli, and minimal adherent cytoplasm. In *b*, several cells wrap around each other, producing the so-called 'onion-skin' effect. When 'oat cells' metastasize and exfoliate into pleural fluid (*c*), many of the characteristics seen in exfoliated samples are retained, such as nuclear molding and Indian filing. The cells may appear somewhat larger than those seen in pulmonary samples, probably because of the excellent cell preservation of actively growing cells in a body cavity fluid. Papanicolaou. *a* = × 340; *b, c* = × 850.

Pitfalls. Oat cells from a brushing or fine needle aspirate will have fewer lymphocyte-like cells, a paler chromatin, and more obvious, albeit scant, cytoplasm (fig. 81). This appearance is no doubt due to the freshness of the sample. Comparison with carcinoids is discussed on pp. 150, 151. Although the cytologic certainty of a diagnosis of oat cell carcinoma is the highest of all primary lung cancers, the list of pitfalls is the longest (table 15, 16). The most common pitfall is to confuse these tumor cells with

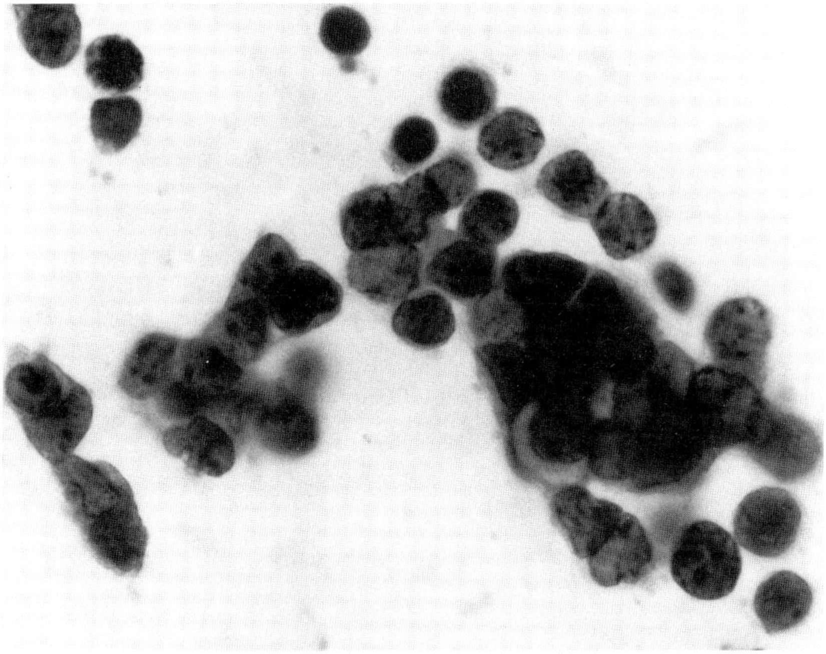

b

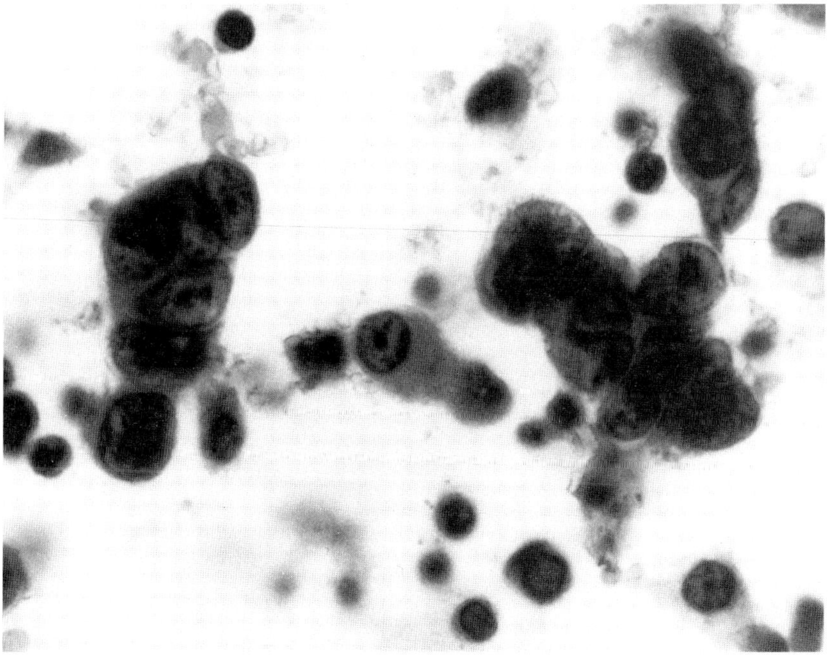

c

lymphocytes. The latter never mold, and while they may occur in streams, do not interrelate intimately to create molding. Groups of *reserve cells,* while small and hyperchromatic, are held together with a uniform amount of cytoplasm. Other small cell tumors, such as *seminoma,* can be distinguished by the open and coarse chromatin network with prominent nucleoli (fig. 82). Such tumor cells will usually be accompanied by lymphocytes.

Small cell adenocarcinomas will have nucleoli, and a three-dimensional arrangement in clusters (fig. 83). Small cell *breast carcinoma* is the most treacherous pitfall as Indian-filing and molding are prominent features, but crush artefact is absent and nucleoli are usually conspicuous. In tissue, Indian-filing in metastatic breast carcinoma is more uniformly arranged and linear than the haphazard Indian-filing in oat cell carcinoma.

Table 15. Pitfalls of small cell undifferentiated carcinoma

1.	*Lymphocytes* – these never mold; while they may occur in streams, they do not interrelate in a shape relationship
2.	*Other small cell tumors,* i.e. seminoma – these tumors have prominent nucleoli, oat cell carcinoma does not
3.	*Oat cells from a brushing* – will have a more consistent and open chromatin network, probably due to freshness of cells – do not overlook this pattern as oat cell carcinoma
4.	*Tumor diathesis* of necrotic debris *from other* type of *tumor,* i.e. squamous carcinoma or adenocarcinoma
5.	*Debris from a bronchiectasis* or other inflammatory process; must have molding, onion-skinning or Indian-filing to make the diagnosis of oat cell
6.	*Small cell breast carcinoma* can closely mimic oat cell especially with Indian-filing and molding; be sure to get clinical history if tumor occurs in a female

Fig. 81. Small cell undifferentiated carcinoma (FNA): Most of the cytologic characteristics of exfoliative material apply to 'oat cells' retrieved in FNA specimens. Tissue patterns are also appreciated, including rosette formation (*b*) and rarely, squamous pearls. These variations of the lesion should not change the final diagnosis. $a = \times 340$, Papanicolaou; $b = \times 850$, MGG.

a

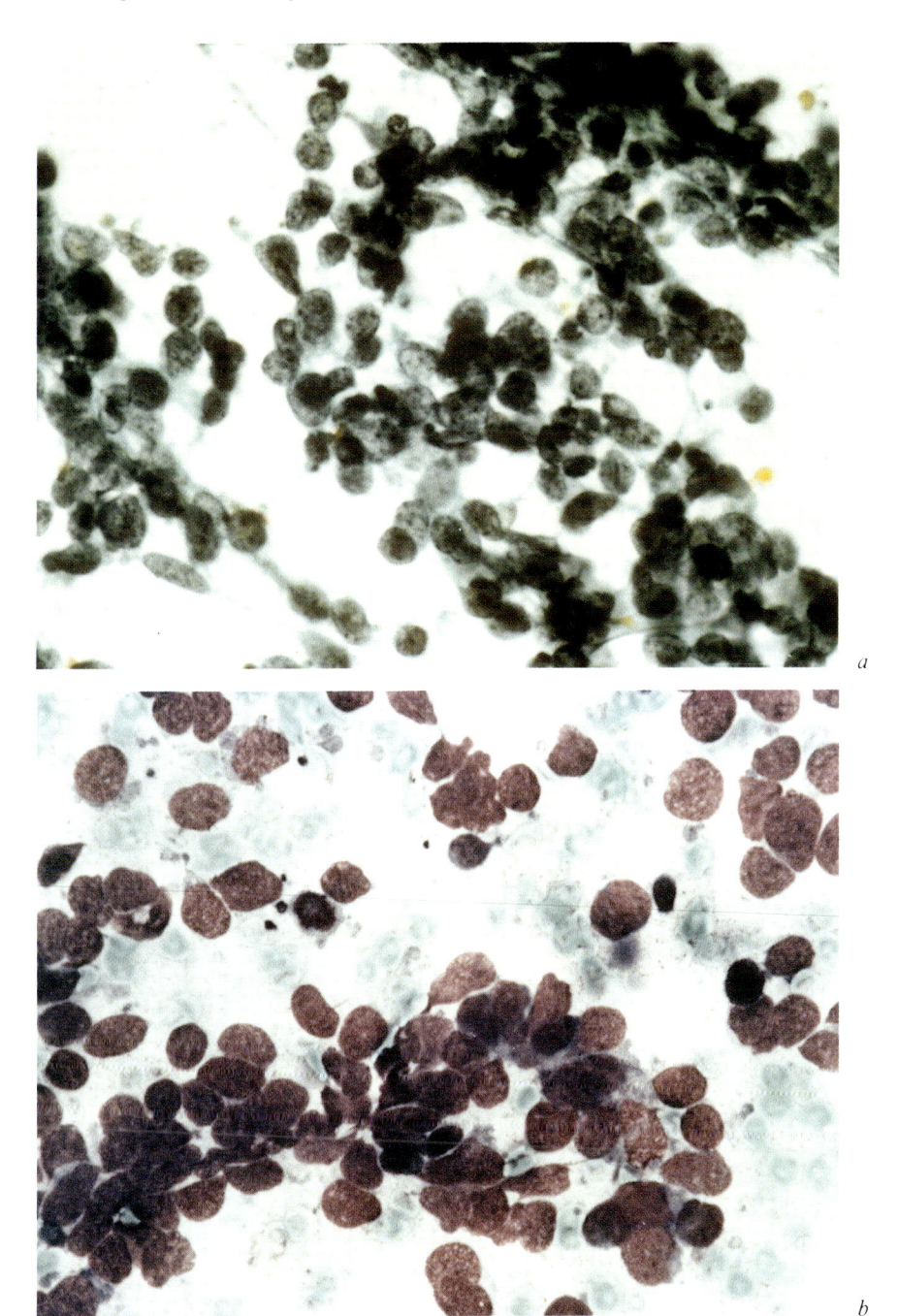

b

Table 16. Small cell undifferentiated carcinoma ('oat cell') (SCUC) – cytologic features which distinguish it from similar lesions

	SCUC	SC[1] adeno-carcinoma	SC squamous	Lymphocytes	Tumor debris	Reserve cell hyperplasia
Cell features						
Cytoplasm	appears absent					
Border		indistinct	distinct	sharp	fragments	sharp
Shape		oval	oval/bipolar	round/oval	irregular	'square'
Quality		delicate	delicate	opaque	opaque	opaque
Relation to other cells		shared borders	separate	very separate	separate	shared borders
N/C ratio	1/1	almost 1/1	almost 1/1	almost 1/1	N/A	almost 1/1
Nucleus						
Border	polygonal	oval	oval	round	irregular	'square'
Chromatin	smudged	finely granular	somewhat coarse	dark-coarse	dark-opaque	dark-opaque
Place in cell	total	eccentric	central	central	N/A	central
Nucleolus						
Size	invisible	small	small	invisible	N/A	invisible
Shape		round	round			
Prominence		visible	indistinct			
Number		usually one	usually one			
Pattern of groups	Indian-file onion skin semicohesive	acinar groups or three-dimensional balls; molding	thick groups occasional, cell within cell pearls	streams – but separate cells	none	tight clusters
Single cells	infrequent	infrequent	frequent	always	cell pieces	rare
Smear background	dirty	dirty	dirty	inflamed	dirty	clean or inflamed

[1] SC = Small cell.

Neoplasms of the Lung

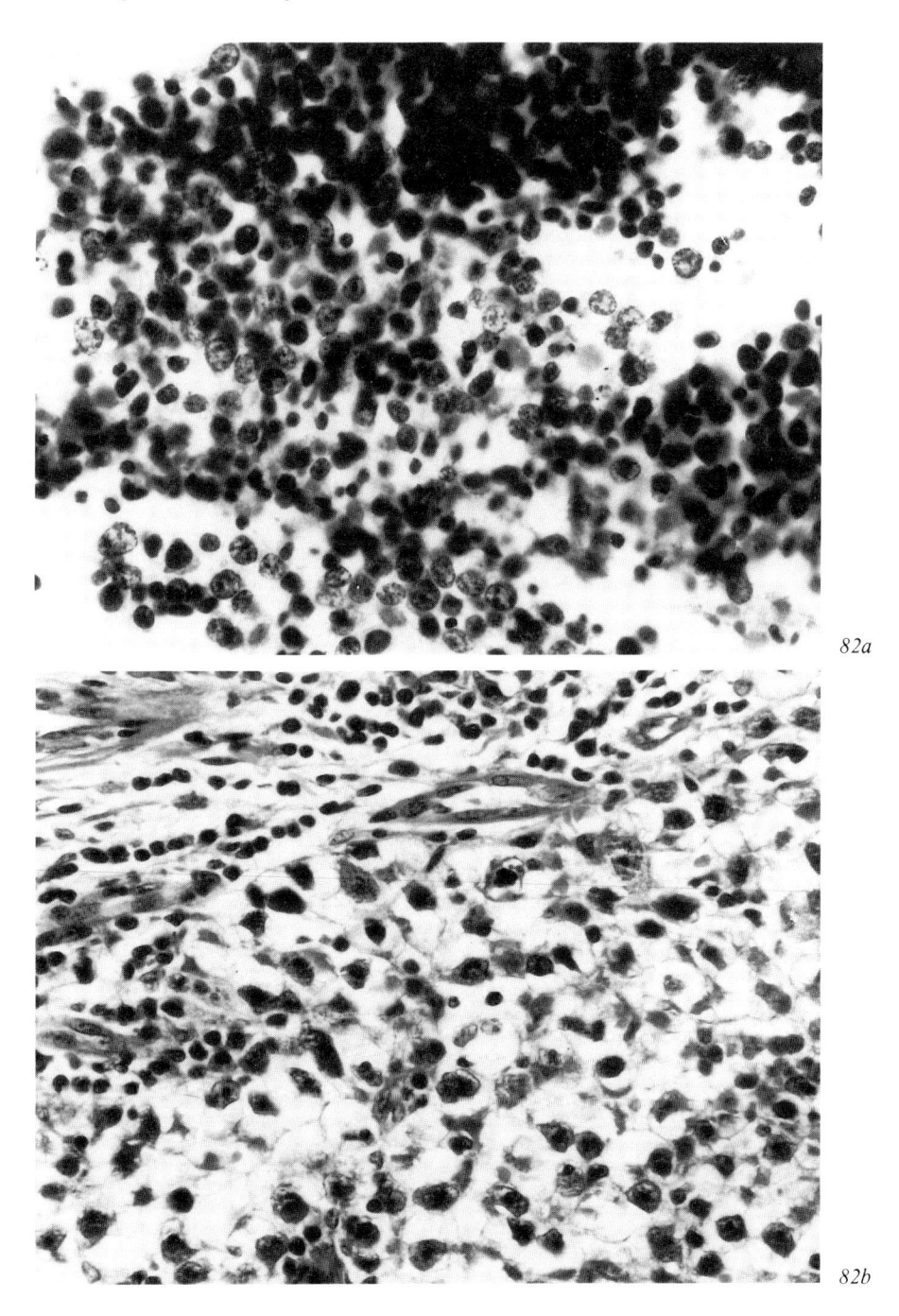

82a

82b

(For legend see page 148.)

Cytopathology of Pulmonary Disease 148

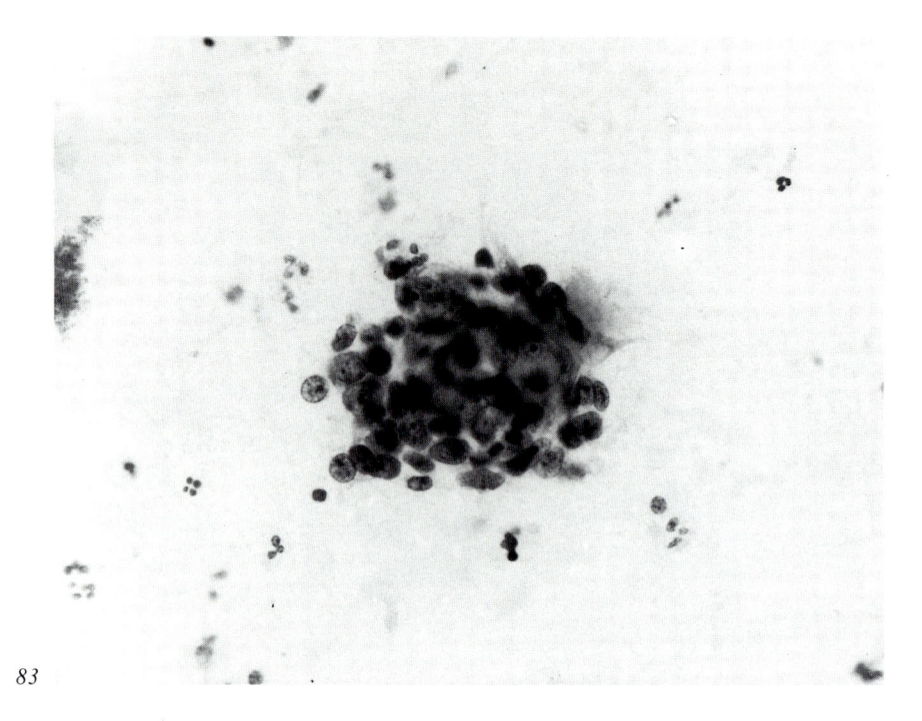

83

Fig. 82. Seminoma, from the mediastinum to the lung (*a* = bronchial wash; *b* = transbronchial biopsy): A small cell tumor, seminoma must be distinguished from 'oat cell' carcinoma in the lung. Prominent nucleoli, more abundant cytoplasm, lack of nuclear molding and accompaniment by numerous lymphocytes, are all features which distinguish the seminoma from 'oat cell' carcinoma. *a, b* = × 340; *a* = Papanicolaou; *b* = HE.

Fig. 83. Small cell adenocarcinoma of the lung (bronchial brush): When small tumor cells are recovered in a respiratory specimen, the differential must include lesions other than 'oat cell' carcinoma. If nucleoli are identified, as in this cell group, the diagnosis of 'oat cell' becomes improbable. Adenocarcinoma is the primary diagnosis until proven otherwise. Electron microscopy and other studies are usually needed to define the cell type, a critical distinction for proper treatment and prognosis. Papanicolaou. × 340.

Fig. 84. Pulmonary blastoma/carcinosarcoma (*a* = FNA; *b* = tissue): The FNA was originally interpreted as consistent with 'oat cell' carcinoma, until the tissue, shown in *b*, and the history were correlated. This patient had a prior resection for a 'carcinosarcoma', and the material illustrated is from the more primitive portion of that tumor, which is now recurrent. *a* = Papanicolaou; *b* = HE. *a, b* = × 340.

Neoplasms of the Lung

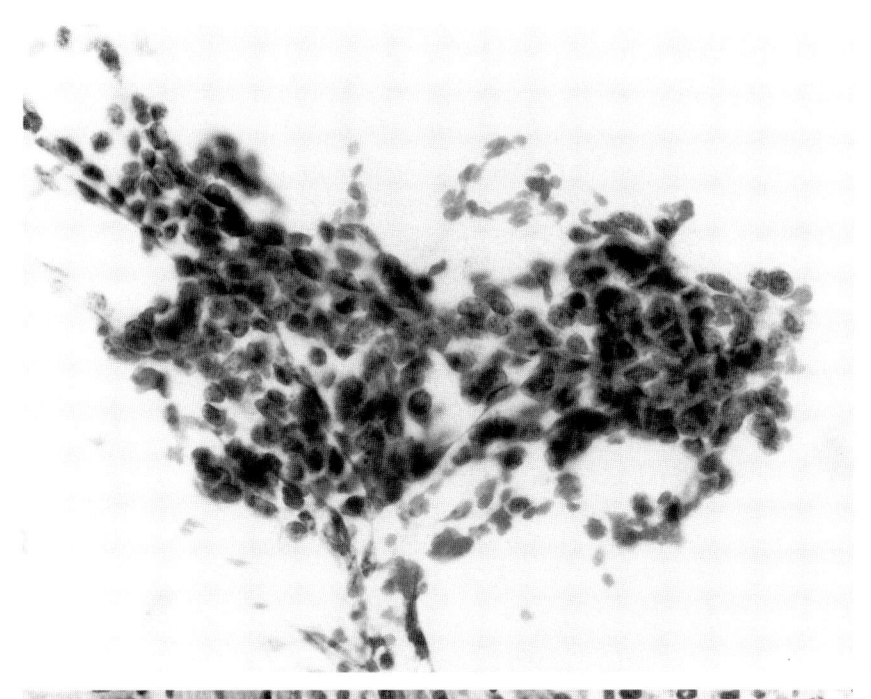

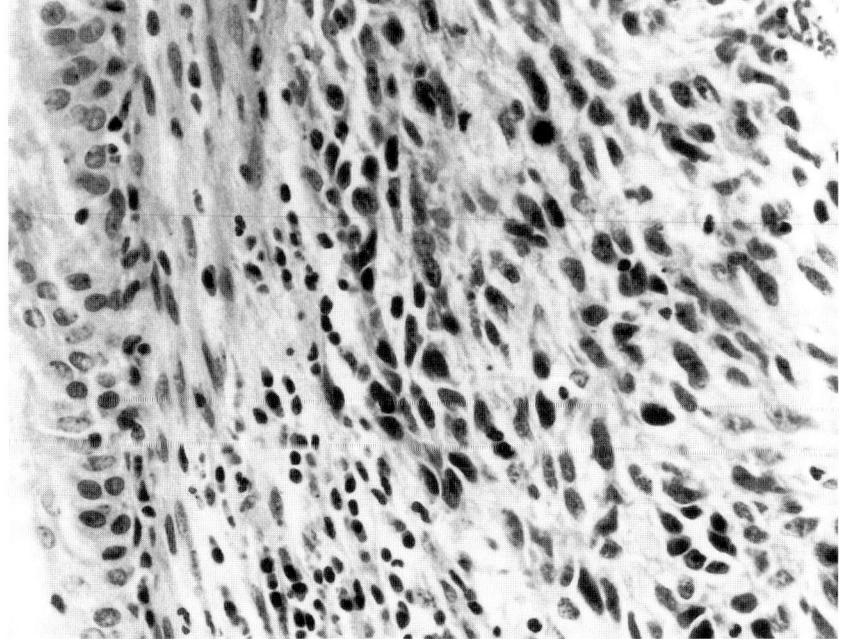

84a

84b

Pulmonary blastomas have undifferentiated (sarcomatous) components which closely resemble oat cell carcinoma but which are slightly more pleomorphic [175, 242] (fig. 84). Unlike oat cell carcinomas, 'blastomas' have columnar cells in branching tubular structures; carcinosarcomas also have two malignant cell lines, usually epidermoid or glandular, and spindle cell or fibrous. Both of these tumors are best diagnosed by multiple samples via FNA to harvest the biphasic components [45, p. 355].

Tumor diathesis, consisting of necrotic debris from a variety of tumors, should not be confused with oat cell carcinoma (fig. 85). Rigid diagnostic criteria of 'oat cell' carcinoma must be followed. Debris from bronchiectasis and other inflammatory processes can also mimic oat cell carcinoma.

Squamous aggregates and rosette formation (fig. 81b) can both be seen within a bonafide oat cell carcinoma. This should not persuade the observer to classify the tumor erroneously as a squamous cell or adenocarcinoma. However, such double primary combinations have been reported [56], and should always be considered when confronted with two malignant cell lines [284].

Large Cell Undifferentiated Carcinoma

Large cell undifferentiated carcinoma is usually located peripherally and in a subpleural location. The tumor commonly presents as a large, bulky, demarcated mass, frequently with cavitation. Access to bronchial lumens is usually not present, so recovery of diagnostic cells in sputum is uncommon.

These tumors comprise approximately 10% of primary lung tumors in most series. However, the diagnosis of 'large cell' varies from pathologist to pathologist, so that these figures are unreliable. Many poorly differentiated squamous carcinomas or poorly differentiated adenocarcinomas are included in this category erroneously; most are adenocarcinomas by electron microscopy [89]. Metastases will be found in the liver, adrenals, brain, and abdominal lymph nodes as well as in the contralateral lung. Treatment of choice is resection if the lesion is determined to be technically curable. A 25% overall 5-year survival rate can be expected.

Cytologic Criteria. Cellular material is very often difficult to distinguish from poorly differentiated epidermoid or adenocarcinoma, in which case electron microscopy can be helpful. The easiest diagnosis to arrive at is 'large cell undifferentiated' if the observer is confronted with a specimen

Neoplasms of the Lung 151

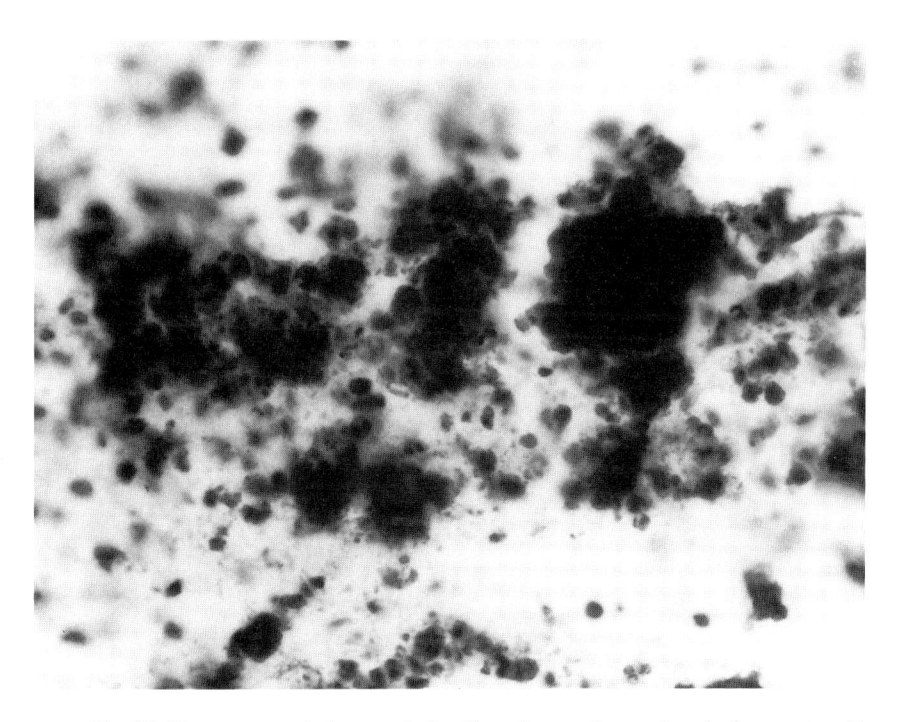

Fig. 85. Tumor necrosis (sputum): Small nuclear and cytoplasmic fragments with inflammatory cells and blood indicate tumor, but the cell type is frequently obscured. While the observer may be tempted to call such debris consistent with 'oat cell' carcinoma, other lesions, especially squamous cell carcinomas, can produce the same cytologic picture (see fig. 56). Definitive, well-preserved tumor cells are necessary for a final diagnosis. Papanicolaou. × 340.

with large undifferentiated cells which happen to show a lack of consistency from one specimen to another, and yet still maintain malignant criteria. The large, variably shaped cells will have ill-defined cytoplasm with inconsistent staining quality. Cells will frequently occur singly, and in cell clusters with or without 3-dimensionality (fig. 86). If cavitation is present, and the specimen is a needle aspirate, extensive tumor diathesis will be evident. The giant cell variant is quite rare and dramatic in its cytology. Huge pleomorphic single cells are the prototypical malignancy, but have little to categorize them other than their epithelial quality [28]. Multinucleation is a consistant feature. Electron microscopy is necessary to appreciate features which will facilitate cell typing.

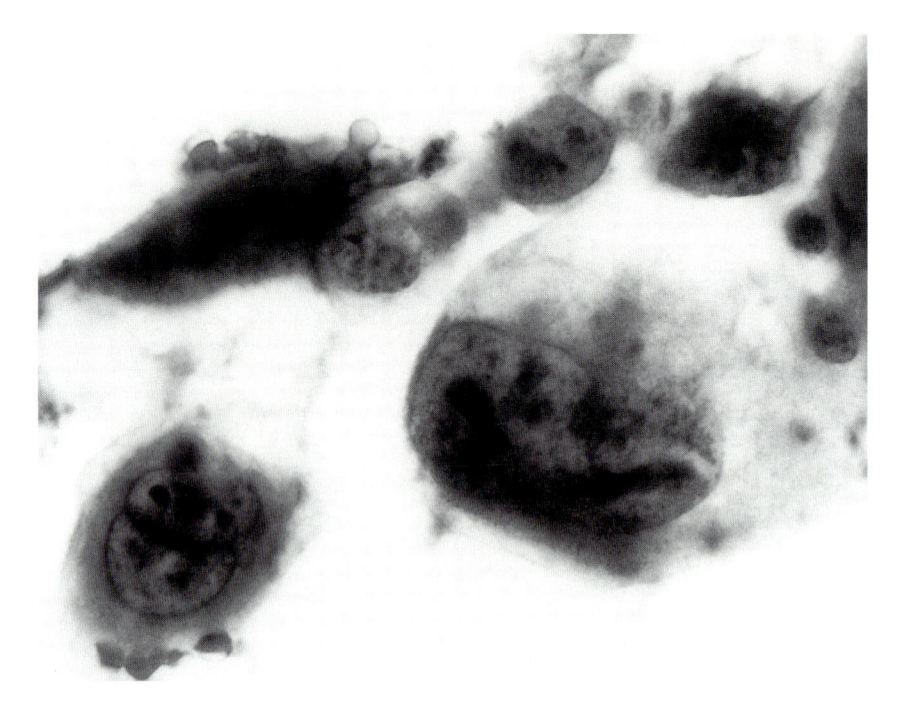

Fig. 86. Large cell undifferentiated carcinoma (FNA): Most 'large cell' undifferentiated carcinomas can be cell typed if careful attention to cytologic criteria is paid. If electronmicroscopy is done, most of these lesions are defined as adenocarcinomas. However, sometimes there are no distinguishing criteria by any modality and the term 'large cell', especially when cells are this large, is the most appropriate designation. Papanicolaou. × 900.

Pitfalls. There is usually little chance of a false-positive since these cells present with definitely malignant criteria. The only problem usually is the cell type, which has been addressed above (also see fig. 103). Another possible confusion would be with a large cell lymphoma. A tumor diathesis may not contain absolutely malignant cells in the first specimen, with the hyperchromatic nuclear fragments mimicking either an oat cell carcinoma or suggesting origin in a bronchiectasis.

Carcinoid Tumors

These rare lesions usually originate in the large bronchi, having an 'iceberg' configuration, with the tip presenting in the lumen, and the bulk of the lesion extending outside of the bronchus (fig. 87). The tumor is considered to originate in Kulchitsky cells of the bronchial epithelium [282]. The tumor may rarely give rise to the carcinoid syndrome or manifest a paraneoplastic syndrome despite the ability to produce a variety of hormones [281]. Carcinoids may also occur peripherally and present as solitary nodules.

These lesions account for less than 5% of all primary lung neoplasms, and have been erroneously termed bronchial adenomas. The age range is 9–73 years with a mean age of 45 years, and equal frequency in males and females. Metastases occur rarely, but will involve regional lymph nodes in 10% of the cases, with distant metastases or recurrence an unusual event. Survival for 5 years can be expected in 82% of the patients. Treatment is most generally surgical.

Cytologic Criteria. This is perhaps the most difficult lesion to diagnose cytologically because of the uniformly small cells which appear in cohesive aggregates and have a very benign, almost normal appearance [80, 142]. These cell groups often present a three-dimensional configuration. Nucleoli are small but present and chromatin is very bland (fig. 88). The cells have features of reserve cells but the more atypical tumors can be mistaken for adenocarcinoma [190] or may appear as undifferentiated neoplastic cells. Current theory holds that there is a continuous spectrum between the carcinoid and the small cell 'oat cell' undifferentiated carcinoma of the lung, with varying gradations of 'atypical carcinoid' in between. The 'atypical carcinoid' cells are often spindle shape. Exfoliated material in sputum is generally scanty and therefore is least reliable for diagnosis; bronchial brush and FNA specimens are most reliable.

Pitfalls. Cells from carcinoids can be mistaken for reactive reserve cells, and the more atypical cells in the atypical carcinoid mistaken for a small cell undifferentiated carcinoma. If nucleoli are prominent, confusion with a seminoma can occur. As the experience with this tumor is generally low, and the cytology usually 'benign', biopsy is the most frequent means of diagnosing such tumors. Immunochemical stain for chromogranin will separate the atypical carcinoid (positive) from 'oat cell' carcinoma (negative) [263].

Other Primary Lung Tumors

The so-called *bronchial adenomas* are unusual tumors which occur in the bronchial submucosal regions, arising from the bronchial glands. Orig-

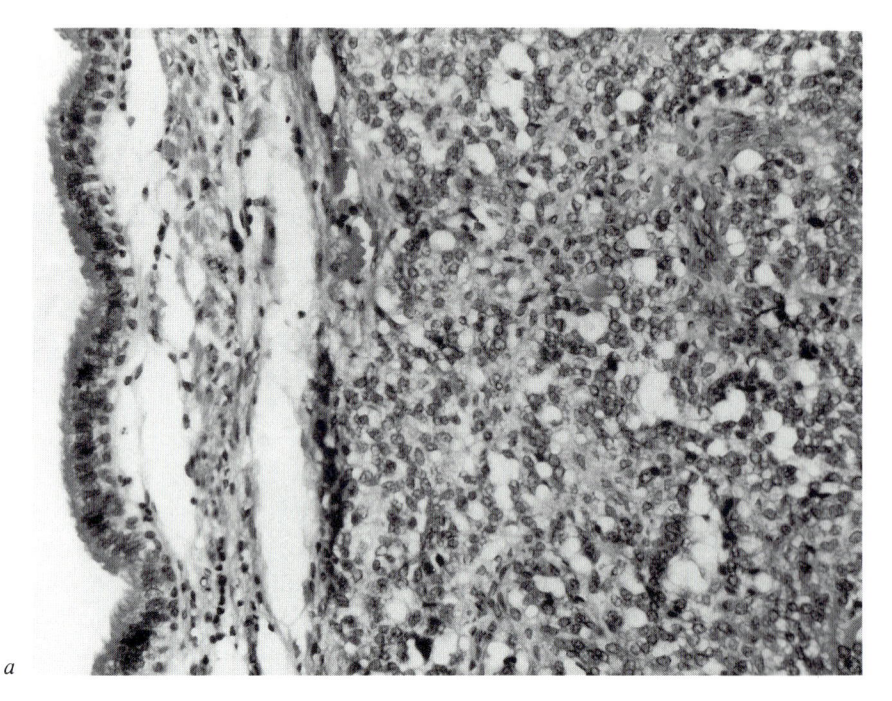

Fig. 87. Carcinoid of the lung (*a* = partial pneumonectomy; *b,c* = FNA): At the benign end of the 'oat cell' spectrum is the carcinoid, usually a large submucosal mass with a smaller protrusion in a 'dumbbell' fashion into the bronchial lumen. Nuclei are uniform, with light chromatin, and the tissue pattern is that of a glandular or trabecular configuration. The aspirate of the lesion in figure *a* contains uniform, small tumor cells with diaphanous cytoplasm. Nucleoli are small but conspicuous. These cells are often so benign appearing that in bronchial brushing specimens, they may be easily mistaken for benign, non-neoplastic respiratory epithelial cells without cilia. Only their large number and monomorphous quality provide the diagnosis. *a* = HE. ×170; *b,c* = Papanicolaou. *b* = ×340; *c* = ×850.

inally thought to be benign, this belief is no longer held as many case reports attest to metastases. Adenoid cystic carcinoma [141], muco-epidermoid carcinoma, pleomorphic adenoma (mixed tumor) and acinic cell tumors have the same histology as their salivary gland counterparts [45, p. 354]. Rare descriptions of cytologic specimens from these tumors document cellular criteria, most frequently and reliably obtained from FNA [250]. Rarely, metastases to the lung from similar salivary gland tumors may confound the picture, but the peripheral site(s) of the metastases will separate them from the peritracheal location of primary lesions [5, 239].

b

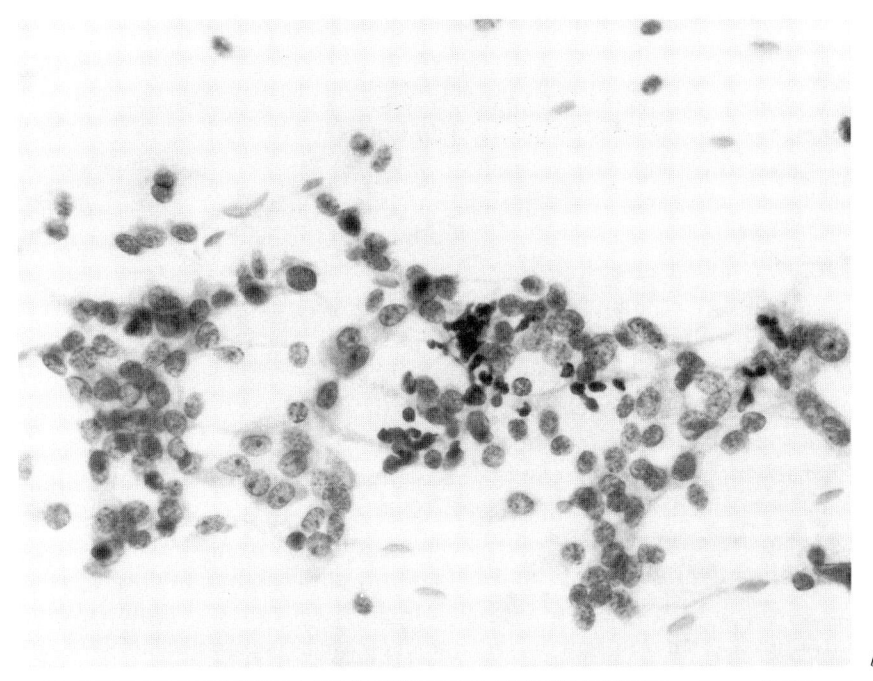

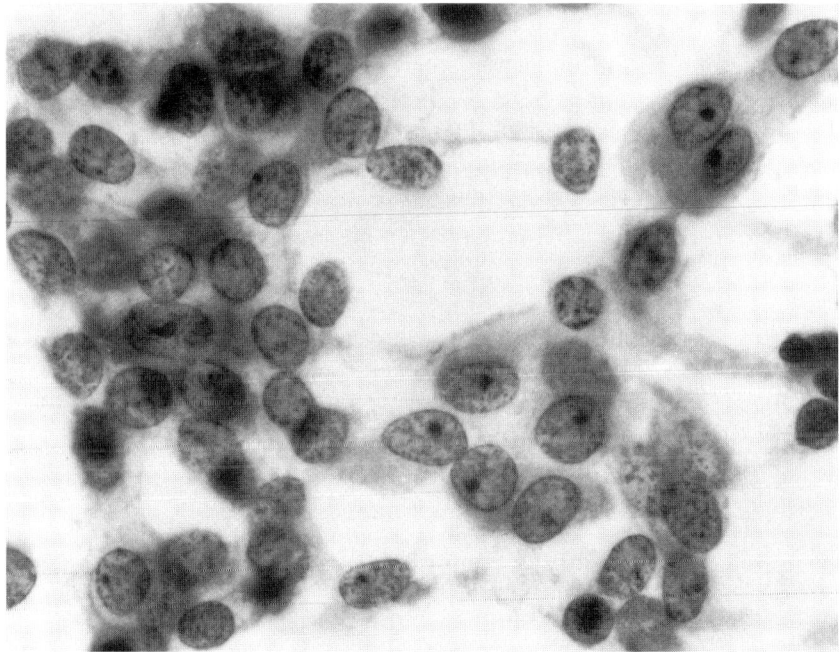

c

Tracheobronchial lesions, such as *papillomatosis,* are rare, but when they occur must be distinguished from more serious squamous lesions of the lower bronchi [274]. *Granular-cell tumor* of the bronchus can clinically mimic a bronchogenic carcinoma; cytologic features, however, are distinctive, with brushings and washings containing large polyhedral cells with uniform bland central nuclei, and granular cytoplasm [251].

Lymphomas and Leukemia

Malignant lymphomas and leukemias may occur de novo or as a result of chemotherapy or other immunosuppressive maneuver in a patient who is threatened by a seemingly unrelated disease [107]. Lymphomas are also common in AIDS patients. The cytopathologist is therefore constantly challenged to recognize malignant lymphoid cells [144, 212, 257] as distinct from otherwise mundane chronic inflammatory cells. Consultation with hematologists is strongly recommended.

Patients with non-Hodgkin's lymphoma (NHL) present with intrathoracic disease 43% of the time but with lung parenchymal involvement in only 3.7% of the cases. Mediastinal or hilar sites are most common (36%). Intrathoracic disease without generalized disease occurs in only 4% of cases (80% mediastinal), while only 3.8% of parenchymal lesions occur without mediastinal or hilar disease. Pleural effusions accompany these lesions in one-third of the patients.

Primary pulmonary lymphomas are rare [134], almost all of which are lymphocytic. They are typically a large (> 3 cm), homogeneous mass, with smooth sharp outlines, most often centrally located. They can, however, simulate infectious consolidation, which makes the diagnosis even more treacherous. Secondary pulmonary NHL are more common, affecting the lung 21%, and pleura 29% of the time. Lesions may present as solitary or multiple 'nodular' lesions (3–7 mm), with fuzzy outlines. The histiocytic type may occasionally rapidly infiltrate. Secondary or primary lymphomas rarely present as endobronchial masses [11, 79].

Hodgkin's lymphoma (HL) at presentation involves the following: intrathorax (67%), lung (11.6%) and mediastinum (50%). At some time in

---

Fig. 88. Carcinoid of the lung (*a* = FNA; *b* = lobectomy): The sample of this carcinoid is more obviously from a neoplasm than that of figure 87. The chromatin is darker and smudged, and rosette formation is apparent. *a* = ×340, Papanicolaou; *b* = ×180, HE.

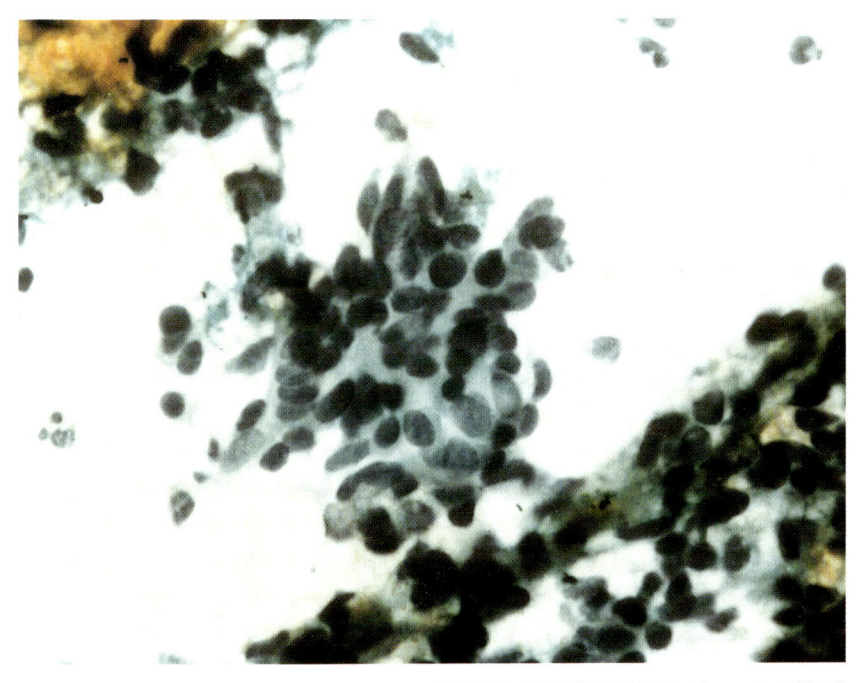

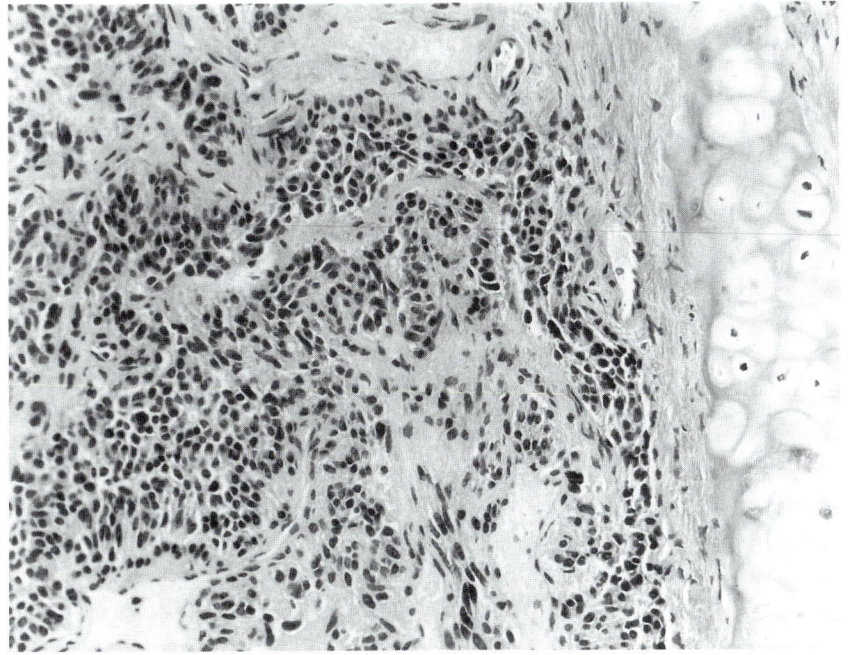

Neoplasms of the Lung

89a

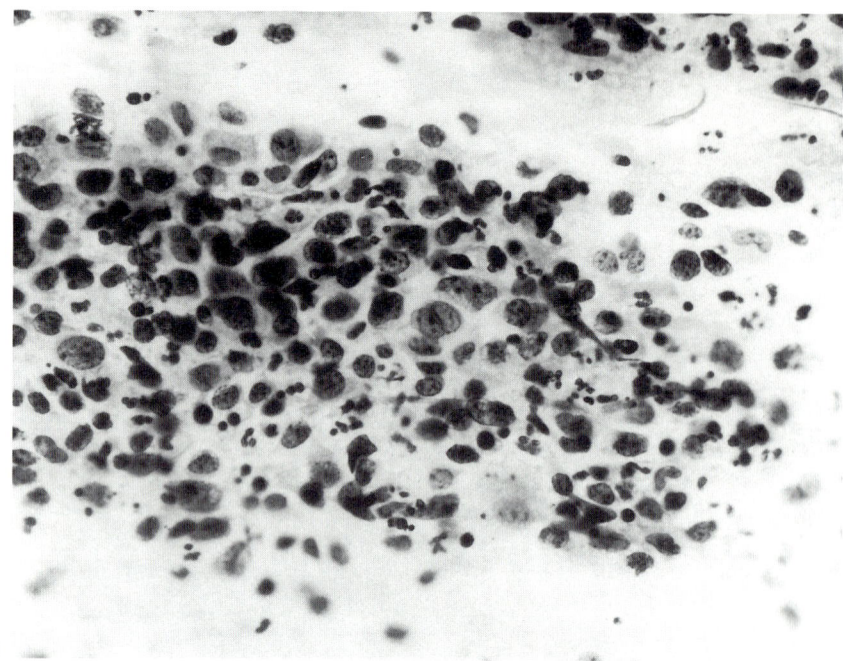

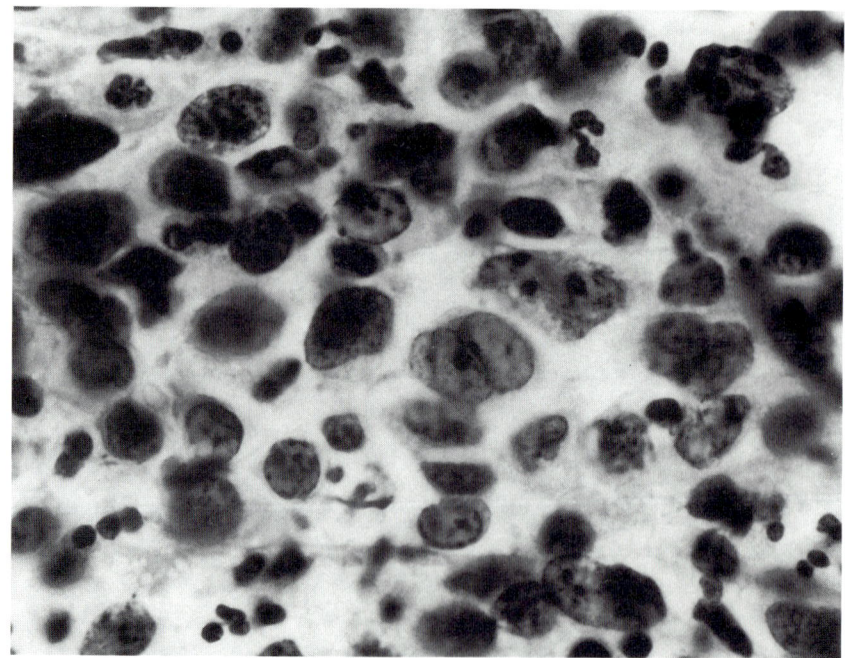

89b

Neoplasms of the Lung

the course of the disease the intrathorax will be affected at a 90% rate. Lung lesions are seen in less than 30% of patients, usually with those having the nodular sclerosing type. The nodules/consolidation are of variable size, and may coalesce to form large masses, with shaggy ill-defined borders. Bronchial obstruction is rare. Pleural effusions are present in one-third of the cases.

While sputa are occasionally diagnostic [82, 199, 226] BAL of diffuse infiltrates and FNA of defined masses [171] are the most productive ways

Fig. 89. Large cell lymphoma (sputum): Abundant cellular material, consisting of pleomorphic and variable size primitive cells, indicates an intraluminal lesion of probable nonepithelial origin. Higher power confirms the mixed character of these cells, ranging from those the size of a small lymphocyte to much larger and often binucleated cells. Chromatin varies considerably, within the largest cells being very fine but unevenly distributed. Nucleoli are often prominent and multiple; nuclear shapes are characteristically cerebroid. Papanicolaou. $a = \times 340$; $b = \times 850$.

Fig. 90. Benign lymphoid hyperplasia (FNA – mediastinal node): These lymphoid cells are large, and relatively monomorphous. The chromatin is very fine. Scattered macrophages and follicular center cells are indicative of a benign process. Papanicolaou. $\times 340$.

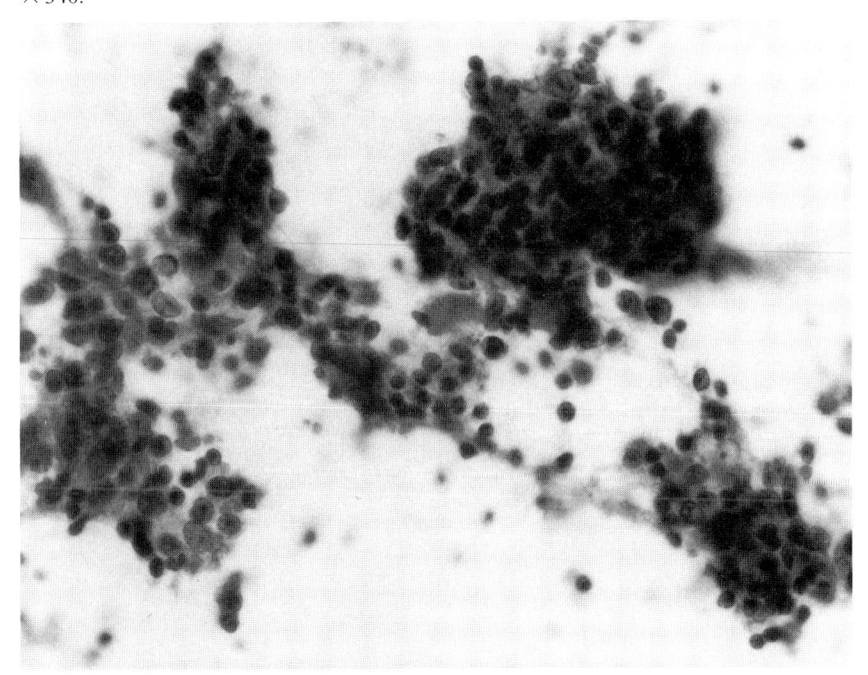

Cytopathology of Pulmonary Disease 160

91

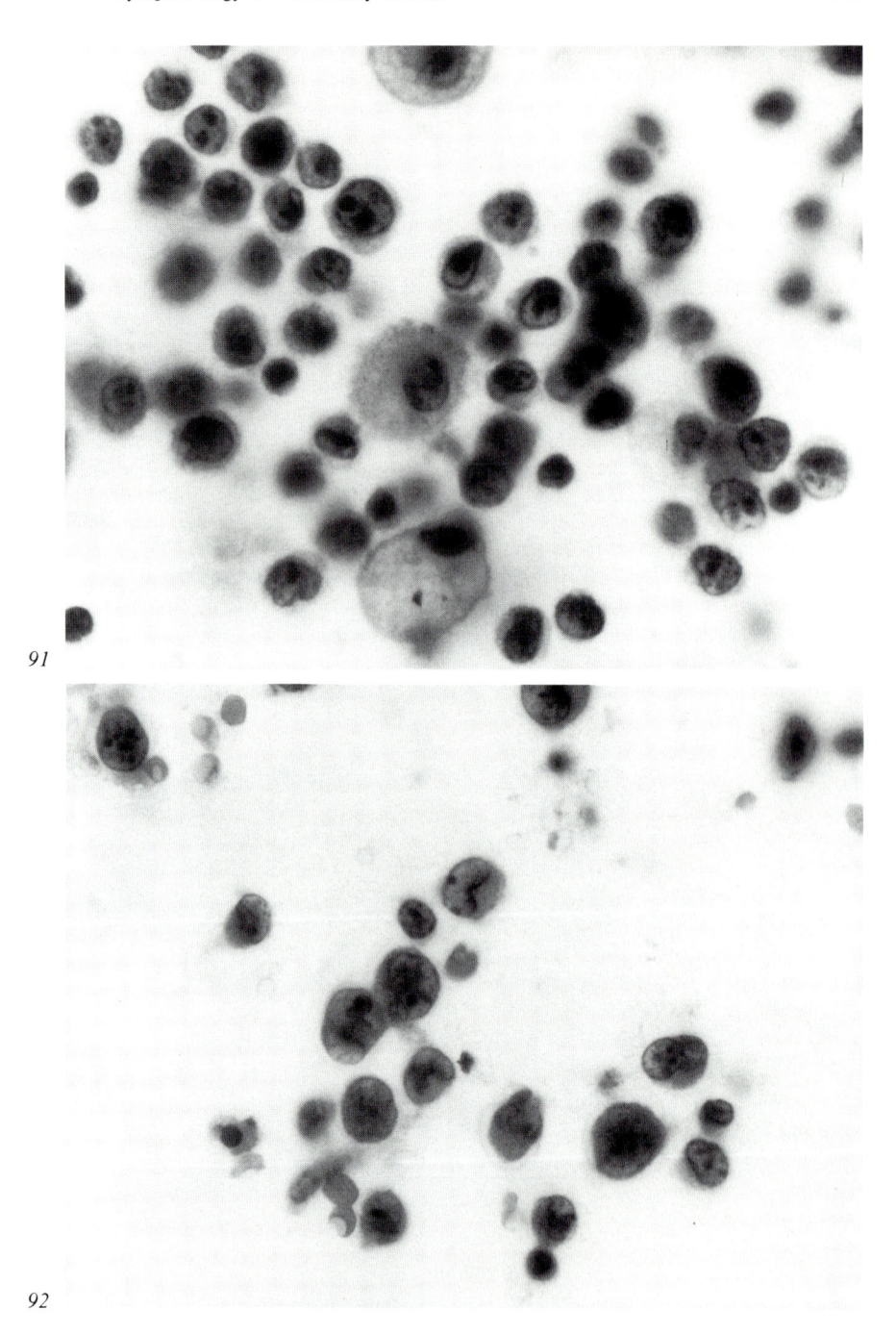

92

(For legends see page 162.)

Neoplasms of the Lung

93a

93b

(For legend see page 162.)

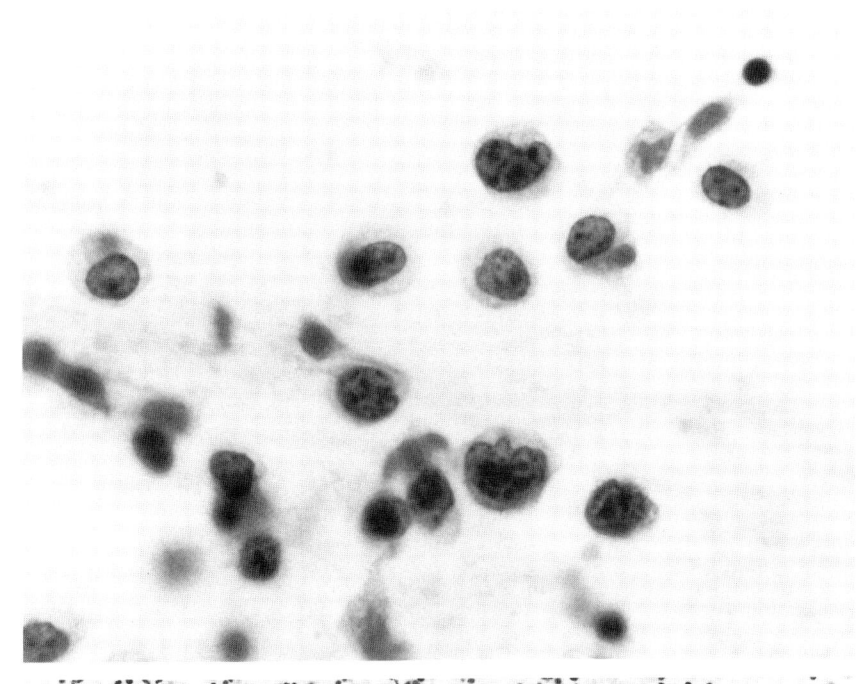

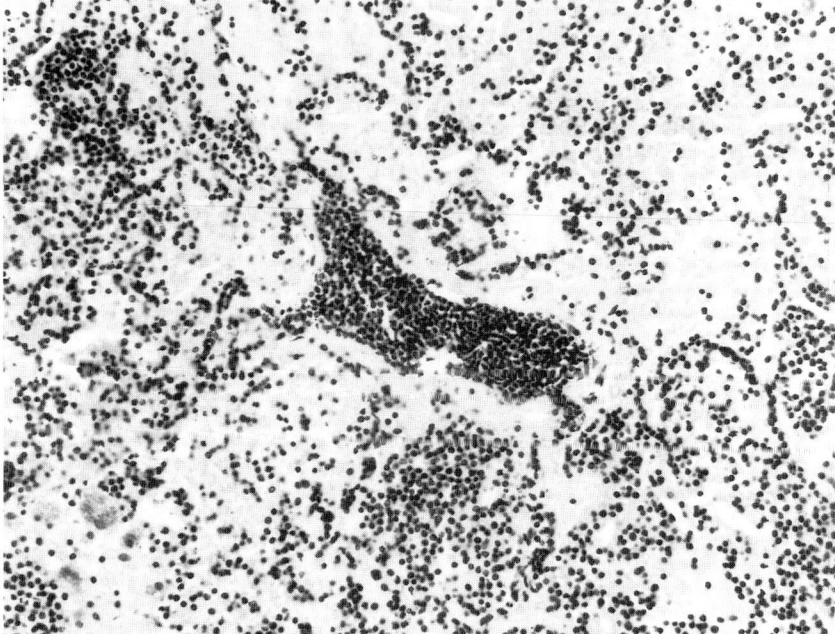

to approach these lesions in our experience. Fiberoptic bronchoscopy with washings, brushings, and TBB are diagnostic if the lesion is more central. Cytologic criteria are the same as for the specific lesions in bone marrow, lymph node or peripheral blood samples (fig. 89–93). Wright stains are mandatory to allow comparison with hematologic samples for confirmation. Sufficient material for a monoclonal antibody panel is advantageous to rule out a polyclonal infiltrate in response to an infectious disease, to which these patients are so prone.

Miscellaneous and Rare Tumors

The possibility of rare tumors, including carcinosarcomas, pulmonary blastomas (fig. 84), metastases from melanomas (fig. 94, 95), primary and secondary sarcomas [125, 140, 172, 173, 232, 283] (fig. 96–99), thymomas [243] (fig. 100, 101), and unusual metastases to the lungs [47, 58, 239] must be considered whenever the cells in question in a sputum or other respiratory specimen do not accurately fit any of the cytologic criteria defined above. Pulmonary hamartomas and endometriosis are two such examples.

Fig. 91. Lymphoma (sputum): Not all lymphoma cells are large and pleomorphic; compare these tumor cells with the benign macrophages for size. However, benign they are not, as indicated by multiple large nucleoli, irregular nuclear outlines, and uneven chromatin distribution. Papanicolaou. × 850.

Fig. 92. Lymphoma (chest tube drainage): Cytologic diagnosis of lymphoma in a pleural effusion is quite difficult, especially with Papanicolaou-stained material. However, careful attention to morphology of these lymphoid cells confirms the suspected clinical diagnosis. Primary diagnosis of a lymphoma on pleural fluid is rare. History of previously diagnosed lymphoma is the rule rather than the exception. Air dried Wright-stained smears of pleural fluid suspected of containing lymphoma cells are of great help in arriving at an accurate diagnosis. Papanicolaou. × 850.

Fig. 93. Acute lymphocytic leukemia (a = sputum; b = lung): Diagnoses of leukemias are usually well-established before a question of pulmonary involvement is asked of the cytopathologist. Cells are usually small, but are readily distinguished from benign lymphocytes and macrophages if cell preservation is good and processing optimal. Stain criteria apply as for other lymphoid malignancies. The section of lung shows the extent of leukemic involvement. a = × 850, Papanicolaou; b = × 85, HE.

Fig. 94. Melanoma metastatic to the lung (bronchial brushing): Large epithelioid cells with obviously malignant nuclei and prominent nucleoli could be from any epithelial malignancy that is poorly differentiated. The lack of cohesiveness and presence of melanin pigment, fully appreciated on high power provide the diagnosis of melanoma. Without the pigment, this could only be considered a poorly differentiated carcinoma; sarcoma must be ruled out. Papanicolaou. a = × 340; b = × 900.

Neoplasms of the Lung

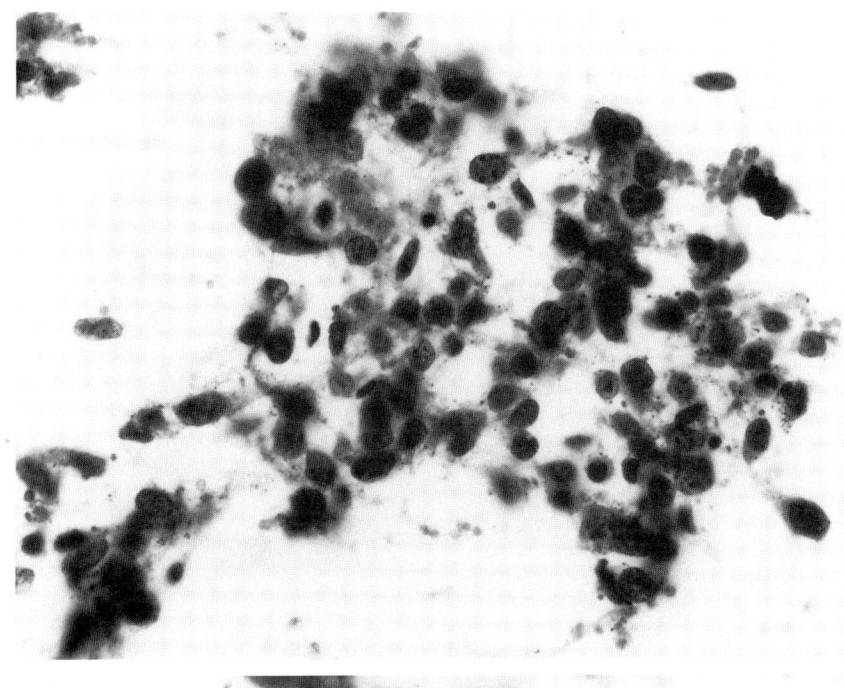

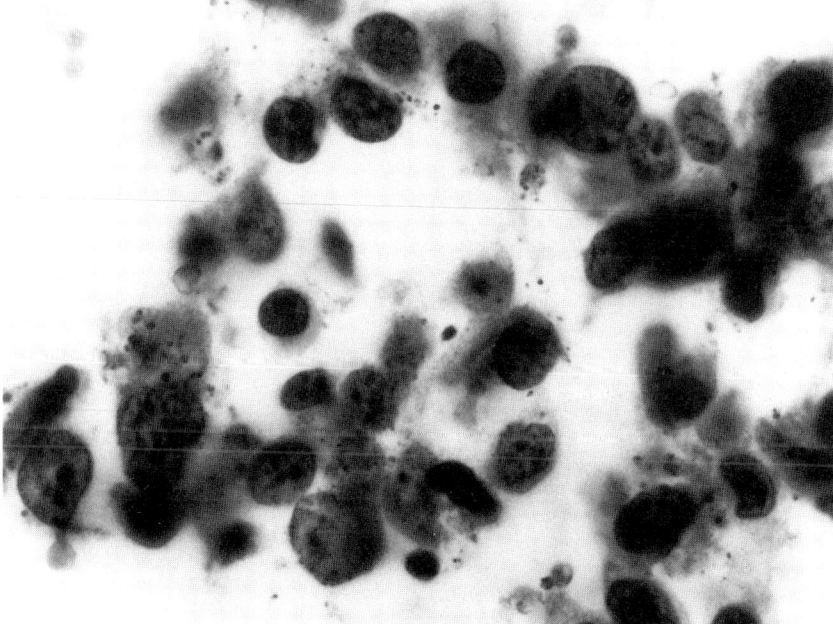

94a

94b

Cytopathology of Pulmonary Disease

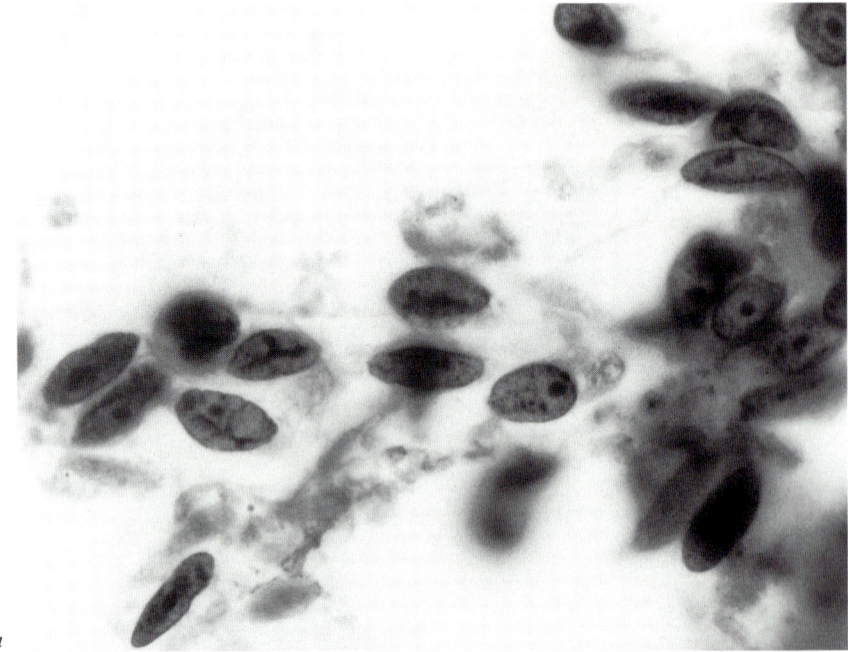

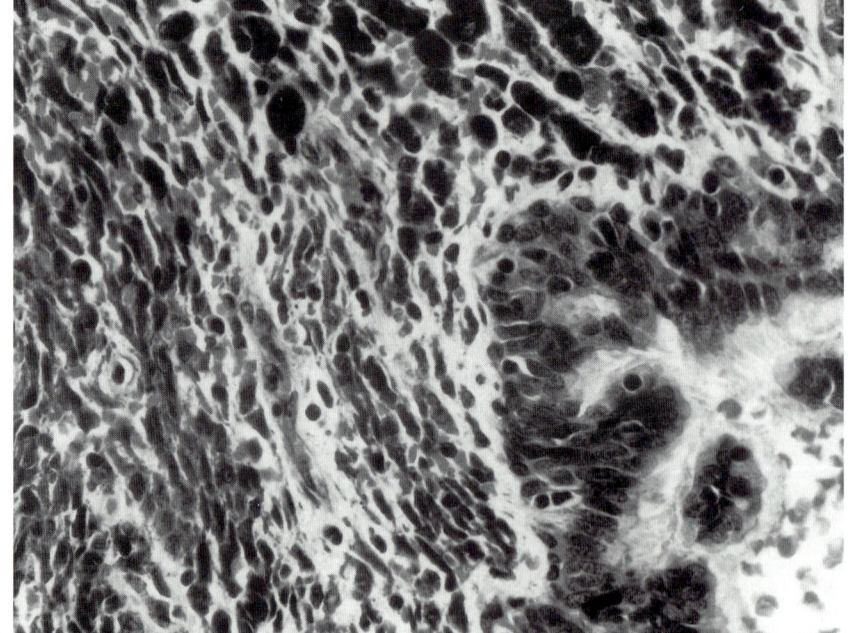

95a

95b

(For legend see page 166.)

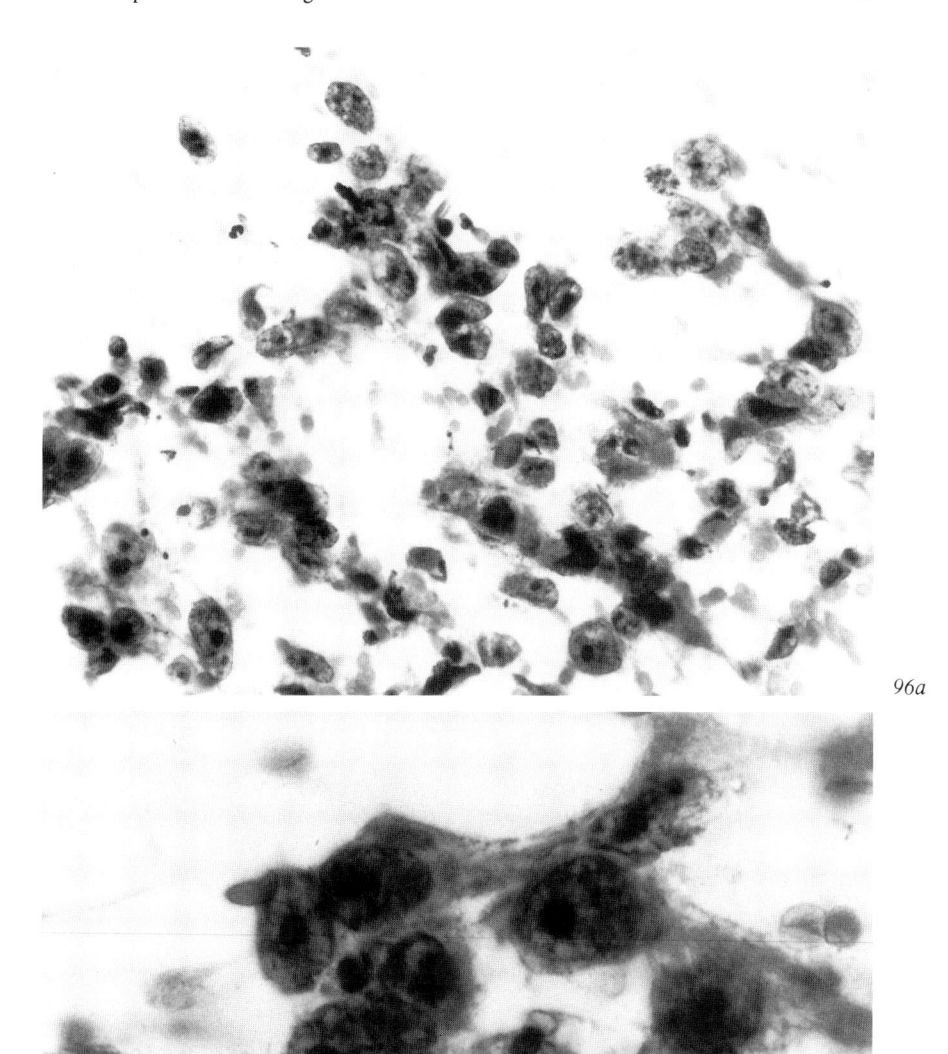

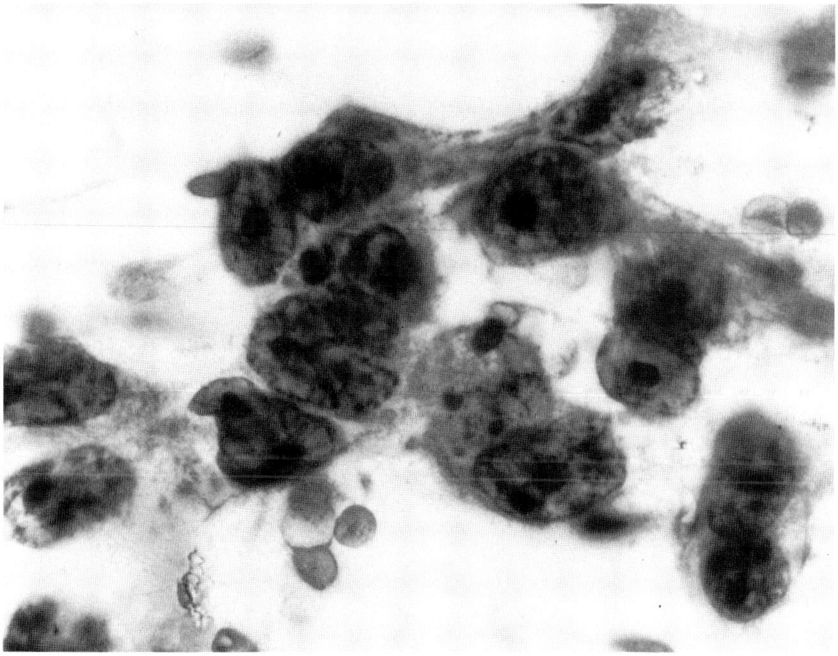

Neoplasms of the Lung

96a

96b

(For legend see page 166.)

FNA is the only way, short of surgical excision, to obtain material from a *pulmonary hamartoma*. Such aspirates are usually sparcely cellular, containing only a few groups of benign respiratory epithelial cells, scattered lymphocytes and histiocytes, and, hopefully, fragments of cartilage. The latter is the hallmark of the lesion, without which the diagnosis cannot be made on cytologic grounds [143, 197].

Endometriosis, a difficult diagnosis for any modality, can perhaps best be reached and defined by FNA, obtaining cells and tissue fragments for cytologic and histologic examination. The smears can be expected to be richly cellular, containing both uniform epithelial cells with prominent nucleoli, and spindle (stromal) cells. Histologic confirmation of endometrioid tissue will avoid mistaking the active glandular cells for a carcinoma [84]. Aside from metastatic carcinoma, all other types of tumors occur with a sufficient infrequency that the day-to-day practice of respiratory cytology will probably never encounter them.

Fig. 95. Melanoma, spindle cell variant, metastatic to the lung (*a* = FNA; *b* = tissue): While most melanomas are of the epithelioid variety, this spindle cell variant is occasionally seen. With or without melanin pigment, the diagnosis should be entertained when the pattern of dissociated pleomorphic cells is encountered. The correlation between the cytology and histology is excellent; pigment can be appreciated as dark overlay to some of the tumor cells and in pigment laden macrophages. Case courtesy of Denise Hidvegi, MD, Northwestern University School of Medicine. *a* = ×850, Papanicolaou; *b* = ×340, HE.

Fig. 96. Embryonal carcinoma of the testes, metastatic to the lung (bronchial wash): When large pleomorphic tumor cells, with impressively prominent nucleoli are seen, a germ cell tumor should be considered. These cells have scant cytoplasm, and dramatic nuclei with a somewhat characteristic owl eye clearing around the prominent nucleolus. Other large cell tumors must be considered. Clinical history is most important to verify the diagnosis as is comparison with any available primary tumor tissue. Papanicolaou. *a* = ×360; *b* = ×850.

Fig. 97. Soft tissue spindle cell sarcoma of leg, metastatic to lung (*a* = FNA; *b* = tissue): Large multinucleated cells could imply the diagnosis of a benign granuloma. However, careful scrutiny of the specimen reveals additional pleomorphic neoplastic cells and a pattern which coincides extremely well with the metastatic lung lesion. Without the original amputation specimen, only a differential diagnosis can be provided: Malignant fibrous histiocytoma, malignant giant cell tumor of tendon sheath, osteogenic sarcoma of soft tissue. HE. ×340.

97a

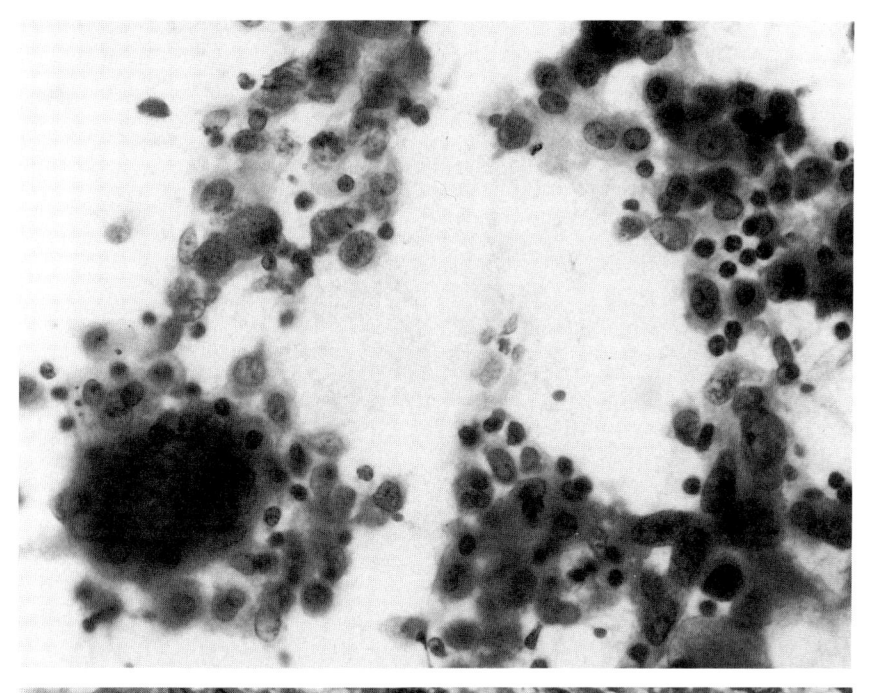

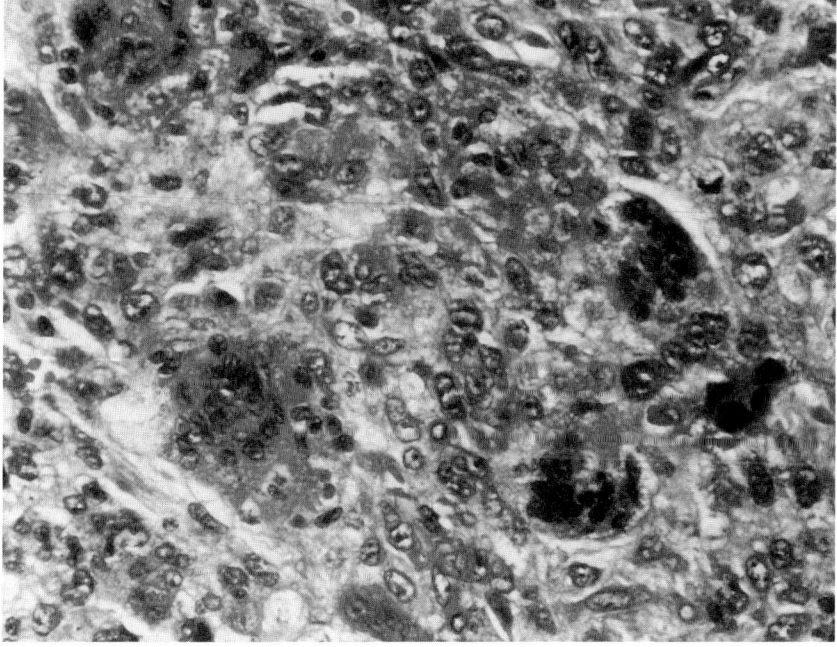

97b

98a

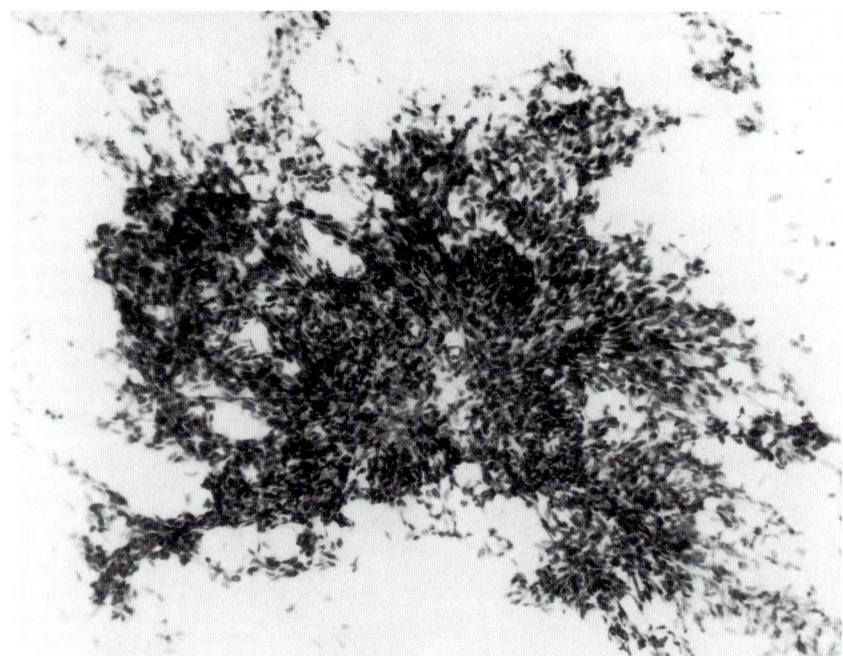

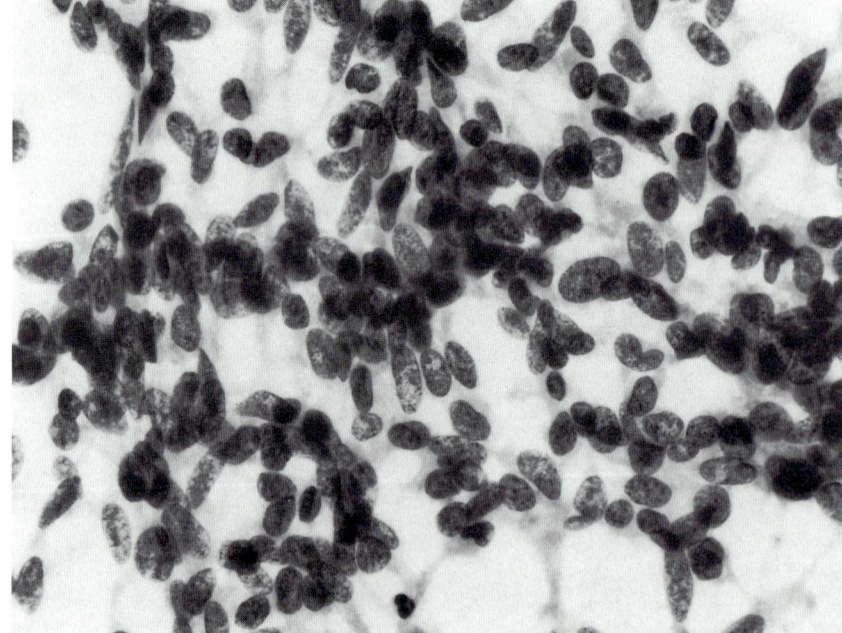

98b

Metastatic Carcinoma to the Lungs

Distinction between primary and secondary lung cancer is essential to optimal patient management. In all instances, careful correlation with any tissue available from other tumor sites is mandatory to define the process within the lung [110] (table 17). Other epithelial tumors, such as squamous carcinoma from other body sites, can be confused as a primary lung tumor. Such a disastrous assumption can be avoided by careful history-taking. Uncommonly, transitional carcinoma of the bladder can travel to the lung and resemble squamous carcinoma (fig. 102).

As the survival of cancer patients increases with more effective therapy and/or earlier diagnosis, a patient's chances of a second primary increases. A lung lesion may be a second primary, and should be managed as such, even with a convincing history of an antedating other malignancy.

Comparative Cytologic Criteria for Lung Tumors

Once the student of cytology learns the basic cytomorphologic patterns of the major types of lung tumors, fine tuning becomes a lifetime challenge. Admittedly, the decision of benign versus malignant is sometimes quite difficult, but usually, if the specimen is adequate and the clinical history and X-ray findings considered, that decision can be made reliably.

Fig. 98. Schwannoma, involving the lung (FNA): A monomorphous spindle cell pattern is characteristic of this tumor. An attempt at pallisading can be appreciated on low power. Higher power reveals a finely granular chromatin pattern, no discernable nucleoli, and fibrillary cytoplasm. The mitotic index is low, indicating a low grade neoplasm. HE. $a = \times 85$; $b = \times 340$. Case courtesy of Denise Hidvegi, MD, Northwestern University School of Medicine.

Fig. 99. Cystosarcoma phyllodes, metastatic to the lung (a = original breast tissue; b and c = FNA of lung, d = lung resection): The original breast lesion contains classic components of a cystosarcoma phyllodes, i.e. atypical epithelium, and neoplastic fibrous stroma. The FNA specimen contains numerous neoplastic spindle cells, with large blunt nuclei and irregular nuclear chromatin. Compare the difference of the tinctorial characteristics on the two stains. The specimen has very few epithelial fragments, so that inspection of the original tumor is essential to make an intelligent diagnosis. $a, d = \times 85$, HE; $b, c = \times 340$, b = Papanicolaou; c = May-Grünwald-Giemsa. Case courtesy of McNeil Memorial Hospital, Berwyn, Ill., via Denise Hidvegi, MD.

Cytopathology of Pulmonary Disease 170

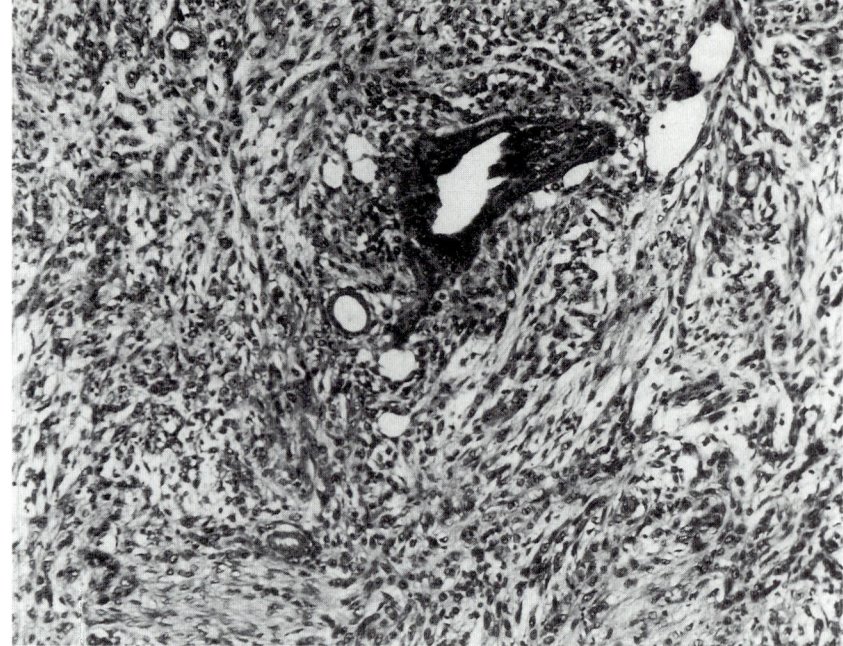

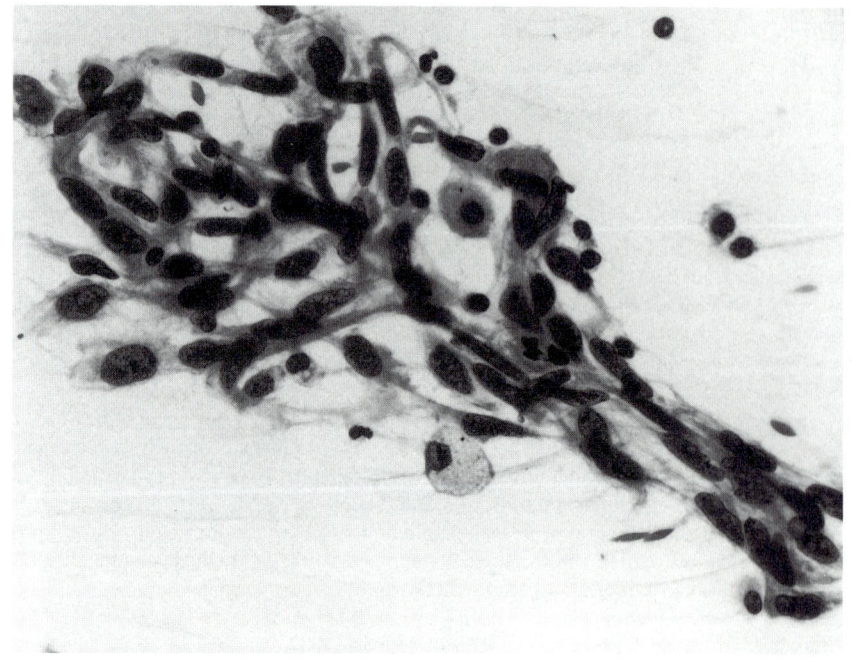

99a

99b

(For legend see page 169.)

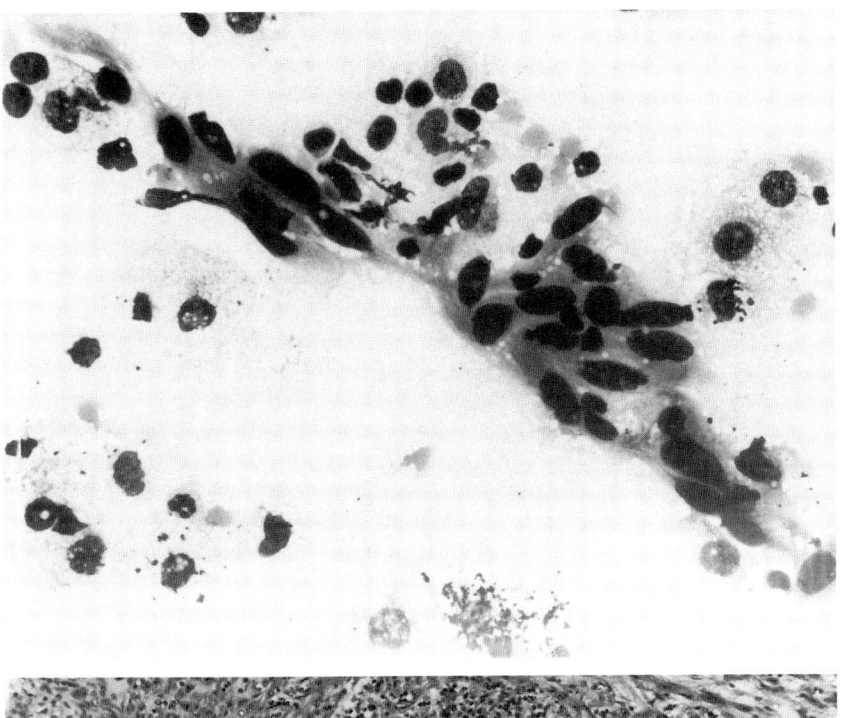

Neoplasms of the Lung

99c

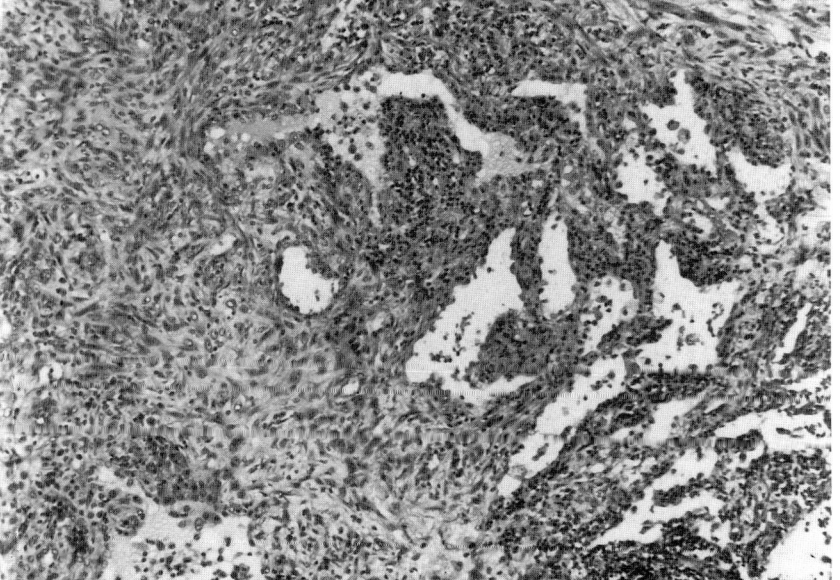

99d

(For legend see page 169.)

Cytopathology of Pulmonary Disease

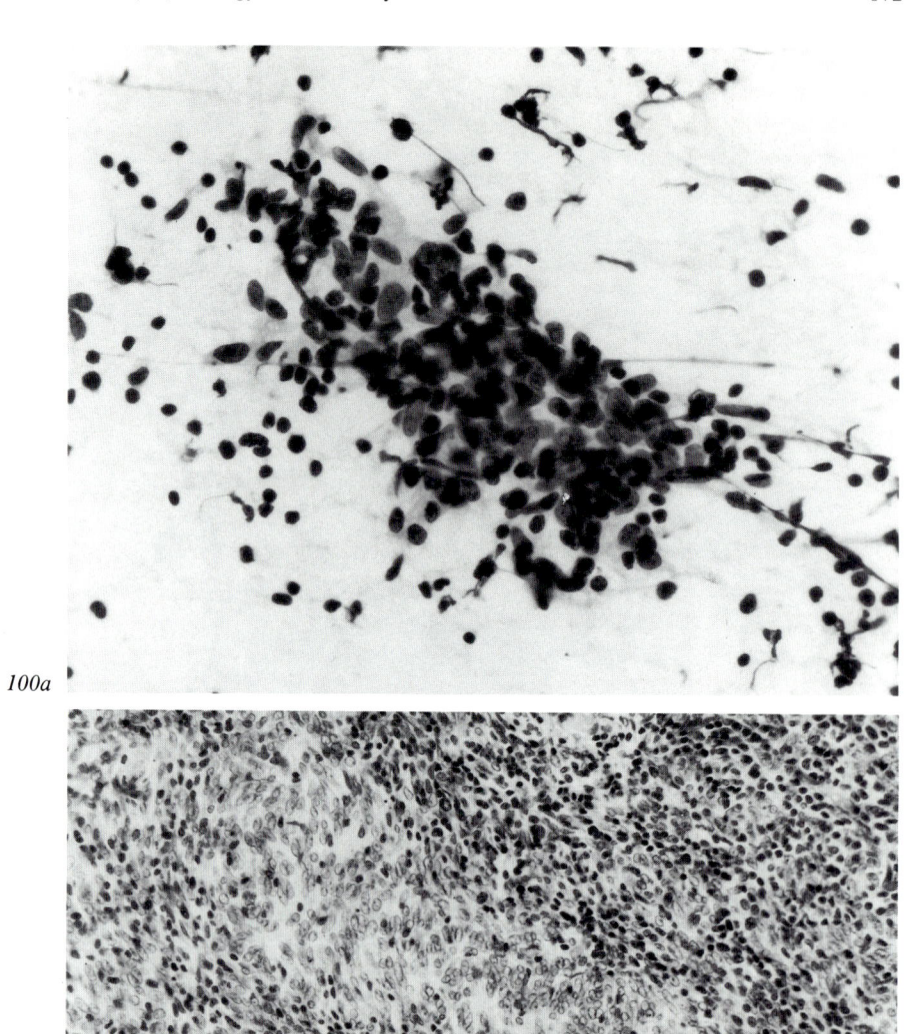

100a

100b

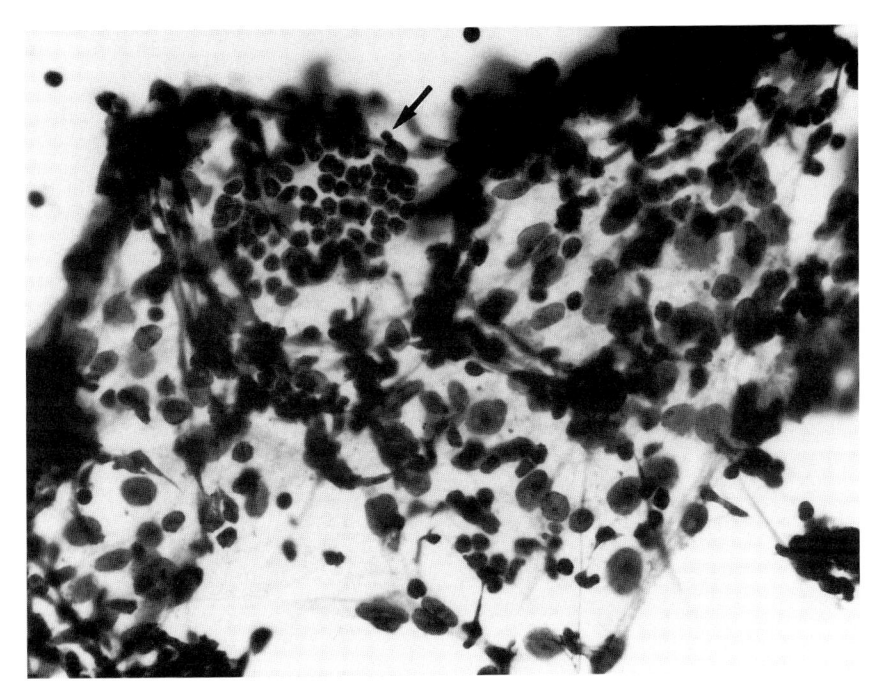

Neoplasms of the Lung

Fig. 100. Spindle cell thymoma (*a* = FNA; *b* = tissue): A thick and therefore fuzzy fragment of spindle cells provides only the diagnosis of a spindle cell neoplasm not otherwise specified. The tissue verifies the diagnosis. *a* = × 360, Papanicolaou stain; *b* = × 170, HE. Case courtesy of Denise Hidvegi, MD, Northwestern University School of Medicine.

Fig. 101. Thymoma, involving the lung (FNA): A mixture of epithelioid cells, and smaller lymphocytes confirm the clinical impression of a thymoma. Size relationship of these epithelial cells compared with a cluster of benign respiratory epithelial cells (arrow), can be appreciated. Papanicolaou stain. × 340. Case courtesy of Denise Hidvegi, MD, Northwestern University School of Medicine.

Fig. 102. Transitional cell carcinoma, metastatic to the lung (*a* = sputum; *b* = transbronchial biopsy): Large, pleomorphic, epithelial cells, associated but disconnected were recovered in sputum. The history of transitional cell carcinoma was obtained, and the tissue diagnosis verified in the transbronchial biopsy. The correlation between the cytologic sample and the tissue was excellent. Without the clinical history, the diagnosis could have been that of a large cell primary carcinoma of the lung. *a* = × 850, Papanicolaou stain; *b* = × 340, HE.

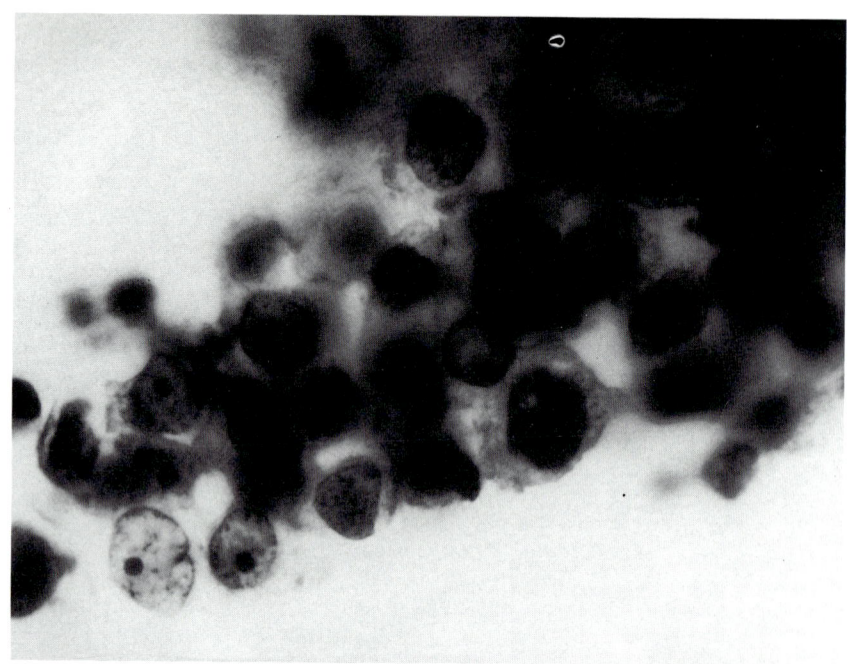

102a

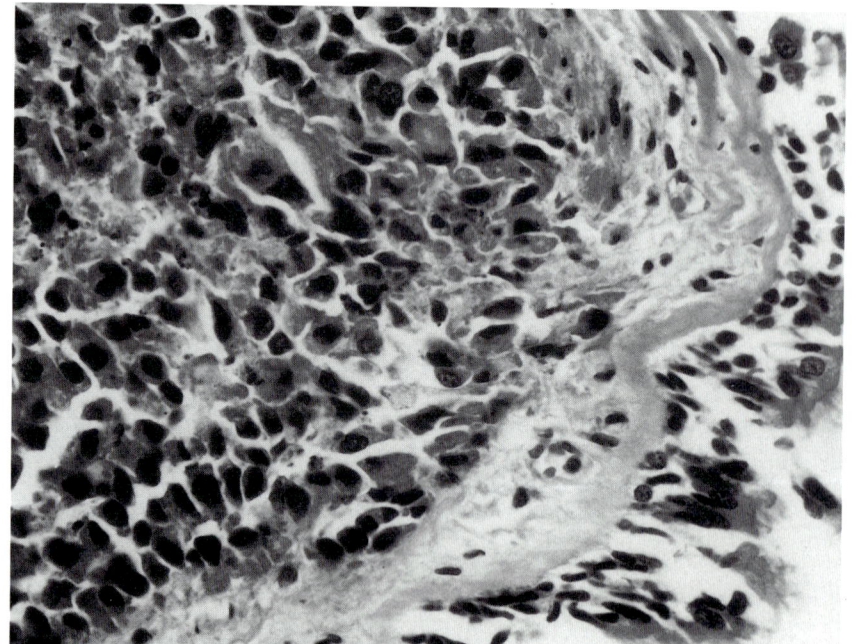

102b

(For legend see page 173.)

Table 17. Neoplasms metastatic to the lungs in FNAB patients [110]

Type of neoplasm or tissue of origin	Patients	
	n	%
Malignant melanoma	34	23.8
Urinary and male genital tract	30	20.9
Transitional cell carcinoma	14	
Adenocarcinoma, kidney	11	
Adenocarcinoma, prostate	4	
Teratocarcinoma, testis	1	
Breast	20	14.0
Female genital tract	18	12.6
Squamous cell carcinoma	15	
Mixed mesodermal tumor	2	
Adenoid cystic carcinoma	1	
Colon-rectum	15	10.5
Bone and soft tissues	12	8.4
Ewing's sarcoma	3	
Osteosarcoma	2	
Fibrosarcoma	2	
Synovial sarcoma	2	
Angiosarcoma	1	
Leiomyosarcoma	1	
Ameloblastoma	1	
Lymphoma	5	3.5
Non-Hodgkin's	3	
Hodgkin's	2	
Mediastinum	3	2.1
Seminoma	2	
Thymoma	1	
Primary unknown	3	2.1
Salivary glands	1	0.7
Adenoid cystic carcinoma	1	
Neuroendocrine	1	0.7
Neuroblastoma	1	
False-positive	1	0.7
	143	100.0

Table 18. Cell features helpful in discriminating among squamous carcinoma[1] (SC), adenocarcinoma[1] (AC) and highly atypical nonmalignant cells

Cell features	SC	AC	Benign (atypical)
Cytoplasm			
Border	defined	poorly defined	defined
Shape	variable	usually oval	round or oval
Quality	opaque	delicate	delicate
Relation to other cells	separate	syncytial	shared
N/C ratio	variable	moderate	low
Nucleus			
Border	irregular	round to oval	round or oval
Chromatin	coarse-variable cell to cell	finely granular-monotonous cell to cell	delicate
Place in cell	central	eccentric/central	variable
Nucleolus			
Size	small	large	small
Shape	round	round/irregular	round
Prominence	visible	prominent	variable
Number	single/multiple	multiple/single	one
Pattern of groups	multilayered	balls or papillae	single/flat clusters
Single cells	usual	rare	rare

[1] Excluding very well differentiated types.

More difficult perhaps is the decision as to cell type. The accuracy with which this can be done in specimens from the lung is addressed in chapter VII. This accuracy depends upon two basic factors: the quality of the preparation and the experience of the microscopist. The following photographs are presented because of their similarities and dissimilarities. When viewed as groups, distinguishing features can be appreciated which provide the real clues as to the cells of origin (table 18). The importance of going through this extra effort cannot be overstressed. In most sophisticated medical settings, treatment and prognosis are dependent upon the typing of the cells. True, tissue is often available. However, at UCLA and in other major medical centers, cytology is frequently relied upon for the 'final diagnosis' before therapy is begun, without the aid of tissue.

As stated earlier in this chapter, this author infrequently uses the category of 'large cell undifferentiated' carcinoma. Figure 103 illustrates three 'large cell' tumors, two of which could be categorized into differentiated tumors. The giant cell lesion is so undifferentiated, that even electron microscopy was of no help. The most convincing evidence favoring adenocarcinoma (fig. 103a) is the occasional cell with eccentrically placed nucleus and apparent terminal plate. Groups of cells with shared cell borders also provide support for an adenocarcinoma.

Figure 104c is included in a group of adenocarcinomas to show the coarser chromatin in the squamous lesion. Nucleoli are usually of no help in separating squamous from adenocarcinomas. The chromatin clearing and relatively thin nuclear membranes of many adenocarcinomas can be useful. Cells of bronchiolo-alveolar carcinoma are frequently difficult to separate from histiocytes (fig. 104d). Any sample that contains large groups of 'histiocytes' should be carefully scrutinized to exclude a bronchiolo-alveolar carcinoma.

The small cell lesions of the lung present the same problems as do small cell lesions everywhere. Figures 105 and 106 contain predominantly small cell lesions of the lung, separated into two groups to contrast the two stains. Figure 106 also includes two larger cell tumors for comparison. The characteristic features of oat cell carcinoma, as depicted in figure 105a, might be mimicked by the pulmonary blastoma (fig. 105e). However, if one appreciates the clinical setting and looks for a mixture of components in the pulmonary blastoma samples, the correct diagnosis may be rendered. However, pulmonary blastomas are so rare that such a mistake, calling one an oat cell carcinoma, would not be unreasonable.

Distinguishing the epithelial lesion from lymphomas (fig. 105d) is usually not difficult, again if one pays attention to strict nuclear criteria. The noses and notches of the lymphoid malignancies provide unique characteristics. Seminomas (fig. 105f) can be distinguished from other small cell lesions by more abundant cytoplasm, prominent nucleoli, and a mixture of lymphocytes.

In this author's experience, while the May-Grünwald-Giemsa stain is excellent for cytoplasmic products and for general patterns, the final diagnosis is most reliable using samples stained with the Papanicolaou stain. If one compares figures 106c–g, great difficulty will be experienced in accurately diagnosing the lesions by May-Grünwald-Giemsa stain. While figure 106c has acinar groups, there is considerable nuclear molding which could be identified as characteristic of oat cell carcinoma.

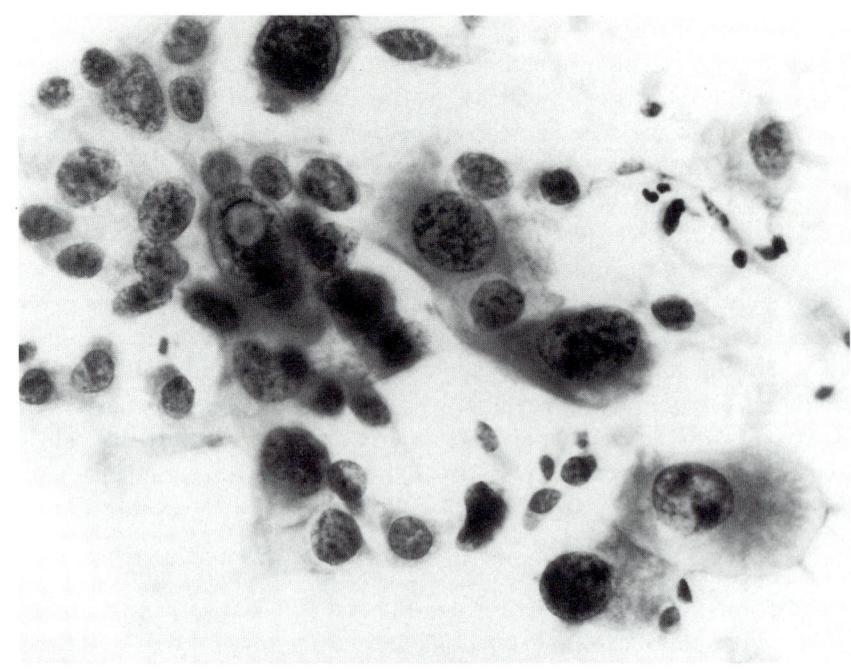

103a

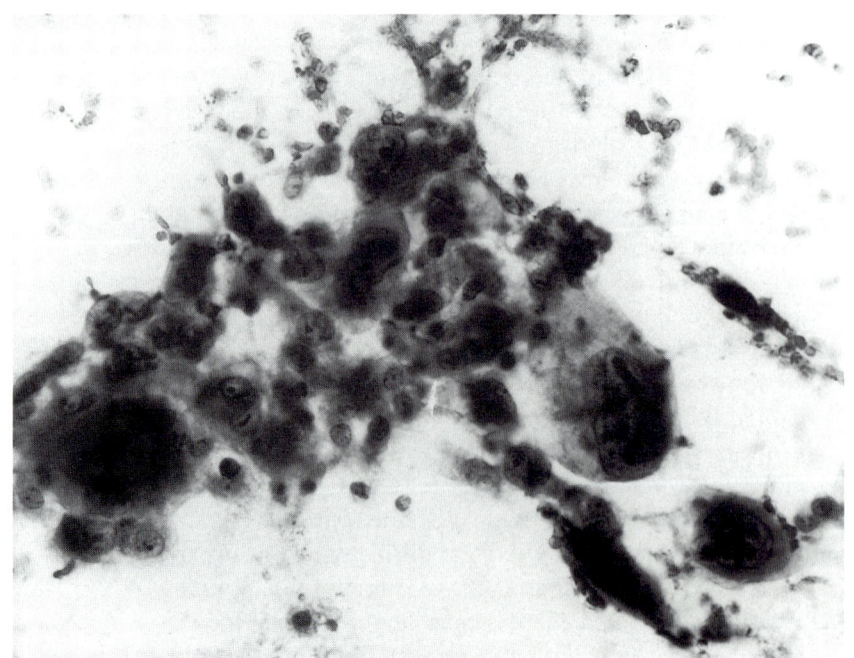

103b

Neoplasms of the Lung 179

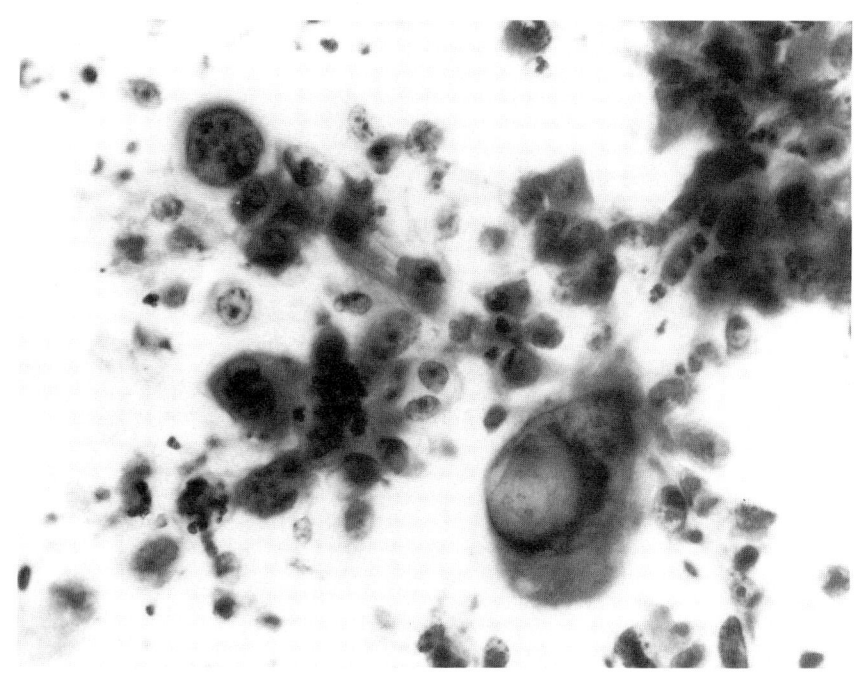

103c

Fig. 103. a Adenocarcinoma (bronchial brushing) × 340. *b* Giant cell carcinoma of the lung (FNA) × 360. *c* Squamous carcinoma of the lung (FNA). Papanicolaou stain. × 360.

The carcinoid in figure 106e is different from figure 106c only in its more uniform chromatin, but is otherwise indistinguishable. The Papanicolaou-stained carcinoid, figure 105b, on the other hand, is clearly different from an adenocarcinoma by virtue of inconspicuous nucleoli. Figure 105c is a small cell adenocarcinoma, complete with vacuoles and small nucleoli.

The best ways for the cytologist to refine diagnostic accuracy are as follows:

(1) Insist on optimal specimen collection, processing and staining. Anything less makes consistently reliable diagnoses impossible.

Fig. 104. a Adenocarcinoma (bronchial wash). *b* Adenocarcinoma (bronchial wash). *c* Squamous carcinoma (bronchial brush). *d* Bronchiolo-alveolar carcinoma (sputum). Papanicolaou. *a–c* × 900; *d* × 360.

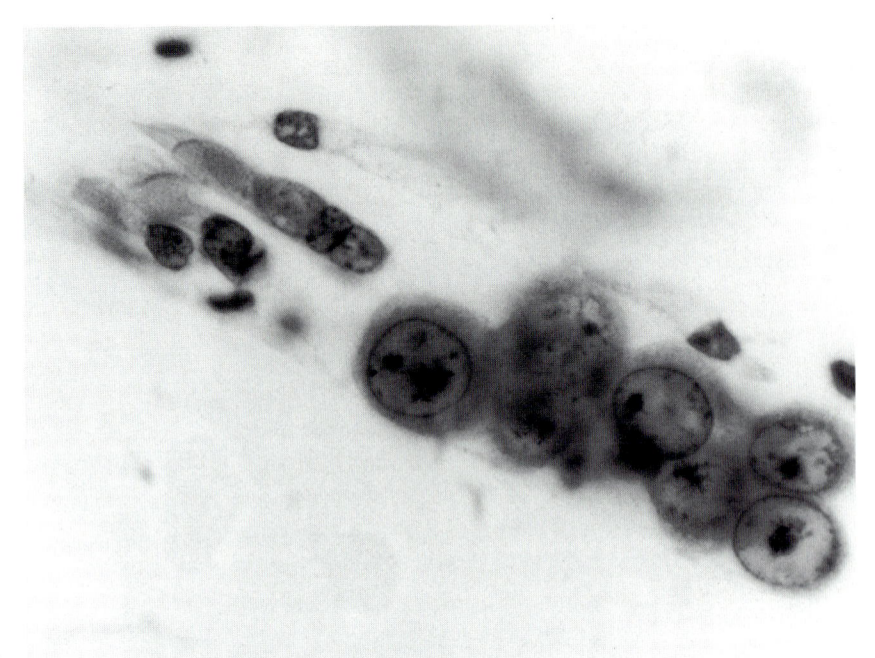

104a

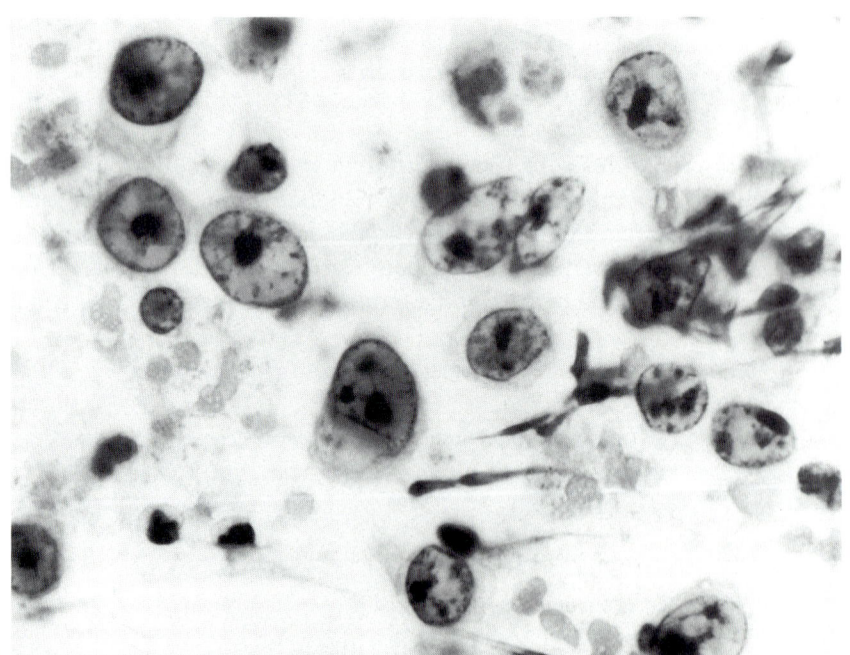

104b

(For legend see page 179.)

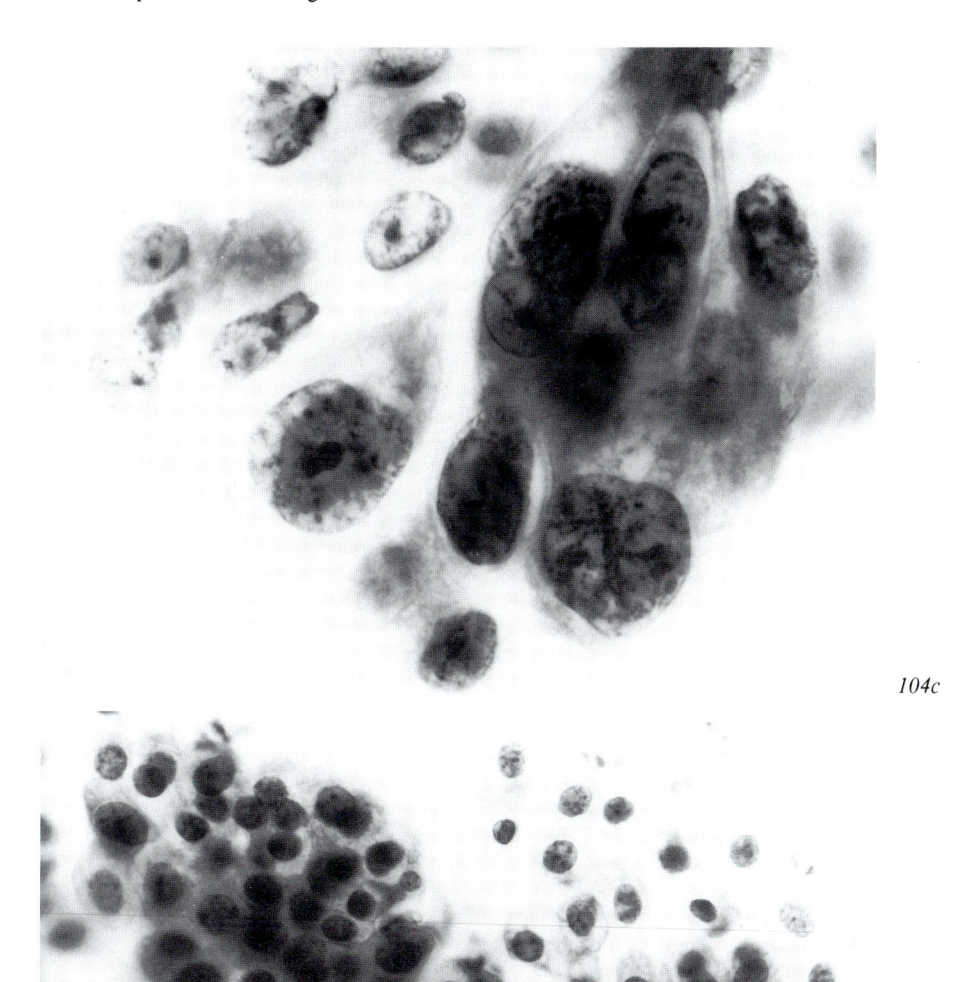

Neoplasms of the Lung 181

104c

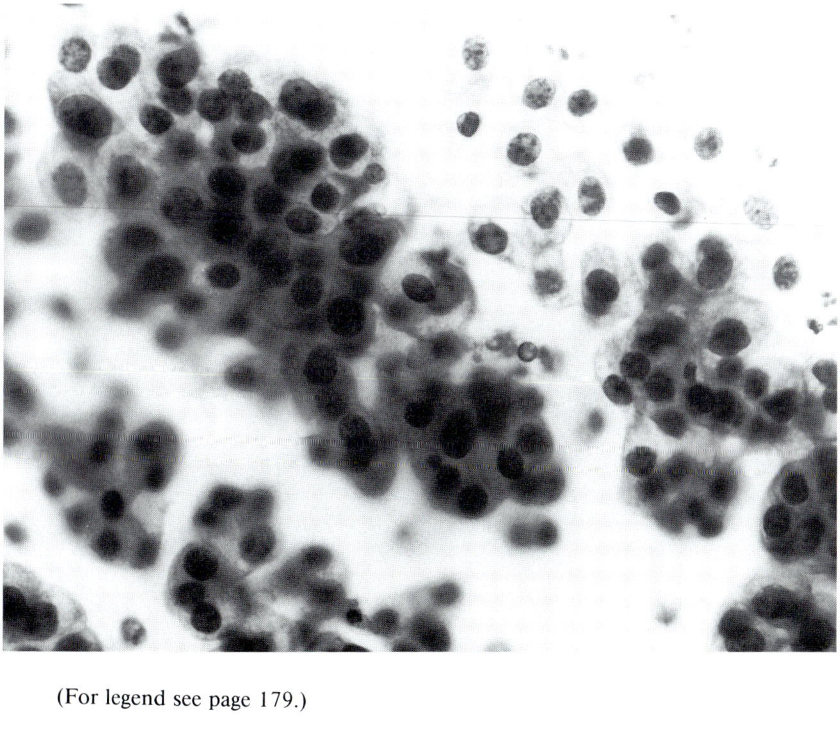

104d

(For legend see page 179.)

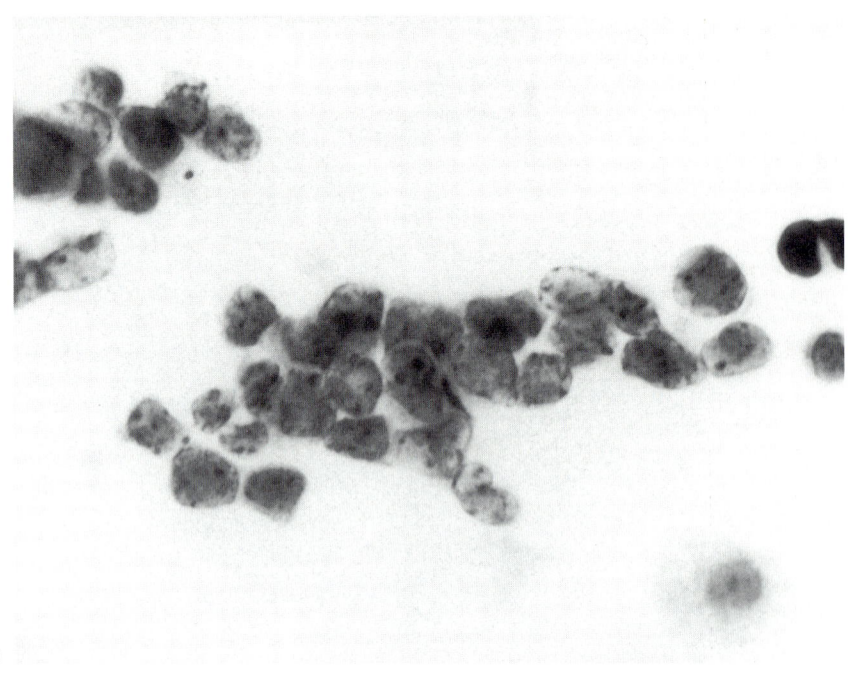

Cytopathology of Pulmonary Disease 182

105a

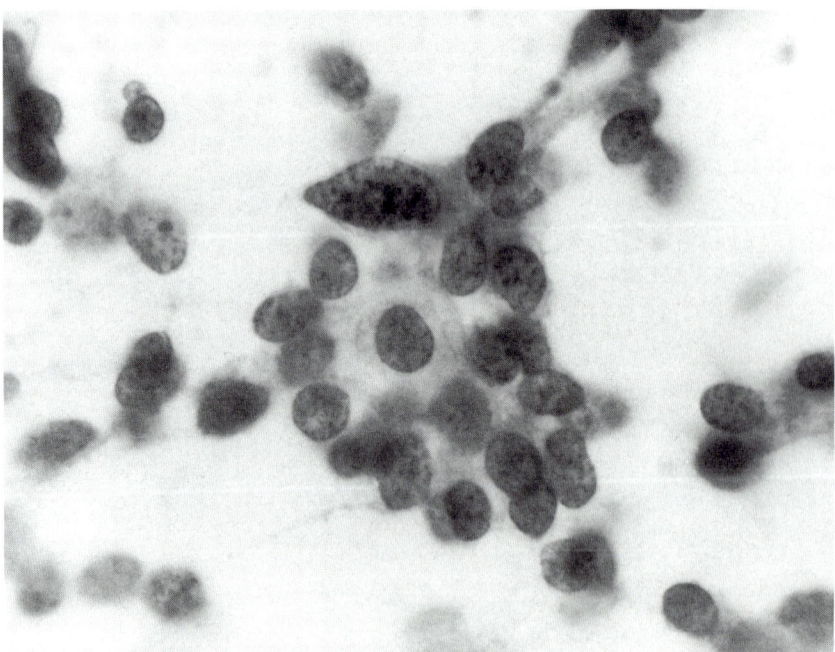

105b

(For legend see page 185.)

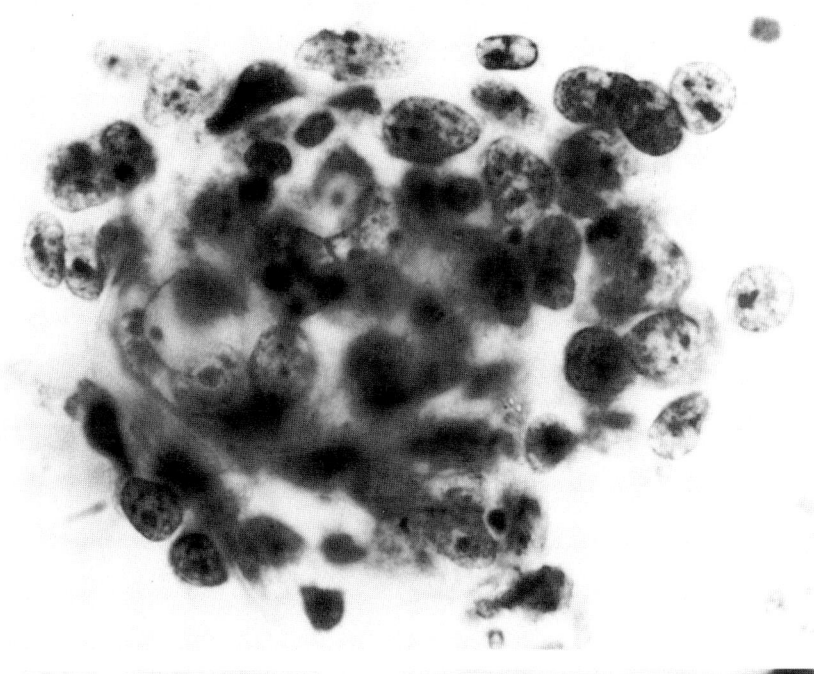

Neoplasms of the Lung

105c

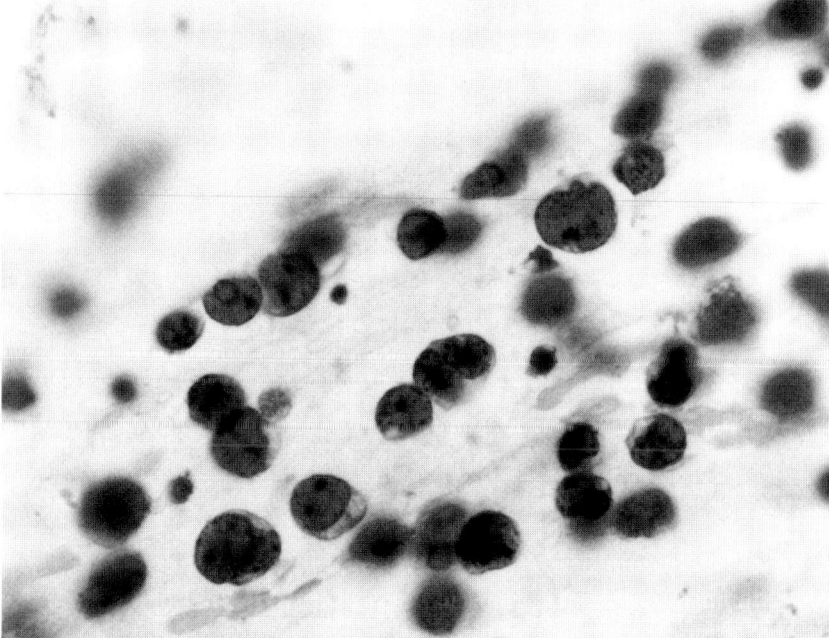

105d

(For legend see page 185.)

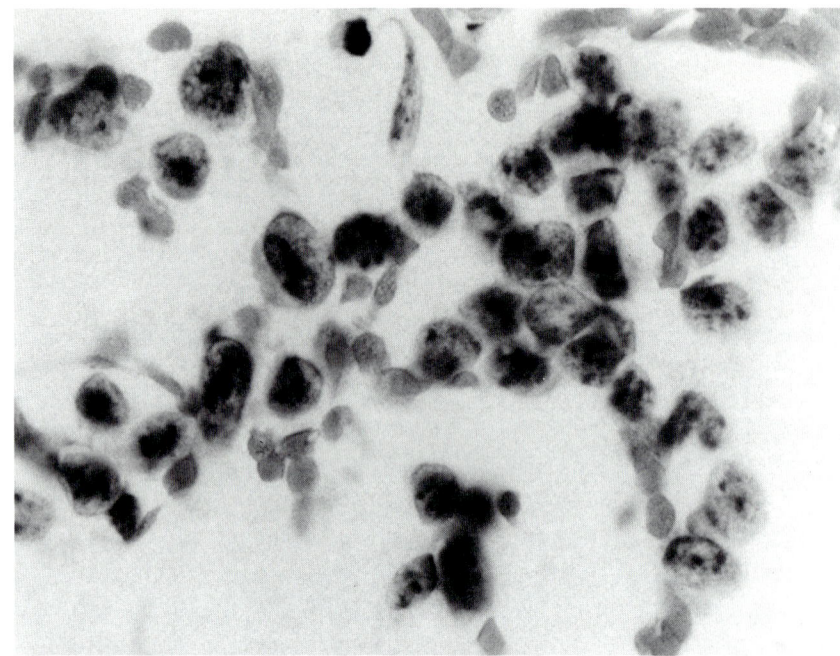

105e

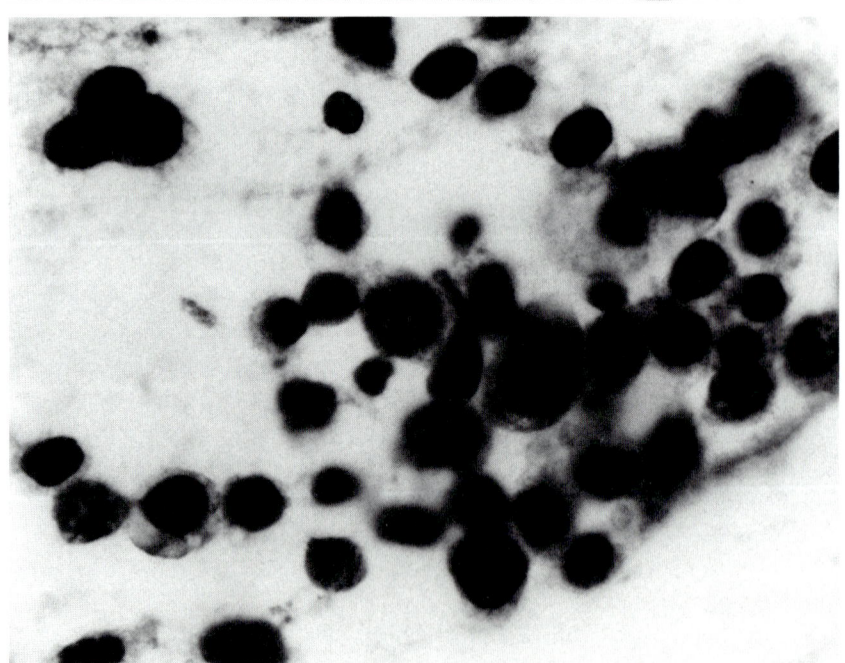

105f

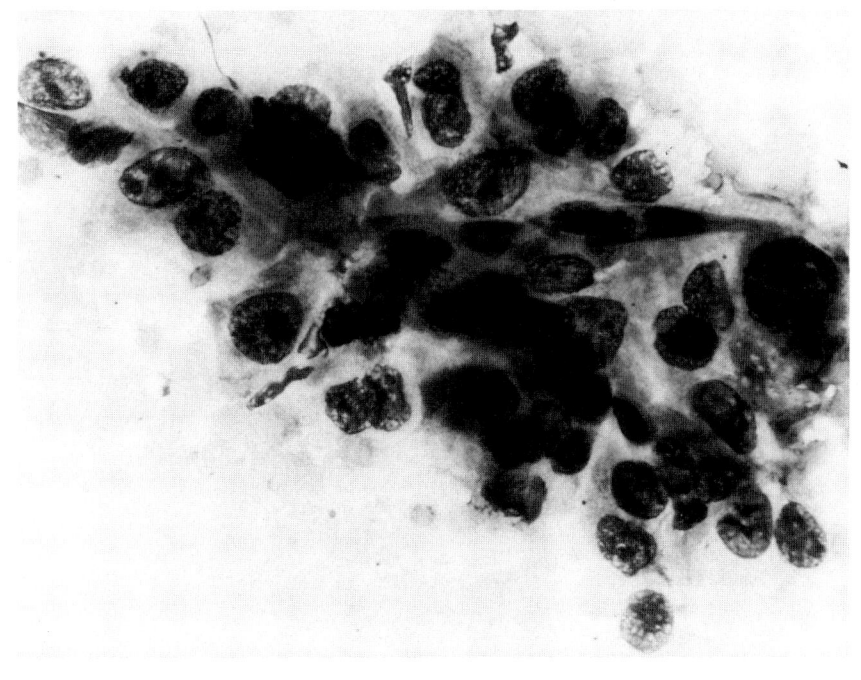

Neoplasms of the Lung

Fig. 106. a Squamous carcinoma (FNA). *b* = × 340. Large cell carcinoma (FNA). *c* Poorly differentiated adenocarcinoma (FNA). *d* Adenocarcinoma (bronchiolo-alveolar type) (FNA). *e* Carcinoid (FNA). *f* 'Oat cell' carcinoma (FNA). *g* Pulmonary blastoma (FNA). MGG. × 360.

(2) Review cytologic and histologic samples from the same or similar cases *before* final sign-out; this provides 'instant' reinforcement of criteria.

(3) Continually consult with the clinicians. Discussing difficult diagnoses can provide further insight into the most probable choice, and will help direct subsequent workup.

(4) An isolated diagnosis on a single sample can be dangerous. A team approach, using carefully selected diagnostic modalities, is the most efficient and accurate way to achieve 'best patient care'.

Fig. 105. a 'Oat cell' carcinoma (sputum). *b* Carcinoid (FNA). *c* Adenocarcinoma (sputum). *d* Lymphoma (sputum). *e* Pulmonary blastoma (FNA). *f* Seminoma (bronchial wash). Papanicolaou. × 900.

Cytopathology of Pulmonary Disease 186

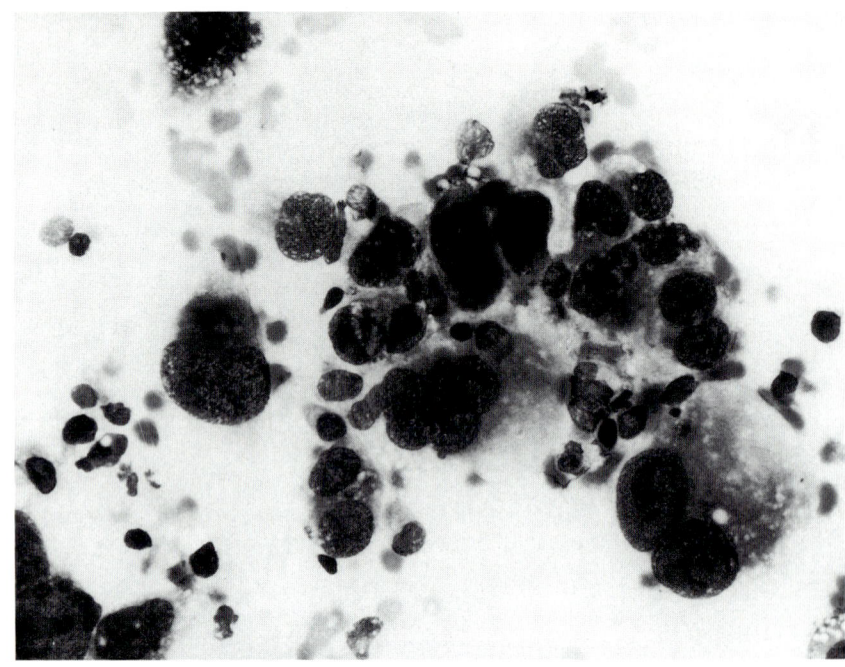

106b

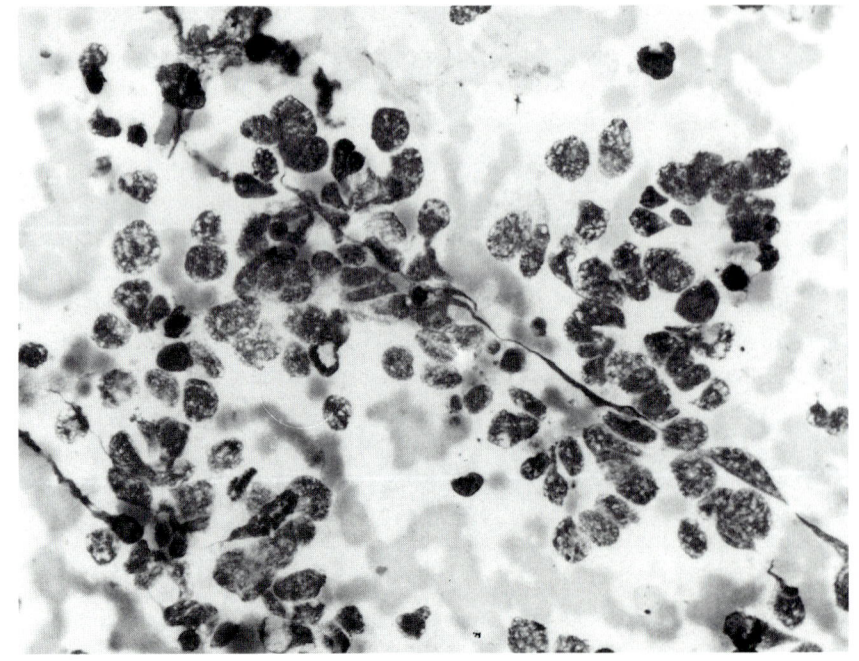

106c

(For legend see page 185.)

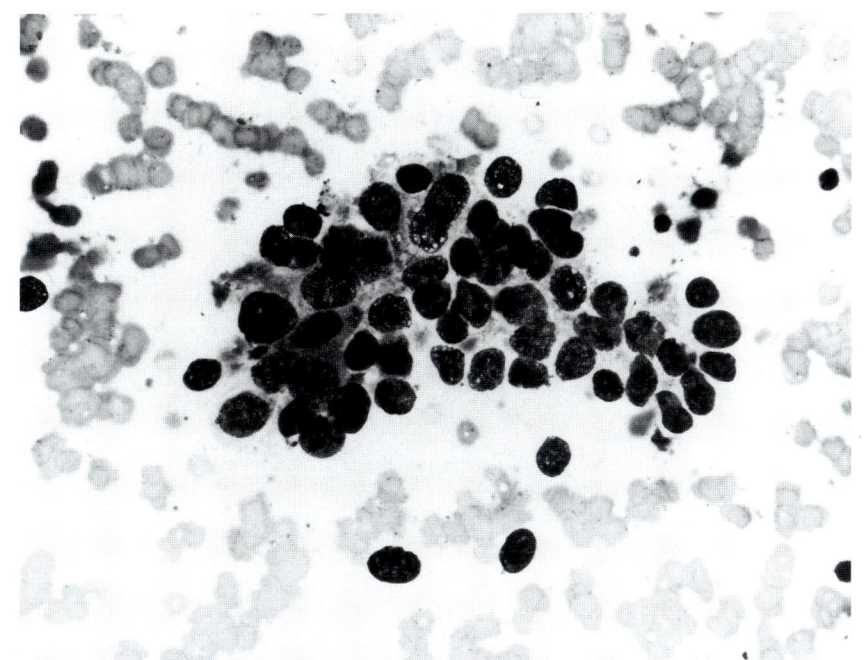

Neoplasms of the Lung

106d

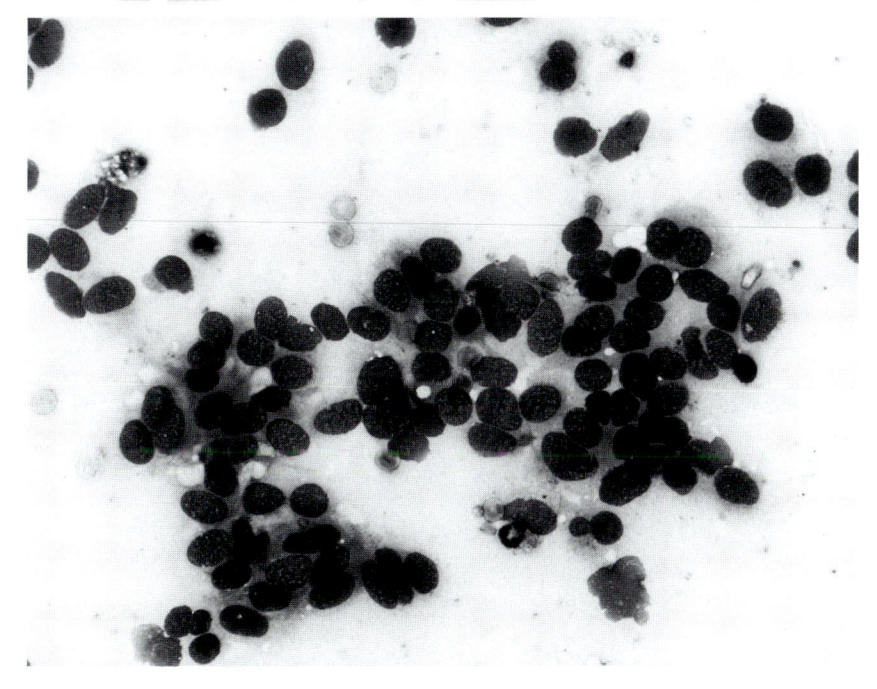

106e

(For legend see page 185.)

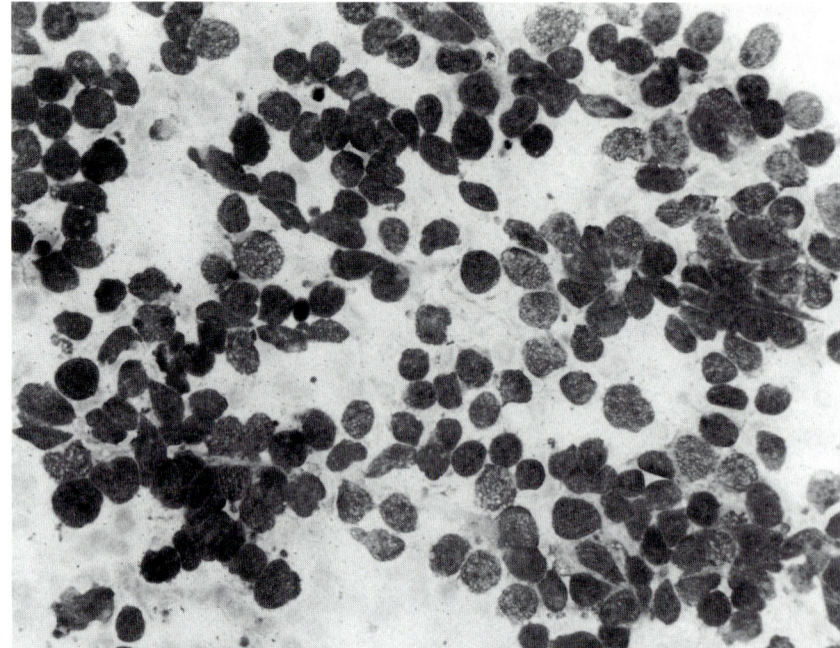

Cytopathology of Pulmonary Disease

106f

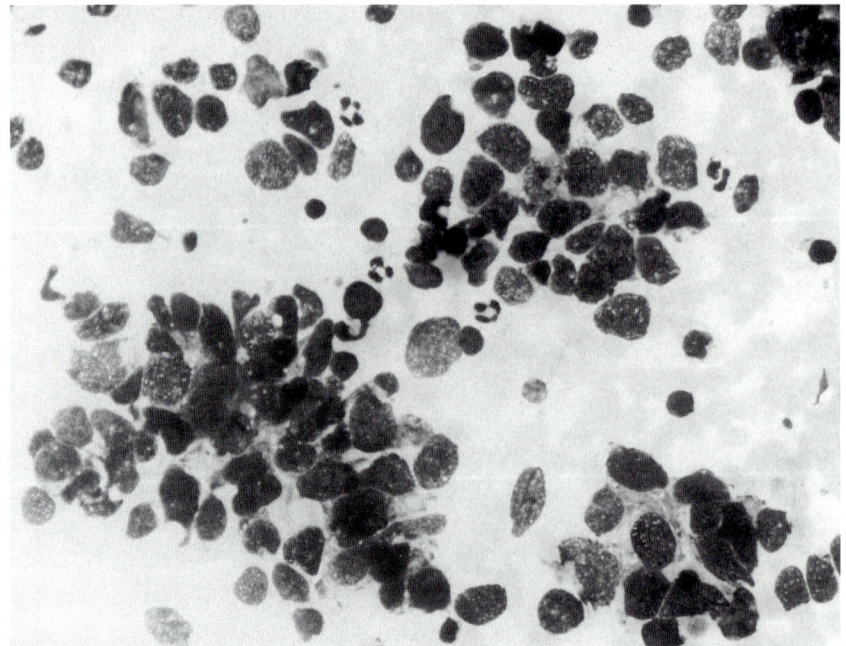

106g

(For legend see page 185.)

VII. Diagnostic Accuracy of Pulmonary Cytology

In order to fully appreciate the worth of cytologic samples from the respiratory tract, their place in the workup of the patient with a pulmonary lesion needs to be detailed. In many medical settings, sputum samples are still regarded as the prime tool for the detection of lung cancer. More sophisticated diagnostic centers can offer fiberoptic bronchoscopy, transthoracic and transbronchial FNA to the patient with evidence of pulmonary disease, neoplastic or infectious. When selecting the 'best' methods for efficient diagnosis, both tumor location and anticipated cell type, as indicated by the radiologist, are important considerations (table 19, 20).

Table 19. Diagnostic rate according to examination method and lesion of lung cancer [118]: January 1973 – August 1980 (614 cases)

Examination methods	Central type (317 cases) n	%	Peripheral type (297 cases) n	%
Cytological methods				
Sputum cytology	223/287	77.70	104/220	47.27
Brushing cytology	249/278	89.56	163/230	70.86
Percutaneous needle cytology	0/0		104/117	88.88
TBAC	10/12	83.33	6/7	85.71
Histological method				
Bronchoscopic biopsy	168/186	90.32	117/163	71.77
Preoperative or pretherapeutic diagnosis	310/317	97.79	278/297	93.60

TBAC = Transbronchial aspiration cytology.

Table 20. Diagnostic accuracy according to histological type and examination method [118]: May 1978 – August 1980 (204 cases)

Histological types and examination method	Squamous cell carcinoma (59 cases)		Adenocarcinoma (99 cases)		Small cell carcinoma (30 cases)		Large cell carcinoma (13 cases)		Mucoepi. ca, adenoid cyst. ca., carcinosarcoma (3 cases)	
	n	%	n	%	n	%	n	%	n	%
Cytological methods										
Sputum cytology	47/59	79.66	45/79	56.96	16/25	64.0	8/11	72.72	0/3	0
Brushing cytology	49/52	94.23	61/77	79.22	24/29	82.75	10/11	90.90	3/3	100
Percutaneous needle cytology	9/11	81.81	18/19	94.73	8/8	100	2/2	100	0/0	
TBAC	4/4	100	5/6	83.33	2/4	50	3/3	100	1/1	100
Histological method										
Bronchoscopic biopsy	37/43	86.01	54/74	72.97	16/19	84.21	11/12	91.66	2/3	66.66

Historic Background

Johnston and Frable [115] provide a brief historic summary, noting that Donné described exfoliated cells from the respiratory tract in 1845. Tissue fragments of a malignant tumor in sputum were described by Walshe in London in 1846. At the end of the 19th century, Hamplen published a case report in which cancer cells were diagnosed in a sputum 5 months before the patient's death; the tumor was confirmed by autopsy. He further published, in 1919, a series of 25 cases of lung cancer in which 13 were diagnosed cytologically. Although such efforts should have established sputum cytology as a valid diagnostic tool, enthusiasm was greatly diminished by the development of cultural methods for micro-organisms and the invention of the microtome, thus establishing surgical pathology as a valid discipline. However, once Papanicolaou and Trout published their landmark monograph in 1943, interest in cytology was revived, and ... the rest is history.

Sputum Cytology

Early studies concerned with the diagnostic accuracy of sputum cytology are reviewed by Johnston and Frable. They note that Koss et al. [132] in 1964, published the largest series to that date on pulmonary cytology. Koss' prophetic statement to follow, reflects what time witnessed. 'It is to be hoped that pulmonary cytology will at some time in the near future become a diagnostic tool as readily accessible and as confidently used and interpreted as cervical cytology appears to be at this time.' The study included 149 patients with known lung cancer in which pulmonary cytology provided 89% accurate detection when 3 or more cytologic specimens were examined [132]. Subsequent studies have confirmed this now well accepted fact that the accuracy of sputum cytology increases with increasing numbers of samples obtained on consecutive mornings [112, 170, 203]. The role of postbronchoscopy sputa (PBS) is generally overlooked. Before the development of the flexible scope, Bibbo et al. [23] recovered tumor cells in sputa from patients whose prebrushing samples were negative in 160 patients with lung tumors. Prebrushing sputa were positive in 17%, whereas postbrushing sputa were positive in 66% of cases. Castella et al. [33] stress that the overall diagnostic yield of multiple types of cytologic samples from an individual is increased with PBS. PBS also is effective in recovering material from tumors beyond the reach of the flexible scope. Bender et al. [19] provide a discussion of the diagnostic effectiveness of pre- and postbronchoscopy sputa. The authors conclude that pre-bronchoscopy sputa contribute no more to the diagnosis than would be found from the bronchoscopy specimens. Risse et al. [204] found just the opposite to be true. PBS occasionally will be positive when the bronchoscopy has been negative, and therefore should still be performed [203].

Erozan and Frost [62], in 1970, further emphasized the importance of multiple specimens and the technique used to obtain samples: of 107 patients with lung cancer, one bronchoscopic examination was positive in 61% of patients, one sputum specimen was diagnostic in 42%, whereas the accuracy rate increased to 82% with 3 sputa and 91% with 5; in a total of 141 cases, the general diagnostic accuracy of sputa, as a screen for lung cancer, was 80% of cases. This accuracy rate varies according to location of the tumor, central versus peripheral, and according to cell type. With the advent of the flexible bronchoscope, the more peripheral lesions can be reached by that instrument, and Hattori et al. [91] accurately diagnosed 83% of peripheral lung tumors through the bronchoscope. Comparison of sampling methods will be discussed below.

The Early Lung Cancer Project was begun in 1969 and was formally established by the National Cancer Institute in 1972. The three participating institutions, Johns Hopkins Medical School [74], The Mayo Foundation [69], and Memorial Sloan-Kettering Cancer Center [65, 149] screened nearly 30,000 subjects with four monthly cytologic examinations of sputum and either yearly or 4-monthly chest X-rays [20]. Data derived from a ten year period of that study revealed the following facts relevant to this discussion:

(1) Regarding chest X-ray detection of occult cancers, 89% of the 31,360 total prevalence chest X-ray exams were considered 'negative for cancer'. Of the remaining 11%, 2% of those (0.2% of the total population) were subsequently diagnosed as having lung cancer. Less than 1% of the patients' X-rays were considered 'suspicious for cancer'; almost half of these eventually were proven to have lung cancer.

(2) Of the 10,233 men screened by chest X-ray only, 63 (0.62%) had subsequent pathologic verification of their lung cancer.

(3) Sputum exam in the group of men who were screened by both X-ray and cytology proved highly specific. Of the 21,127 men, only 300 (1.4%) had sputum cytologies reported as at least 'moderate atypia'. Of the 79 men (0.4%) whose sputa contained cells with evidence of marked atypia

or carcinoma cells, 55 had lung cancer, and 12 had cancer of the upper respiratory tract. These results provide a predictive value of 85%.

(4) In the dual screen group, 67 of the 160 cases with detected lung cancer would have been diagnosed by cytology alone, and 123 by X-ray alone.

The members of the Early Lung Cancer Cooperative Study regarded their data with the following conclusions:

(1) 'If screening for lung cancer is to be carried out it should be done within the framework of general health care; that is, in the private practitioner's office, health maintenance organization, or a general medical clinic.'

(2) 'The chest roentgenogram is the most sensitive method of detecting lung cancer currently available. Approximately 40% of radiologically visible cancers in a screening program are found in stage I (AJCC), where the chances for lung-term survival are excellent.'

(3) 'Sputum cytology is the most effective method of detecting early squamous cell carcinomas of the lung. The technique is highly specific, and the patients with radiologically occult cancer detected by this method can usually be treated with expectation of long survival' [76].

Hope was raised by the Early Lung Cancer Project that screening programs using sputum cytology would cost-effectively identify patients with early mucosal alterations. While the study did discover potentially fatal lesions in males at high risk at an earlier stage, the overall long-term survival rate was the same as for the control group. Of utmost importance to note is that the cell type detected in any significant numbers was squamous cell carcinoma. This leaves the other common types of primary lung cancer beyond the reach of this type of screening program.

Since sputum sampling has been the easiest to obtain and longest used type of cytologic evaluation of the respiratory tract, should its use be discarded in the face of such discouraging results [279]? Several large studies, in addition to that cited above, support the use of mass screening programs to detect occult bronchial mucosal alterations. Implicit in the programs are their well-controlled and structured plan. Usually one center is used to gather the specimens and demographic data, and direct followup. Such programs obviously require support from a large agency, usually governmental. The reasons for their scarcity are obvious: they are very expensive, and the results have been similar to the Early Lung Cancer Project.

A long-standing sputum screening program has just ended with the retirement of its founder, Geno Saccomanno. The target population was uranium miners, particularly cigarette smokers, without evidence of lung disease. Saccomanno and co-workers contributed significantly to our knowledge of the development of squamous carcinoma of the lung, and illustrated its parallelity to squamous carcinoma of the uterine cervix [7, 217, 221]. The need for a convenient method of collecting and transporting the enormous number of sputum samples to their laboratory resulted in the 'Saccomanno method', and the Saccomanno fixative, both in widespread, although not universal, use today.

A similar project was conducted by three universities in The Netherlands [202]. The study was designed to determine the reliability and applicability of the Saccomanno method, and relate the accuracy as a function of the number of sputum samples obtained per patient. The major difference from the Uranium miners study is that these patients were already suspected of having lung cancer, including probable metastases to the lung. Sensitivity of the Saccomanno sputum method was calculated as the probability of a true positive diagnosis expressed as a function of the number of sputa examined. The results emphasize the importance of collecting multiple specimens from the same patient. A single sputum is equivalent to a coin toss for detecting primary lung cancer, even if the lesion is clinically suspected. However, when four or more samples are collected, the sensitivity increases to an acceptable rate (77–87%). However, the false negative rate for patients with 'a malignant process' is 45.8%. The cost-effectiveness of these serial specimens with such low accuracy should be considered.

Perhaps the most regulated study is the annual mass survey performed on high-risk employees of Tokyo Metropolitan Government, and centered at Tokyo Medical College [93]. Through a nationwide patient education program, the adult population is encouraged to obtain sputum collection kits, containing Saccomanno fixative, and instructions for a 3- to 5-day deep-cough collection. The specimens are mailed to Tokyo Medical College, where they are processed and diagnosed. The positive diagnostic rate of their mail-in sputum program is 59.8%. Anyone with any cytologic abnormalities is notified and requested to appear for fiberoptic bronchoscopy. Depending upon the gross findings at bronchoscopy, patients are either treated for infection and then asked to repeat the sputum collection, or brushings, washings and biopsies are obtained. If these be positive, then staging is carried out. If the lesion is considered to be carcinoma in situ, hematoporphyrin localization and laser treatment of the tumor is utilized to prevent invasion.

The experience of this program is obviously extensive, and has a discouragingly low yield by sputum cytology. Chest X-ray has proved more diagnostic. Begun in 1953, a total of almost 2 million patients has been screened with 198 cases of lung cancer detected by 1982. The screened patients clearly have an improved outcome when compared to a control population. Their curative resectability was 33.8%, compared with 10.7% of the unscreened population. The results emphasize the importance of such screening programs if carried out under controlled circumstances. Combined X-ray and sputum cytology, as in the Early Lung Cancer Project, still provide the best noninvasive method of screening the patient at risk. In the face of medical cost-containment, such programs may be less frequently funded than in the past.

Johnston and Frable [114] analyzed their false-positive rates in a comprehensive article. At Medical College of Virginia (MCV), 15 false-positive diagnoses were made over 5 years, providing a false-positive rate of 4.8%. Duke University Medical Center, also for a 5-year period, experienced an overall detection rate of 60.2% (253 patients out of 420), with 7 false-positive cases, calculated at 2.7% false-positive rate. In the early part of the 1970s, the trend toward treatment based solely on cytologic diagnosis was seen at Duke and MCV, as well as other institutions. 'The authors would recommend this only in those situations in which the highest quality of respiratory cytopathology practice is available.'

Frable [70] stressed as early as 1968 that the routine cytologic diagnosis of cancer by sputa failed to improve the survival rate. What is missing from all subsequent studies, except for the Early Lung Cancer Project, is an analysis of the effect of such efforts on the quality and quantity of life for all patients studied. Such an analysis must include long-term follow-up of patients who were diagnosed as having bronchial dysplasia, the findings of which persuaded them to quit smoking.

Fiberoptic Bronchoscopy

While the worth of sputum cytology is not menial, the development of the flexible bronchoscope by Ikeda [103] in the 1960s revolutionized the diagnosis of pulmonary lesions. Brushings, washings, transbronchial biopsies and transbronchial FNA provide the diagnosis and staging of the pulmonary lesion with minimal morbidity, cost and time, compared with surgical diagnosis.

In a paper soon after the advent of the flexible bronchoscope, Skitarelic and Von Haam [236] compared brushings and washings obtained by both the flexible and rigid bronchoscopes. They found that the diagnostic accuracy of specimens obtained by the flexible bronchoscope was 91.67% whereas with the rigid bronchoscope only 80.2% diagnostic accuracy was possible. The bronchial biopsy, considered the gold standard, gave an accuracy of only 60.76%; this low yield could reflect the fact that only 79 cases out of 204 had biopsy material that was considered adequate for evaluation. Bronchial washings yielded a higher accuracy rate than sputa, 81.1% with no false-positives. Brushings gave an accuracy rate of 85.1% with no false-positives. There were no significant differences among the types of cytologic procedures but a definitive difference between the cytologic procedures and the bronchial biopsy with the cytologic procedures being higher. Of 188 cases studied, the cytologic procedures yielded an overall accuracy rate of 84.57% [236].

Series in which all diagnostic techniques are compared are rare [38, 73, 106, 245]. An early study by Francis and Borgescov [73] studied 40 patients in whom transthoracic fine needle aspiration and bronchoscopy were performed. Because of the inconsistency in types of specimens obtained, the data is difficult to interpret. However, diagnostic yields of approximately 70% or greater are quoted throughout the paper.

Chopra et al. [38] studied 70 UCLA patients with bronchoscopically obtained brushings, washings, biopsies, and pre- and postbronchoscopy sputa. Brushings and biopsies gave the greatest diagnostic yield in cases with definite carcinoma, (67% brushing, 66% biopsy). Bronchial washings were never positive when the other specimens were negative. Pre- and postbronchoscopy sputa, while not of great diagnostic yield (18%) were diagnostic in 4 cases, 2 proven cases of bronchogenic carcinoma in which all other specimens were reported as either negative or atypical (prebronchoscopy sputa) and 2 patients when the biopsy was either atypical or negative (PBS). The authors conclude that of all the specimens, the washing is the least diagnostic by itself. Essentially the same study, repeated at UCLA 10 years later, analyzing data from over 800 patients, has produced similar results.

Although the bronchial washing is considered by some to be least helpful of all the bronchoscopically obtained material, Ng and Horak [169], in a study of bronchial washings, disclosed an overall accuracy of 74% in a study of 276 cases of proven primary lung cancer in which bronchial washings were performed. They combined specimen categories with 'definitely malignant cells' and 'abnormal cells consistent with malignancy' together. If the former group is taken by itself, the accuracy rate is 67.8%. Only 8.3% were considered unsatisfactory. Jay et al. [106], analyzing all collection methods found that bronchial washing and PBS were exclusively responsible for definitive diagnosis in 12% of a series of 69 lung cancer patients.

Fine Needle Aspiration of the Lung

Depending on the location of the lesion and the skills of the invasive thoracic radiologist and bronchoscopy team, an FNA may be the technique of choice. Whether transthoracically or transbronchially, the position of the aspirating needle must be confirmed to be within the lesion. In our experience, the ideal situation is to have the cytopathologist or cytotechnologist present during the aspiration to observe the location of the lesion and the needle within, to prepare the direct smears, and with use of a rapid stain, to microscopically evaluate the adequacy of the material for diagnosis. With experience, gross evaluation of the material as it smears on the slide will indicate if a sufficient sample has been obtained. However, even the most practiced can be fooled, so we advocate the use of the microscope to avoid disappointment after the patient has left the room. A definitive diagnosis cannot and should not always be made on the spot. However, an indication of malignant, infectious, or benign lesion can usually be given, with the final diagnosis forthcoming, just as with a frozen section from the operating room. This practice should considerably reduce the number of inadequate specimens, the most frequent source of false positive diagnoses, in this author's experience. Smith et al. [238] improved their inadequate rate (22–2%) by rinsing the needle and preparing membrane filters of the solution; this technique also increased their malignant diagnosis rate by 24%.

Table 21 is compiled from the available, recent literature. The data is often sketchy in the papers reviewed, with very little attention being given to false negatives. Most of the reviews did indicate the inadequate rate, which as noted above, is an important index of the success of the technique. When developing the skill at one's institution, this parameter should be monitored closely. If the inadequate rate does not fall within the collective experience of similar institutions within a reasonable time, the

Table 21. Diagnostic accuracy rates of FNA of the lung

Authors	Patients	Dates	Sensitivity, %	False-negative, %	Inadequate, %
Dahlgren and Lind [50]	125	1972	93	13	NG
Hayata et al. [95]	113	1967–1971	85	NG	NG
Horsley et al. [100]*	171	1981–1982	81	4	5
Johnston [110]	1,015	1973–1983	83.8	14.6	NG
Michel et al. [153]	239	1968–1980	92	5	4
Mitchell et al. [154]	272	1976–1980	99	<1	<1
Nasiell [162]	144	1960–1965	72	17	7
Pilotti et al. [186]	130	1982	91	5	7
Pilotti et al. [187]	271	1979–1983	89	3	10

NG = Not given; * = TBr-FNA. Dates: If only 1 year is given, this is the year of publication; series years were not indicated in paper.

aspirator should seek further training, so that this excellent diagnostic modality is available to the patients of that hospital.

In a study of 1,015 patients undergoing fine needle aspiration biopsy of the lung, Johnston [110] found that of 123 patients in whom tissue confirmation was obtained within a short period following aspiration, 83.8% of malignant lesions could be definitively detected, 14.6% would be missed and 1.6% were incorrectly diagnosed. Further, 11.7% of patients without lung cancer (316 of the 1,015) were diagnosed as having infectious organisms or morphologic criteria sufficient to diagnose a specific type of inflammation. Of importance to this discussion is the singular case report of a 'possible spread of bronchogenic carcinoma to the chest wall' after a transthoracic FNA. The patient survived for 26 months following the FNA with widespread pulmonary metastases from his prostatic carcinoma [158].

Bronchoalveolar Lavage

The above cited paper by Johnston [110] pays attention to the underplayed role of FNA, and of cytology in general, in the detection of non-neoplastic diseases. The newest sampling technique, the BAL, has gained increasing prominence in the realm of infectious disease diagnosis. Originally intended to harvest the benign immunocompetent cells of the lung for study, the technique has proven invaluable in diagnosis of infectious disease among the immunocompromised population. This minimally invasive bedside technique is described in chapter II and in the 'Appendix'.

The diagnostic yield for certain infectious diseases, especially pneumocystis, approaches 100% in most studies [66, 85, 174, 180, 210]. Not only can fungi and viruses be identified by routine Papanicolaou processing, but DNA probes are now being employed to identify the rare cell infected with virus, especially before viral hallmarks are obvious [97]. Cell population profiles, for which the study was originally designed, are currently being analyzed, so that eventually BAL may replace open lung biopsy to define interstitial and cryptogenic 'benign' lung diseases [102].

Accuracy of Cell Typing

Not only do the clinicians wish to know whether a specimen contains benign or malignant cells, but if the sample is 'positive', the cell type is equally important. Besides being an academic question, the cell type will dictate the kind of therapy, once staging is considered. In the case of 'oat cell' carcinoma, cell type is *the* most important issue, for except in experimental protocols, surgery is not a consideration, once the diagnosis has been made. In our experience, and that of others [113], a single sputum is often the definitive study of an 'oat cell' carcinoma patient, after which therapy is begun. The responsibility of the diagnostic cytopathology team is obviously monumental.

Table 22 lists the collective experience of numerous groups relative to accuracy of cell typing. The most frequently misclassified are the poorly differentiated adenocarcinomas [237], and the large cell carcinomas [89]. At UCLA, vigorous attempts are made to avoid designating a tumor 'large cell undifferentiated'. In order to accurately define all tumors, the bronchoscopy team is instructed to obtain a transbronchial or endobronchial biopsy for electron microscopy, which is fixed in glutaraldehyde. If the diagnosis is obvious on light microscopy, the additional biopsy is discarded. If the diagnosis is uncertain, the electron microscopy specimen is processed. If the light microscopy diagnosis is handicapped by insufficient or crushed material, then the tissue fixed for electron microscopy is processed for light microscopy. Our series thus has far fewer inconclusive designations, and very few lesions categorized as 'large cell undifferen-

Table 22. Accuracy of cell typing of lung tumors by cytology

Reference	Patients	SCC	SCUC	AC	LC	Spec	Year
Gupta [87]	320	100	92	N/A	55	Sp and Br	1982
Lange and Høeg [135]	91	86	100	20	N/A	Sp and Br	1971
Ng and Horak [169[	276	93	93	93	77	BrWash	1959–1974
Ng and Horak [170]	449	95	95	80	80	Sputa	1959–1974
Pilotti et al. [188]	400	65	58	50	42	Sputa	1974–1978
Pilotti et al. [189]	252	79	76	43	19	Bronch	1974–1978
Suprun et al. [245]	232	81	91	53	59	All	1975–1977

All numbers under cell types refer to % accurately typed. SCC = Squamous cell carcinoma; SCUC = small cell undifferentiated carcinoma; AC = adenocarcinoma; LC = large cell undifferentiated carcinoma; Sp = sputa; Br and Bronch = obtained by bronchoscopy; All = sputa, bronchoscopy, FNA.

tiated carcinoma'. While electron microscopy is considered expensive, the difference to patient management is significant, and if processed on an 'as needed' basis, can prove to be very cost-effective, especially when evaluated in relation to best patient care.

Cytologic detection of bronchiolo-alveolar carcinoma has been notoriously poor, not only because these lesions occur generally peripherally, but also because of their somewhat benign cytologic appearance and their close resemblance and admixture with pneumocytes and pulmonary macrophages. Tao et al. [249] decided to improve their diagnostic rate and provided an extensive and scholarly review of 101 patients with bronchiolo-alveolar carcinoma. Upon reassessment of the criteria for cytologic diagnosis their detection rate increased remarkably; they conclude that FNA is the primary diagnostic test for this tumor. This lesion, with its variations [41, 249], will no doubt continue to provide diagnostic challenges to even the most expert cytopathologist. However, if the radiographic appearance is considered along with the cytomorphology of the cells in either sputum cytology or fine needle aspiration material, the diagnosis becomes much easier and more reliable.

The importance of sampling the entire lesion when correlating cytology with histology is stressed by Tanaka et al. [247]. Diagnoses of 154 patients whose tumors were completely resected were compared with the cytologic diagnoses obtained by sputa and bronchial brushings. Compared to other papers, this paper had an overall cytologic typing accuracy of 64.3% (83.6% for squamous cell carcinomas to 25.0% in large cell carcinomas) versus Gagneten [77] (57.4%), Kanhouwa and Matthews [116] (77.5%), Pilotti [189] (77%), and Suprun [245] (75%). Tanaka et al. [247] feel that the differences may depend upon the methodology and partly on the materials used for pathologic examination, and stress the importance of examining the largest available resection when correlating cytologies with histologies.

The most comprehensive evaluation of respiratory cytology has been undertaken by Johnston from Duke University Medical Center [108, 112, 113]. The first of the series paid particular attention to the number of specimens obtained and the ultimate diagnosis of cancer. The study concluded that 50% of 357 patients had an unequivocal diagnosis of cancer made by cytologic methods. In order to achieve that diagnostic rate, multiple specimens from the lower respiratory tract were needed. In those patients who were able to provide sufficient cytologic material five specimens were necessary to make a definitive diagnosis in over 85% of those cases. The authors further emphasized that 'no one specimen type is of exclusive importance in lung cancer diagnosis. Both sputum and bronchial material are essential for maximum diagnostic accuracy.' They further point out that sputum examination was equal if not superior to material obtained through the bronchoscope. Conversely, if bronchoscopic material had not been obtained, 26% of the cancers would have been missed.

The second portion of the 10-year study compared cytologic diagnosis with histopathology, with a special attention to cell type. Their results emphasize the reliability of cell identification of small cell undifferentiated carcinoma in which there is 95.5% agreement with histology. Johnston and Bosen [113] declare that small cell undifferentiated carcinoma has cytologic features which are so characteristic and diagnostic that therapy is able to be instituted based on the cytologic findings without subjecting the patient to additional biopsy or thoracotomy. This author concurs with that statement. A futuristic concept relates to the current controversy of combination diagnoses of lung tumors or multiple tissue patterns in the same lesion. Johnston and Bosen plead for cytopathologic interpretation being considered as correct as the tissue diagnosis, another statement with which this author could not agree more.

The final portion of their study [108] considers the inconclusive diagnoses of 218 patients. When a diagnosis of atypical metaplasia was made in 70 patients, 40% proved to have cancer by tissue confirmation. Of the remaining 60%, follow-up studies revealed only non-neoplastic diseases, usually inflammatory. Pneumonia was the most frequent type of disease. An additional 135 patients had been given a diagnosis of 'atypical cells suspicious for malignancy'. 68% of these patients were subsequently proven to have cancer. Approximately 32% had no cancer, and, again, pneumonia was the underlying disease. Although the article does not break down the specimens into types, one statement indicates that most of the inconclusive diagnoses were encountered in sputum samples rather than bronchoscopically obtained specimens. This also happens to be the experience at UCLA.

VIII. Into the Future (circa 1987)

'Never has so much been expected from so little!' Not a political campaign slogan, but an observation concerning the amount of pulmonary material contemporary pathologists have available for categorizing lung lesions. When the original criteria for classifying lung tumors were established by light microscopy, the tissue examined usually came from a lobectomy or from an autopsy. Adequate and multiple samples easily revealed any mixtures of histologic patterns. Currently, many critical decisions categorizing lung lesions are made on fragments of tissue less than 0.5 cm in greatest dimension, frequently partially crushed by the biopsy forceps. Further, cytologic diagnosis has become so sophisticated and reliable that definitive diagnoses and therapeutic decisions are based on exfoliated or aspirated material consisting of approximately 100,000 cells.

Because of therapeutic implications, surgeons and oncologists demand that lung tumors be placed in specific categories. This insistence reflects our accumulated knowledge of pulmonary neoplasms, especially their natural history and response to therapy [31]. In order to continue expanding our experience with this vitally important group of human neoplasms, not only accuracy but precision in classification must be maintained. To confound the issue, light microscopy is no longer the only valid parameter for evaluating tissues and cells. Electron microscopy has established its place in the workup of controversial lesions. Numerous articles have been published attesting to the discrepancy between light and electron microscopy categorization of lung cancers [152, 216]. In fact, certain tumors are now found to have squamous, glandular and endocrine features by electron microscopy [89]. Recently, immunochemistry has added further knowledge about the cytochemical properties of these cells [13], but has significantly added to the confusion [61, 83]. Keratin, the sine qua non of squamous carcinoma, is now demonstrable in most epithelial cells, including glandular and mesothelial cells. 'Oat cells', which were once considered 'undifferentiated', have been found to be highly sophisticated, capable of producing a variety of hormones [133], and have consequently been included in the APUD classification of tumors.

Table 23. Electron microscopic criteria in lung cancer diagnosis [152]

Criteria	Squamous cell carcinoma	Adenocarcinoma	Oat cell carcinoma	Mesothelioma
Cell size	variable – 10–60 μm in maximum dimension; usually large	variable – 30–60 μm in maximum dimension	usually small – 10–20 μm in dimension	usually relatively uniform – 20–30 μm
Cell shape	variable; usually ovoid or polygonal but may be spindle shaped	highly variable – cuboidal, columnar, ovoid, polygonal	usually ovoid or spindle shaped; may have prominent cell processes	usually ovoid or polygonal but may be spindle shaped
Nucleus	large; ovoid or elliptical but may be convoluted or multilobulated; nucleoli frequently large	size and shape variable; frequently convoluted or multilobulated; nucleoli large with prominent nucleolonemma	usually ovoid or slightly spindle shaped; prominent heterochromatin; nucleoli often inconspicuous	large; ovoid or convoluted; nucleoli may be prominent
Cytoplasm	number and type of organelles variable; generally have prominent microfilaments often aggregated to form tonofilaments which insert into desmosomes	frequently have very active cytoplasm with numerous organelles; mucus vacuoles may be present in cytoplasm and, if so, usually associated with prominent terminal web and intracellular microfilaments; intracellular neolumen formation common	generally few organelles; sparse, rough endoplasmic reticulum; dense core membrane bound neurosecretory granules characteristic; some microfilaments	rough endoplasmic reticulum prominent and often oriented circumferentially around nucleus; numerous microfilaments often in form of tonofilaments – insert into desmosomes; neolumen formation frequent
Cell surface and cell junctions	short cytoplasmic projections which interdigitate with adjacent cell processes; numerous desmosomes connect cell processes to each other	apical or free surface of cell has microvilli of variable length; microvilli covered by fibrillar glycocalyx; junctional complexes connect cells to each other; lateral surfaces often interdigitate	generally smooth cell surfaces; occasional desmosome connects cells together	Characteristically have long, thin microvilli on free surfaces; microvilli smooth – not covered by glycocalyx; prominent desmosomes attach cells to each other

Table 24. Results of histochemical immunoperoxidase and electron microscopic studies in 54 cases of lung tumors[1] [225]

Histologic diagnosis	Mucin[2]	CEA[3]	Keratin[4]	Secretion[5]	Neurosecretory granules[6]	Tonofilaments[7]
Squamous cell carcinoma (n = 8)	7/8	6/8	8/8[9]	0/7	0/7	5/7
Adenocarcinoma (n = 6)	6/6	6/6	2/6	6/6	0/6	0/6
Adenosquamous carcinoma (n = 3)	3/3	3/3	3/3	3/3	0/3	3/3
Large cell undifferentiated carcinoma (n = 10)	7/10	8/10	7/10[10]	8/10	0/10	1/10
Large cell undifferentiated giant cell type (n = 3)	0/3	0/3	0/3	0/3	0/3	0/3
Small cell anaplastic carcinoma (n = 12)[8]	5/12	4/12	1/12	2/12	11/12	0/12
Carcinoid tumor (n = 4)	0/4	0/4	0/4	0/4	4/4	0/4
Malignant mesothelioma (n = 8)	1/8	2/8	8/8[11]	0/3	0/3	3/3

CEA = Carcinoembryonic antigen.
[1] Results given as number of positive cases relative to total in each group.
[2] Presence of determined by mucicarmine stain and PAS following diastase digestion.
[3] CEA staining determined by immunoperoxidase.
[4] Keratin staining determined by immunoperoxidase.
[5] Evidence of secretion determined by electron microscopy.
[6] Neurosecretory granules determined by electron microscopy.
[7] Tonofilaments determined by electron microscopy.
[8] Cases of small cell anaplastic carcinoma comprising intermediate cell type (10 cases) and oat cell type (2 cases).
[9] Positive keratin staining significantly more often in squamous carcinoma than in adenocarcinoma ($p = 0.01$).
[10] Positive keratin staining significantly more often in large cell undifferentiated carcinoma than in small cell anaplastic carcinoma ($p = 0.03$).
[11] Positive keratin staining significantly more often in mesothelioma than in adenocarcinoma ($p = 0.01$).

If one agrees that continued accuracy and precision are necessary for therapeutics, prognostics, and for epidemiologic data gathering, then the pathologist is faced with a dilemma. On what basis should lung tumors be classified? Clearly, light microscopy has received the longest experience, and established itself as reliable and relatively reproducible. Electron microscopy is excellent for settling controversy but expensive in time and equipment. The fledgling and exciting field of immunochemistry currently needs more experience to refine techniques, to reveal as yet undiscovered cross-reactivity, and to explore new and more reliable markers.

Will the classification of lung tumors undergo 20 years of seismic convulsions such as have rocked lymphology? Sobin [240], in a thoughtful editorial, advocates considering these diagnostic modalities as complimentary techniques, and reporting the results in tandem. 'In this way, different classifying features would be separated, just as they are when topographic site, behavior, histologic type, differentiation, and extent of spread are used in conventional classifications of tumors. This separation would promote the study of the biologic significance of individual features, help identify subsets of major established categories, facilitate stratification of cases in clinical trials, and enhance precision in statistical tabulation.'

While this monograph deals basically with morphology assessed at the light microscopic level, the enhancement of diagnosis by the techniques just described cannot be ignored. In our daily practice of cytopathology at UCLA, electron microscopy, immunochemistry and DNA probes [97, 227] are performed on pulmonary specimens that are contentious. We hope to soon add image analysis [74, 246]. Tables 23 and 24 are provided for the service pathologist as additional diagnostic guides, as well as to stimulate the search for other ways of clarifying and characterizing this fascinating group of pathologic lesions. Clearly, the same techniques apply to specimens from all other body sites. Rather than complicate one's day, these studies should be looked upon as providing the variety that not only prevents boredom, but results in finer diagnosis, and ultimately, better patient care.

IX. Appendix: Preparatory and Staining Procedures

The recipes that follow are directly from the procedure manuals of the UCLA Cytology and Surgical Pathology Histology Laboratories. They are included in the belief that most procedures as described in texts do not provide the reader with the details needed for success. These methods have been constantly reworked until, in our opinion, they have been optimized. If you try them, and experience difficulties or improve upon them, please share that information with us.

I. Processing of sputum, bronchial washing, bronchial brush, BAL specimens

A. Sputum
1. Specimens should be fresh. No preservative is required (24-hour collections or specimens older than 5 h are unsatisfactory)
2. Materials required for smear preparation:
    a. Labeled slides (3 for sputum and bronchial wash, 4 for BAL)
    b. 95% ethyl alcohol (fixative) in a Coplin jar
    c. Plastic gloves, paper mask, plastic apron
    d. Petri dish, glass rod, pipette, wooden stick
    e. Chlorine
3. Sputum preparation procedure is done under the biological hood; mask, gloves and apron are always worn when working with unfixed specimens
4. Examine the specimen, which has been placed into a petri dish against a light background. Pick out any bloody particles with a pipette or glass rod. If the material is thick a wooden stick may be used to tease the particles apart. Examine the specimen against a dark background and pick out any white string-like flecks or solid material
5. Place the selected material on the slide. Use only a small amount of material on a slide
6. Smear the material on the slides, spreading out the very thick mucus to make a fairly even smear (monolayer)
7. Immediately place the prepared slides in the fixative jar
8. The remaining specimen is mixed with a prepared chlorine solution for decontamination and discarded along with the gloves, apron and mask into a plastic bag which is then placed in the bag used to discard contaminated material

Cytopathology of Pulmonary Disease

B. Bronchial washing
1. If the specimen is small in volume, it can be treated in the same fashion as a sputum
2. If a large amount of bloody material is received then the specimen should be poured into a centrifuge tube and spun at 3,500 rpm for 5 min. Use a disposable tube with screw-top lid
3. The supernatant is poured/pipetted off, and smears prepared. If blood is prominent, take care to make very thin smears

C. Bronchial brushing
Specimens are usually prepared at the time of bronchoscopy and are then submitted in fixative. Check for correct labeling as to location of brush and patient's name

D. Bronchoalveolar lavage
1. Prepare 4 slides under biological hood using the same technique as used for bronchial washing
   (a) 2 frosted slides for Papanicolaou stain
   (b) 2 frosted end slides for silver stain
2. Slides for silver are prepared on all immunocompromised patients. Do not use paper clips to separate slides for silver stain; the material in conventional paper clips contaminates staining interpretation – use separate bottle of fixative for silver stain

II. Preparation of stains

General instructions: All supplies for staining should be labeled as to date of expiration and date opened.

A. Papanicolaou stain
1. Papanicolaou stain stock solutions
   a. Hematoxylin (Mayer's)
   (1) Ingredients
      (a) Distilled water   1,000 ml
      (b) Hematoxylin   1.0 g (putty colored powder)
      (c) Ammonium
          (or potassium alum)   50 g (small white crystals)
      (d) Sodium iodate   0.2 g (white powder-like baking soda)
      (e) Citric acid   1.0 g (white powder-like laundry detergent)
      (f) Chloral hydrate   50.0 g (clear crystal-like ice)
   (2) Preparation
      (a) Dissolve the hematoxylin in the distilled water which has been heated to 55–60 °C and rotate until all stain is in solution
          (mixture will look like orange tea in color; if color is incorrect, check purity of the distilled water)

Appendix: Preparatory and Staining Procedures

- (b) Add the alum* (the mixture appears to thicken and turns a deeper purple color)
- (c) Add the citric acid* (the mixture turns to deep red wine color; the solution is opaque)
- (d) Add chloral hydrate* (the mixture runs down the side of the flask as the solution is rotated)
- (e) Allow the solution to stand overnight before use. Pour the hematoxylin into dark brown stock solution bottles. As a stock solution, this stain is stable indefinitely. As a working solution it can be stable up to 2 months if the length of staining time is increased after prolonged use

b. Orange G
(1) Ingredients
- (a) 95% ethyl alcohol   380 ml
- (b) Orange G   1.0 g
- (c) Phosphotungstic acid   0.4 g
- (d) Glacial acetic acid   3.0 ml

(2) Preparation
- (a) Heat the 95% alcohol to boiling point (until you see large bubbles on the surface of the liquid)
- (b) Pour the alcohol into the Waring blender glass container (labeled OG) until the blades are covered. Cover the blender and turn on the motor to 'slow'
- (c) Add the OG through the hole in the lid of the blender
- (d) Add the rest of the heated alcohol
- (e) Mix for 3 min. at medium speed
- (f) When the motor is turned off, the blades should be visible if the stain has completely gone into the solution. If not, the alcohol was probably not hot enough. Repeat the process and re-warm the alcohol and the orange G to boiling
- (g) Cool the OG and alcohol solution overnight
- (h) In the morning, filter the prepared solution of OG. There will be a slight precipitate since the stain is in excess
- (i) Add the phosphotungstic acid and the glacial acetic acid to the filtered OG solution
- (j) The OG working solution is then ready for use and is stable for 4–6 weeks. Store the excess working solution in amber colored bottles to prolong its stability

c. Eosin azure
(1) Ingredients
- (a) 95% ethyl alcohol   380 ml
- (b) Eosin Y   2.0 g (brown, maroon powder)
- (c) Light green SF yellowish 1.0 g
- (d) Phosphotungstic acid   0.4 g
- (e) Glacial acetic acid   3.0 ml

* Be sure that all the crystals are in solution before adding the next ingredient.

(2) Preparation
   (a) Pour a sufficient amount of 95% alcohol to cover the blades into the Waring blender glass container (marked for EA) and put on the lid (the alcohol is not heated for the EA)
   (b) Turn on the motor to 'slow'
   (c) Add the eosin and the light green stains
   (d) Add the remaining alcohol
   (e) Turn the motor to 'fast' for 3 min
   (f) Turn off the motor. Allow the solution to stand overnight. Do not filter. Seal the flask with paraffin film
   (g) The next day, add the phosphotungstic acid and the glacial acetic acid
   (h) The EA working solution is stable for 4–6 weeks if it is poured back into a dark bottle after use

Reference: Phar, S.L.; Wood, D.A.; Traut, H.F.: A simplified method of preparing EA and orange G stains for use in Papanicolaou staining procedure. Am. J. clin. Pathol. *24:* 239–242 (1954).

2. Care of the Papanicolaou staining run
   The length of time a stain is useable is dependent on many factors: number of slides, care taken in staining, etc.
   (a) Filter each dish daily
   (b) Each Friday the hematoxylin, the OG and the EA are stored in brown bottles and the dishes are washed
   (c) New stains are prepared every other month; at the beginning of each month new hematoxylin, new orange G and new eosin-azure are used
   (d) When the 70% alcohol becomes greenish yellow, throw it away
   (e) When the absolute alcohol (100%) becomes pink, throw it away
   (f) If the xylol becomes cloudy while staining, this probably indicates that there is water in the ½ and ½. Discard the ½ and ½ and thoroughly dry the dish or take a dry new dish. Make new ½ and ½. Discard the cloudy xylol

3. Papanicolaou staining procedure (UCLA modification)
   Remove slides from fixative (95% ethyl alcohol)

1.	70% ethanol	10 dips
2.	Distilled water	10 dips
3.	Mayer's hematoxylin	4 min
4.	Tap water (gentle stream of running tap water)	15 min
5.	70% ethanol	10 dips
6.	95% ethanol	10 dips
7.	Orange G	1 min
8.	95% ethanol	10 dips
9.	95% ethanol	10 dips
10.	Eosin azure	1.5 min
11.	95% ethanol	10 dips

   (avoid prolonged standing in alcohol washes which results in decolorization of both eosin and light green)

12.	95% ethanol	10 dips

Appendix: Preparatory and Staining Procedures

13.	Absolute ethanol	10 dips
14.	Absolute ethanol	10 dips
15.	Absolute ethanol:xylol (1:1)	1 min
16.	Xylol	10 dips
17.	Xylol	10 dips
18.	Xylol	10 dips
19.	Mount with permount	

B. May-Grünwald-Giemsa stain
1. MGG stain stock solutions
   a. Methyl alcohol–stock solution
   b. May-Grünwald–stock solution
   c. Giemsa 1:8 with Vol-U-Sol
2. MGG procedure

a.	Methyl alcohol	5 min
b.	May-Grünwald	10 min
c.	Running distilled water	rinse clear
d.	Giemsa	15 min
e.	Running distilled water	rinse clear

3. Care of MGG stain
   a. Methyl alcohol is changed daily
   b. May-Grünwald is changed daily
   c. Giemsa is prepared once in the early morning and then again between 2 and 3 p.m. in the afternoon

C. Modified Grocott's methenamine silver stain (GMS) for fungus and pneumocystis
   (used for both histologic and cytologic specimens)

1. Fixative: any fixative
2. Reagents
   a. 5% aqueous chromic acid
   b. 1% aqueous sodium bisulfite
   c. Methenamine silver solution
      (1) 35 ml   3% hexamethenamine
      (2) 2.5 ml   5% silver nitrate
      (3) 6 ml   5% borax
   d. 0.1% gold chloride
   e. 2% sodium thiosulfate
   f. Light green *stock* solution
      (1) Light green   0.2 g
      (2) Distilled water   100 ml
      (3) Acetic acid, concentration   0.2 ml
   g. Light green *working* solution
      (1) Light green stock   10 ml
      (2) Distilled water   50 ml

3. Procedure
    (a) Hydrate
    (b) Oxidize in 5% chromic acid   60 min
    (c) Wash in tap water   10 min
    (d) Remove residual chromic acid with 2% sodium thiosulfate
        (Hypo)   1 min
    (e) Wash in tap water
    (f) Rinse in distilled water   2 changes
    (g) Place in silver methenamine solution, 60 °C oven. Check control and slide microscopically for adequate impregnation every 15 min. Fungi and mucin will begin to stain yellowish brown in about 10 min
                                            15–60 min
    (h) Rinse in distilled water   4 changes
    (i) Tone in gold chloride
    (j) Rinse in distilled water
    (k) Remove unreduced silver by treating in 2% sodium thiosulfate (Hypo)
    (l) Wash in tap water
    (m) Counterstain with light green
    (n) Dehydrate starting in 95% ETOH
    (o) Mount with permount

4. Results
    Fungi and pneumocystis – sharply delineated in *black*
    Mucin – brownish grey
    Background – light green

References

1 Ahmed, M.N.; Feldman, M.; Seemayer, R.A.: Cytology of epithelioid sarcoma. Acta cytol. *18:* 459–461 (1974).
2 Aisner, J.; Aisner, S.C.; Ostrow, S.; Govindan, S.; Mummert, K.; Wiernik, O.: Meningeal carcinomatosis from small cell carcinoma of the lung. Acta cytol. *23:* 292–296 (1979).
3 Aisner, S.C.; Gupta, P.K.; Frost, J.K.: Sputum cytology in pulmonary sarcoidosis. Acta cytol. *21:* 394–398 (1977).
4 Allen, A.; Fullmer, C.: Primary diagnosis of pulmonary echinococcosis by the cytologic technique. Acta cytol. *16:* 212–216 (1972).
5 Anderson, R.J.; Johnston, W.W.; Szpak, C.A.: Fine needle aspiration of adenoid cystic carcinoma metastatic to the lung. Acta cytol. *29:* 527–532 (1985).
6 An-Foraker, S.; Haesaert, S.: Cytomegalic virus inclusion body in bronchial brushing material. Acta cytol. *21:* 181–182 (1977).
7 Auerbach, O.; Saccomanno, G.; Kuschner, M.; Brown, R.D.; Garfinkel, L.: Histologic findings in the tracheobronchial tree of uranium miners and non-miners with lung cancer. Cancer *42:* 483–489 (1978).
8 Ayres, S.M.: Cigarette smoking and lung diseases: an update. Resp. Care *21:* 632–640 (1976).
9 Baily, T.M.; Akhtar, M.; Ali, M.A.: Fine needle biopsy in the diagnosis of tuberculosis. Acta cytol. *29:* 732–736 (1985).
10 Baker, R.R.; Tockman, M.S.; Marsh, B.R.; Stitik, F.P.; Ball, W.C.; Eggleston, J.C.; Erozan, Y.; Levin, M.L.; Frost, J.K.: Screening for bronchogenic carcinoma. J. thorac. cardiovasc. Surg. *78:* 876–882 (1979).
11 Banks, D.E.; Castellan, R.M.; Hendrick, D.J.: Lymphocytic lymphoma recurring in multiple endobronchial sites. Thorax *35:* 796–797 (1980).
12 Bartlett, J.G.: Diagnosis of bacterial infections of the lung. Clin Chest Med. *8:* 119–134 (1987)
13 Battifora, H.: Recent progress in the immunohistochemistry of solid tumors. Semin. Diagn. Path. *1:* 251–271 (1984).
14 Bauer, T.W.; Erozan, Y.S.: Psammoma bodies in small cell carcinoma of the lung. A case report. Acta cytol. *26:* 327–330 (1982).
15 Baylin, S.B.: Ectopic production of hormones and other proteins by tumors. Hosp. Prac. *10:* 117–126 (1975).
16 Bedrossian, C.W.M.; Accetta, P.A.; Kelly, L.V.: Cytopathology of nonneoplastic pulmonary disease. Lab. Med. *14:* 86–95 (1983).
17 Bedrosian, C.W.M.; Corey, B.J.: Abnormal sputum cytopathology during chemotherapy with bleomycin. Acta cytol. *22:* 202–207 (1978).

18 Bell, W.R., Jr.; Johnston, W.W.; Bigner, S.H.: Cytologic diagnosis of occult small-cell undifferentiated carcinoma of the lung. Acta cytol. 26: 73–77 (1982).
19 Bender, B.L.; Cherock, M.A.; Sotos, S.N.: Effective use of bronchoscopy and sputa in the diagnosis of lung cancer. Diagn. Cytopathol. 1: 183–187 (1985).
20 Berlin, N.I.; Buncher, C.R.; Fontana, R.S.; Frost, J.K.; Melamed, M.R.: The National Cancer Institute Cooperative Early Lung Cancer Detection Program. Results of the initial screen (prevalence). Early lung cancer detection: Introduction. Am. Rev. resp. Dis. 130: 545–549 (1984).
21 Bewtra, C.; Dewan, N.; O'Donahue, W.J., Jr.: Exfoliative sputum cytology in pulmonary embolism. Acta cytol. 27: 489–496 (1983).
22 Bhatt, O.; Miller, R.; Le Riche, J.; King, E.: Aspiration biopsy in pulmonary opportunistic infections. Acta cytol. 21: 206–209 (1977).
23 Bibbo, M.; Fennessy, J.J.; Lu, C.-T.; Straus, F.H.; Variakojis, D.; Wied, G.L.: Bronchial brushing technique for the cytologic diagnosis of peripheral lung lesions. A review of 693 cases. Acta cytol. 17: 245–251 (1973).
24 Bienenstock, J.: Immunology of the lung and upper respiratory tract. (McGraw-Hill, New York 1964).
25 Blackmon, J.A.; Paris, A.L.: Infectious diseases of the lung. Lab. Med. 14: 77–85 (1983).
26 Bloom, W.; Fawcett, D.W.: A textbook of histology; 11th ed. (Saunders, Philadelphia 1986).
27 Bonfiglio, T.: Cytopathologic interpretation of transthoracic fine-needle biopsies (Masson, Paris 1983).
28 Broderick, P.A.; Corvese, N.L.; LaChance, T.; Allard, J.: Giant cell carcinoma of lung: A cytologic evaluation. Acta cytol. 19: 225–230 (1975).
29 Brown, S.E.S.; Kim, K.J.; Goodman, B.E.; Wells, J.R.; Crandall, E.D.: Sodium-amino acid cotransport by type II alveolar epithelial cells. J. appl. Physiol. 59: 1616–1622 (1985).
30 Buhaug, J.N.: Therapy induced atypias (TIA) of benign pulmonary cells. Common Probl. Cytol. 1: 1–18 (1983).
31 Carr, D.T.: Lung cancer. Curr. Pulmonol. 4: 129–139 (1982).
32 Carr, D.T.; Rosenow, E.C., III: Bronchogenic carcinoma. Basics RD 5: 92–97 (1977).
33 Castella, J.; de la Heras, P.; Puzo, C.; Martinez, C.; Lopez, A.; Cornudella, R.: Cytology of postbronchoscopically collected sputum samples and its diagnostic value. Respiration 42: 116–121 (1981).
34 Chalon, J.; Tang, C.-K.; Gorstein, F.; Turndorf, H.; Katz, J.S.; Klein, G.S.; Patel, C.: Diagnostic and prognostic significance of tracheobronchial epithelial multinucleation. Acta cytol. 22: 316–320 (1978).
35 Chaudhuri, B.; Nanos, S.: Disseminated Strongyloides stercoralis infestation detected by sputum cytology. Acta cytol. 24: 360–362 (1980).
36 Chen, K.T.K.: Cytology of tracheobronchial amyloidosis. Acta cytol. 28: 133–135 (1984).
37 Chopra, S.K.; Ben-Isaac, F.: Transbronchial lung biopsy using fiberoptic bronchoscope. Sth. med. J. 70: 302–304 (1977).
38 Chopra, S.K.; Genovesi, M.G.; Simmons, D.H.; Gothe, B.: Fiberoptic bronchoscopy in the diagnosis of lung cancer: Comparison of pre- and postbronchoscopy sputa, washings, brushings and biopsies. Acta cytol. 21: 524–527 (1977).

References

39 Chopra, S.K.; Simmons, D.H.; Cassan, S.M.; Becker, S.; Ben-Isaac, F.E.: Bronchial obstruction by incorporation of aspirated vegetable material in the bronchial wall. Am. Rev. resp. Dis. *112:* 717–720 (1975).

40 Chovil, A.C.: Occupational lung cancer and smoking. A review in the light of current theories of carcinogenesis. Can. med. Ass. J. *121:* 548–555 (1979).

41 Clayton, F.: Bronchioloalveolar carcinomas. Cell types, patterns of growth, and prognostic correlates. Cancer *57:* 1555–1564 (1986).

42 Collan, Y.; Sainio, P.: Relation of bacteria to exfoliated oral cells. An electron microscopy study. Acta cytol. *14:* 570–573 (1970).

43 Cooney, W.; Dzuira, B.; Harper, R.; Nash, G.: The cytology of sputum from thermally injured patients. Acta cytol. *16:* 433–437 (1972).

44 Costabel, U.; Matthys, H.; Guzman, J.; Freudenberg, N.: Multinucleated cells in bronchoalveolar lavage. Acta cytol. *29:* 189–190 (1985).

45 Coulson, W.F.: Surgical pathology; 2nd ed. (Lippincott, Philadelphia 1988).

46 Covell, J.L.; Feldman, P.S.: Fine needle aspiration diagnosis of aspiration pneumonia (phytopneumonitis). Acta cytol. *28:* 77–80 (1984).

47 Craig, I.D.; Shum, D.T.; Desrosiers, P.; McLeod, C.; Lefcoe, M.S.; Paterson, N.A.M.; Finley, R.J.; Woods, B.; Anderson, R.J.: Choriocarcinoma Metastatic to the Lung. A cytologic study with identification of human choriogonadotropin with an immunoperoxidase technique. Acta cytol. *27:* 647–650 (1983).

48 Csako, G.; Chandra, P.: Bronchioloalveolar carcinoma presenting with meningeal carcinomatosis. Cytologic diagnosis in cerebrospinal fluid. Acta cytol. *30:* 653–656 (1986).

49 D'Ablang III, G.; Bernard, B.; Zaharov, I.; Barton, L.; Kaplan, B.; Schwinn, C.P.: Neonatal pulmonary cytology and bronchopulmonary dysplasia. Acta cytol. *19:* 21–27 (1975).

50 Dahlgren, S.E.; Lind, B.: Comparison between diagnostic results obtained by transthoracic needle biopsy and by sputum cytology. Acta cytol. *16:* 53–58 (1972).

51 DeFine, L.A.; Saleba, K.P.; Gibson, B.B.; Wesseler, T.A.; Baughman, R.: Cytologic evaluation of bronchoalveolar lavage specimens in immunosuppressed patients with suspected opportunistic infections. Acta cytol. *31:* 235–242 (1987).

52 Delage, G.; Brochu, P.; Robillard, L.; Jasmin, G.; Joncas, J.H.; Lapointe, N.: Giant cell pneumonia due to respiratory syncytial virus. Occurrence in severe combined immunodeficiency syndrome. Archs Pathol. Lab. Med. *108:* 623–625 (1984).

53 Donaldson, J.C.; Kaminsky, D.B.; Elliot, R.C.: Bronchiolar carcinoma. Cancer *41:* 250–258 (1978).

54 Doshi, N.; Kanbour, A.; Fujikura, T.; Klionsky, B.: Tracheal aspiration cytology in neonates with respiratory distress. Histopathologic correlation. Acta cytol. *26:* 15–21 (1982).

55 Dupont, R.L.: Marijuana smoking. A national epidemic. Am. Lung Ass. Bull. *66:* 2–7 (1980).

56 Ebihara, Y.; Fukushima, N.; Asakuma, Y.: Double primary lung cancers. With special reference to their exfoliative cytology and to the rare, malignant 'mixed' tumor of the salivary-gland type. Acta cytol. *24:* 212–223 (1980).

57 Ebihara, Y.; Sagawa, H.: Mucin-producing bronchioloalveolar-cell carcinoma. With special reference to a characteristic structure revealed by phosphotungstic acid-hematoxylin staining. Acta cytol. *30:* 643–647 (1986).

58 Ehya, H.: Cytology of mesothelioma of the tunica vaginalis metastatic to the lung. Acta cytol. *29:* 79–84 (1985).
59 Emerson, G.; Phillips, C.; Bennett, J.M.; Rubin, P.: Lung cancer. chap. IX in Rubin, Clinical oncology for medical students and physicians, a multidisciplinary approach; 5th ed. (American Cancer Society, Washington 1978).
60 Enders, J.F.; McCarthy, K.; Mitus, A.; Cheatham, W.J.: Isolation of measles virus at autopsy in cases of giant cell pneumonia without rash. New Engl. J. Med. *261:* 875–881 (1959).
61 Erlandson, R.A.: Diagnostic immunohistochemistry of human tumors. An interim evaluation. Am. J. surg. Path. *8:* 615–624 (1984).
62 Erozan, Y.S.; Frost, J.K.: Cytopathologic diagnosis of cancer in pulmonary material: A critical histopathologic correlation. Acta cytol. *14:* 560–565 (1970).
63 Farley, M.L.; Greenberg, S.D.; Shuford, E.H., Jr.; Hurst, G.A.; Spivey, C.G.; Christianson, C.S.: Ferruginous bodies in sputa of former asbestos workers. Acta cytol. *21:* 693–700 (1977).
64 Farley, M.L.; Mabry, L.; Munoz, L.A.; Diserens, H.W.: Crystals occurring in pulmonary cytology specimens. Association with Aspergillus infection. Acta cytol. *29:* 737–744 (1985).
65 Flehinger, B.J.; Melamed, M.R.; Zaman, M.B.; Heelan, R.T.; Perchick, W.B.; Matini, N.: Early lung cancer detection. Results of the initial (prevalence) radiologic and cytologic screening in the Memorial Sloan-Kettering study. Am. Rev. resp. Dis. *130:* 555–560 (1984).
66 Fleury, J.; Escudier, A.; Pocholle, M.-J.; Carre, C.; Bernaudin, J.F.: Cell population obtained by bronchoalveolar lavage in *Pneumocystis carinii* pneumonitis. Acta cytol. *29:* 721–726 (1985).
67 Fontana, R.S.: Screening for lung cancer; in Miller, Screening for cancer, pp. 377–395 (Academic Press, New York 1985).
68 Fontana, R.S.; Sanderson, D.R.; Miller, W.E.; Woolner, L.B.; Taylor, W.F.; Uhlenhopp, M.A.: The Mayo lung project: preliminary report of 'early cancer detection' phase. Cancer *30:* 1373–1382 (1972).
69 Fontana, R.S.; Sanderson, D.R.; Taylor, W.F.; Woolner, L.B.; Miller, W.E.; Muhm, J.R.; Uhlenhopp, M.A.: Early lung cancer detection: Results of the initial (prevalence) radiologic and cytologic screening in the Mayo Clinic study. Am. Rev. resp. Dis. *130:* 561–565 (1984).
70 Frable, W.J.: The relationship of pulmonary cytology to survival in lung cancer. Acta cytol. *12:* 52–56 (1968).
71 Frable, W.; Frable, M.; Seney, F., Jr.: Virus infections of the respiratory tract. Acta cytol. *21:* 32–36 (1977).
72 Frable, W.; Kay, S.: Herpesvirus infection of the respiratory tract: Electronmicroscopic observation of the virus in cells obtained from a sputum cytology. Acta cytol. *21:* 391–393 (1977).
73 Francis, D.; Borgeskov, S.: Progress in preoperative diagnosis of pulmonary lesions. Acta cytol. *19:* 231–234 (1975).
74 Frost, J.K.; Ball, W.C.; Levin, M.L.; Tockman, M.S.; Baker, R.R.; Carter, D.; Eggleston, J.C.; Erozan, Y.S.; Gupta, P.K.; Khouri, N.F.; Marsh, B.R.; Stitik, F.P.: Early lung cancer detection: Results of the initial (prevalence) radiologic and cytologic screening in the Johns Hopkins study. Am. Rev. resp. Dis. *130:* 549–554 (1984).

75 Frost, J.K.; Ball, W.C.; Levin, M.L.; Tockman, M.S.; Erozan, Y.S.; Gupta, P.K.; Eggleston, J.C.; Pressman, N.J.; Donithan, M.P.; Kimball, A.W.: Sputum cytopathology. Use and potential in monitoring the workplace environment by screening for biological effects of exposure. J. occup. Med. *28:* 692–703 (1986).

76 Frost, J.K.; Fontana, R.S.; Melamed, M.R.; Buncher, C.R.; Berlin, N.I.: Early lung cancer detection. Summary and conclusions. Early lung cancer cooperative study. Am. Rev. resp. Dis. *130:* 565–570 (1984).

77 Gagneten, C.B.; Geller, C.E.; del Carmen Saenz, M.: Diagnosis of Bronchogenic carcinoma through the cytologic examination of sputum, with special reference to tumor typing. Acta cytol. *20:* 530–536 (1976).

78 Gal, A.A.; Koss, M.N.; Hawkins, J.; Evans, S.; Einstein, H.: The pathology of pulmonary cryptococcal infections in the acquired immunodeficiency syndrome. Archs Pathol. Lab. Med. *110:* 502–507 (1986).

79 Gallagher, C.J.; Knowles, G.K.; Habeshaw, J.A.; Green, M.; Malpas, J.S.; Lister, T.A.: Early involvement of the bronchi in patients with malignant lymphoma. Br. J. Cancer *48:* 777–781 (1983).

80 Gephardt, G.N.; Belovich, D.M.: Cytology of pulmonary carcinoid tumors. Acta cytol. *26:* 434–438 (1982).

81 Gleason, T.H.; Hammar, S.P.; Barthas, M.; Kasprisin, M.; Bockus, D.: Cytological diagnosis of pulmonary cryptococcosis. Archs Pathol. Lab. Med. *104:* 384–387 (1980).

82 Goldstein, J.; Leslie, H.: Immunoblastic lymphadenopathy with pulmonary lesions and positive sputum cytology. Acta cytol. *22:* 165–167 (1978).

83 Gould, V.E.: Histogenesis and differentiation. A re-evaluation of these concepts as criteria for the classification of tumors. Human Pathol. *17:* 212–215 (1986).

84 Granberg, I.; Willems, J.S.: Endometriosis of lung and pleura diagnosed by aspiration biopsy. Acta cytol. *21:* 295–297 (1977).

85 Greaves, T.S.; Stigle, S.M.: The recognition of *Pneumocystis carinii* in routine Papanicolaou-stained smears. Acta cytol. *29:* 714–720 (1985).

86 Gupta, P.K.; Verma, K.: Calcified (psammoma) bodies in alveolar cell carcinoma of the lung. Acta cytol. *16:* 59–62 (1972).

87 Gupta, R.K.: Value of sputum cytology in the diagnosis and typing of bronchogenic carcinomas, excluding adenocarcinomas. Acta cytol. *26:* 645–648 (1982).

88 Gupta, R.K.: Diagnosis of unsuspected pulmonary cryptococcosis with sputum cytology. Acta cytol. *29:* 154–156 (1985).

89 Hammar, S.P.; Bolen, J.W.; Bockus, D.; Remington, F.; Friedman, S.: Ultrastructural and immunohistochemical features of common lung tumors. An overview. Ultrastruct. Pathol. *9:* 283–318 (1985).

90 Hattori, S.; Matsuda, M.; Nishihara, H.; Horai, T.: Early diagnosis of small peripheral lung cancer. Cytologic diagnosis of very fresh cancer cells obtained by the TV-brushing technique. Acta cytol. *15:* 460–467 (1971).

91 Hattori, S.; Matsuda, M.; Sugiyama, T.; Matsuda, H.: Cytologic diagnosis of early lung cancer: Brushing method under X-ray television fluoroscopy. Dis. Chest *45:* 129–142 (1964).

92 Hawkins, A.G.; Hsiu, J.-G.; Smith, R.M., III; Stitik, F.P.; Siddiky, M.A.; Edwards, O.E.: Pulmonary dirofilariasis diagnosed by fine needle aspiration biopsy. A case report. Acta cytol. *29:* 19–22 (1985).

93 Hayata, Y.: Lung cancer diagnosis (Igaku-Shoin, Tokyo 1982).
94 Hayata, Y.; Kato, H.; Konaka, C.; Ono, J.; Matsushima, Y.; Yoneyama, K.; Nishimiya, K.: Fiberoptic bronchoscopic laser photoradiation for tumor localization in lung cancer. Chest 82: 10-14 (1982).
95 Hayata, Y.; Oho, K.; Ichiba, M.; Goya, Y.; Hayashi, T.: Percutaneous pulmonary puncture for cytologic diagnosis. Its diagnostic value for small peripheral pulmonary carcinoma. Acta cytol. 17: 469-475 (1973).
96 Hellberg, D.; Valentin, J.; Nilsson, S.: Smoking and cervical intraepithelial neoplasia. An association independent of sexual and other risk factors? Acta obstet. gynec. scand. 65: 625-631 (1986).
97 Hilborne, L.H.; Nieberg, R.K.; Cheng, L.; Lewin, K.J.: Direct in-situ hybridization for rapid detection of cytomegalovirus in bronchoalveolar lavage. Am. J. clin. Path. 87: 766-769 (1987).
98 Hoffman, P.C.; Albain, K.S.; Bitran, J.D.; Golomb, H.M.: Current concepts in small cell carcinoma of the lung. CA Cancer J. Clinicians 34: 269-281 (1984).
99 Horai, T.; Sone, H.; Takenaga, A.; Ikegami, H.; Matsuda, M.; Hattori, S.: Cytologic characteristics of oat-cell carcinoma of the lung in relation to the effect of chemotherapy. Cancer 47: 22-26 (1981).
100 Horsley, J.R.; Miller, R.E.; Amy, R.W.M.; King, E.G.: Bronchial submucosal needle aspiration performed through the fiberoptic bronchoscope. Acta cytol. 28: 211-217 (1984).
101 Humphreys, K.; Hieger, L.: Strongyloides stercoralis in routine Papanicolaou-stained sputum smears. Acta cytol. 236: 471-476 (1979).
102 Hunninghake, G.W.; Gadek, J.E.; Kawanami, O.; Ferrans, V.J.; Crystal, R.G.: Inflammatory and immune processes in the human lung in health and disease: Evaluation by bronchoalveolar lavage. Am. J. Path. 97: 149-198 (1979).
103 Ikeda, S.: Flexible bronchofiberscope. Ann. Otol. Rhinol. Lar. 79: 916-923 (1970).
104 Ives, J.C.; Buffler, P.A.; Greenberg, S.D.: Environmental associations and histopathologic patterns of carcinoma of the lung. The challenge and dilemma in epidemiologic studies. Am. Rev. resp. Dis. 128: 195-209 (1983).
105 Jain, U.; Mani, K.; Frable, W.: Cytomegalic inclusion disease. Cytologic diagnosis from bronchial brushing material. Acta cytol. 17: 467-468 (1973).
106 Jay, S.J.; Wehr, K.; Nicholson, D.P.: Smith, A.L.: Diagnostic sensitivity and specificity of pulmonary cytology. Comparison of techniques used in conjunction with flexible fiber optic bronchoscopy. Acta cytol. 24: 304-312 (1980).
107 Jenkins, P.F.; Ward, M.J.; Davies, P.; Fletcher, J.: Non-Hodgkin's lymphoma, chronic lymphatic leukaemia and the lung. Br. J. Dis. Chest 75: 22-30 (1981).
108 Johnston, W.: Ten years of respiratory cytology at Duke University Medical Center III. The significance of inconclusive cytopathologic diagnoses during the years 1970 to 1974. Acta cytol. 26: 759-766 (1982).
109 Johnston, W.: The cytopathology of opportunistic infection of the lungs and other body sites; in Compendium on diagnostic cytology; 5th ed., pp. 282-294 (Tutorials of Cytology, Chicago 1983).
110 Johnston, W.: Percutaneous fine needle aspiration biopsy of the lung. A study of 1,015 patients. Acta cytol. 28: 218-224 (1984).
111 Johnston, W.; Amatull, J.: The role of cytology in the primary diagnosis of North American blastomycosis. Acta cytol. 14: 200-204 (1970).

112 Johnston, W.; Bossen, E.H.: Ten years of respiratory cytology at Duke University Medical Center. I. The cytopathologic diagnosis of lung cancer during the years 1970 to 1974, noting the significance of specimen number and type. Acta cytol. *25:* 103–107 (1981).

113 Johnston, W.; Bossen, E.H.: Ten years of respiratory cytology at Duke University Medical Center II. The cytopathologic diagnosis of lung cancer during the years 1970 to 1974, with a comparison between cytopathology and histopathology in the typing of lung cancer. Acta cytol. *25:* 499–505 (1981).

114 Johnston, W.W.; Frable, W.J.: The cytopathology of the respiratory tract. A review. Am. J. Path. *84:* 372–413 (1976).

115 Johnston, W.R.; Frable, W.J.: Diagnostic respiratory cytopathology (Masson, Paris 1979).

116 Kanhouwa, S.B.; Matthews, M.J.: Reliability of cytologic typing of lung cancer. Acta cytol. *20:* 229–232 (1976).

117 Kato, H.; Konaka, C.; Hayata, Y.; Ono, J.; Iimura, I.; Matsushima, Y.; Tahara, M.; Lei, J.; Nasiell, M.; Auer, G.: Lung cancer histogenesis following in vivo bronchial injections of 20-methylcholanthrene in dogs; in Recent results in cancer research, vol. 82, pp. 69–86 (Springer, Berlin 1982).

118 Kato, H.; Konaka, C.; Ono, J.; Takahashi, M.; Hayata, Y.: Cytology of the lung. Techniques and interpretation (Igaku-Shoin, Tokyo 1983).

119 Kato, H.; Nishimiya, K.; Lay, J.; Ono, J.; Yoneyama, K.; Kawate, N.; Iimura, I.; Hayashi, T.; Iwahashi, H.; Kawamura, I.; Hayata, Y.: Transbronchial needle aspiration biopsy via fiberoptic bronchoscope; in Nakhosteen, Proceedings of the Second World Congress for Bronchology, 2–4 June 1980, pp. 307–309. Bronchology: research, diagnostic and therapeutic aspects (Martinus Nijhoff, The Hague 1981).

120 Kato, H.; Ono, J.; Niizuma, M.; Seo, Y.; Konaka, C.; Hayashi, N.; Kawamura, I.; Oho, K.; Hayata, Y.: Transbronchofiberscopic aspiration biopsy using a special catheter. Jap. J. thorac. Dis. *16:* 774–780 (1978).

121 Katzenstein, A.; Askin, F.: Surgical pathology of non-neoplastic lung disease. Major problems in pathology, No. 13 (Saunders, Philadelphia 1982).

122 Kenney, M.; Webber, C.: Diagnosis of strongyloidiasis on Papanicolaou stained sputum smears. Acta cytol. *18:* 270–273 (1974).

123 Kern, W.H.; Schweizer, C.W.: Sputum cytology of metastatic carcinoma of the lung. Acta cytol. *20:* 514–520 (1976).

124 Kilburn, K.H.: Medical screening for lung cancer: perspective and strategy. J. occup. Med. *28:* 714–718 (1986).

125 Kim, K.; Naylor, B.; Han, I.H.. Fine needle aspiration cytology of sarcomas metastatic to the lung. Acta cytol. *30:* 688–694 (1986).

126 Kleinerman, J.: Pathology standards for coal workers' pneumonconiosis. Archs Pathol. Lab. Med. *103:* 375–432 (1979).

127 Koizumi, J.; Hidvegi, D.: Seaweed *(Undaria pinnatifida)* mimicking fungus. Acta cytol. *25:* 198–199 (1981).

128 Konaka, C.; Auer, G.; Nasiell, M.; Hayata, Y.; Kato, H.; Caspersson, T.; Ono, J.: Sequential cytomorphological and cytochemical changes during development of bronchial carcinoma in beagle dogs exposed to 20-methylcholanthrene. Acta histochem. *15:* 779–797 (1982).

129 Konaka, C.; Auer, G.; Nasiell, M.; Kato, H.; Hayashi, N.; Ono, J.; Hayata, Y.; Cas-

persson, T.: Pathogenesis of squamous bronchial carcinoma in 20-methylcholanthrene-treated beagle dogs. Analyt. Quant. Cytol. *4:* 61–71 (1982).
130 Koss, L.G.: Diagnostic cytology and its histopathologic bases; 3rd ed., pp. 544–686, 1069–1075 (Lippincott, Philadelphia 1979).
131 Koss, L.G.: Aspiration biopsy. Cytologic interpretation and histologic bases, pp. 287–330 (Igaku-Shoin, Tokyo 1984).
132 Koss, L.G.; Melamed, M.R.; Goodner, J.T.: Pulmonary cytology. A brief survey of diagnostic results from July 1st, 1952 until December 31st, 1960. Symposium on Diagnostic Accuracy of Cytology Technics. Acta cytol. *8:* 104–113 (1964).
133 Krauss, S.; Macy, S.; Ichiki, A.T.: A study of immunoreactive calcitonin (CT) adrenocorticotropic hormone (ACTH) and carcinoembryonic antigen (CEA) in lung cancer and other malignancies. Cancer *47:* 2485–2492 (1981).
134 Lambird, P.A.; Ashton, P.R.: Exfoliative cytopathology of a primary pulmonary malignant histiocytoma. Acta cytol. *14:* 83–86 (1970).
135 Lange, E.; Høeg, K.: Cytologic typing of lung cancer. Acta cytol. *16:* 327–330 (1972).
136 Lavoie, R.R.; McDonald, J.R.; Kling, G.A.: Cavitation in squamous carcinoma of the lung. Acta cytol. *21:* 210–214 (1977).
137 Lazzari, G.; Vineis, C.; Cugini, A.: Cytologic diagnosis of primary pulmonary actinomycosis. Acta cytol. *25:* 299–301 (1981).
138 Lillington, G.A.: The utility of needle aspiration biopsy of the lung. Mayo Clin. Proc. *55:* 516–517 (1980).
139 Linsk, J.A.; Franzen, S.: Clinical aspiration cytology, pp. 139–167 (Lippincott, Philadelphia 1983).
140 Lozowski, M.S.; Mishriki, Y.Y.; Epstein, H.: Metastatic malignant fibrous histiocytoma in lung examined by fine needle aspiration. Case report and literature review. Acta cytol. *24:* 350–354 (1980).
141 Lozowski, M.S.; Mishriki, Y.; Solitaire, G.B.: Cytopathologic features of adenoid cystic carcinoma. Case report and literature review. Acta cytol. *27:* 317–322 (1983).
142 Lozowski, W.; Hajdu, S.I.; Melamed, M.R.: Cytomorphology of carcinoid tumors. Acta cytol. *23:* 360–365 (1979).
143 Ludwig, M.E.; Otis, R.D.; Cole, S.R.; Westcott, J.L.: Fine needle aspiration cytology of pulmonary hamartomas. Acta cytol. *26:* 671–677 (1982).
144 Ludwig, R.A.; Balachandran, I.: Mycosis fungoides. The importance of pulmonary cytology in the diagnosis of a case with systemic involvement. Acta cytol. *27:* 198–201 (1983).
145 Lundgren, R.: A flexible thin needle for transbronchial aspiration biopsy through the flexible fiberoptic bronchoscope. Endoscopy *12:* 180–182 (1980).
146 Marchevsky, A.; Nieburgs, H.E.; Olenko, E.; Kirschner, P.; Teirstein, A.; Kleinerman, J.: Pulmonary tumorlets in cases of 'tuberculoma' of the lung with malignant cells in brush biopsy. Acta cytol. *26:* 491–494 (1982).
147 Markowitz, S.; Leiman, G.: Cytologic detection of *Pneumocystis carinii* by ultraviolet light examination of Papanicolaou-stained sputum specimens. Acta cytol. *30:* 79–80 (1986).
148 McTighe, A.H.: Association of Kaposi's sarcoma and opportunistic infections in homosexuals. Lab. Med. *13:* 633–636 (1982).

References

149 Melamed, M.R.; Flehinger, B.J.; Zaman, M.B.; Heelan, R.T.; Perchick, W.A.; Martini, N.: Screening for early lung cancer. Results of the Memorial Sloan-Kettering study in New York. Chest 86: 44–53 (1984).

150 Melamed, M.R.; Koss, L.G.; Cliffton, E.E.: Roentgenologically occult lung cancer diagnosed by cytology. Report of 12 cases. Cancer 16: 1537–1551 (1963).

151 Melamed, M.R.; Zaman, M.B.; Flehinger, B.J.; Martini, N.: Radiologically occult in situ and incipient invasive epidermoid lung cancer. Am. J. surg. Path. 1: 5–16 (1977).

152 Mennemeyer, R.; Hammar, S.P.; Bauermeister, D.E.; Wheelis, R.F.; Jones, H.W.; Bartha, M.: Cytologic, histologic and electron microscopic correlations in poorly differentiated primary lung carcinoma. A study of 43 cases. Acta cytol. 23: 297–302 (1979).

153 Michel, R.P.; Lushpihan, A.; Ahmed, M.N.: Pathologic findings of transthoracic needle aspiration in the diagnosis of localized pulmonary lesions. Cancer 51: 1663–1672 (1983).

154 Mitchell, M.L.; King, D.E.; Bonfiglio, T.A.; Patten, S.F., Jr.: Pulmonary fine needle aspiration cytopathology. Acta cytol. 28: 72–76 (1984).

155 Mitchell, M.L.; Ryan, F.P., Jr.; Shermer, R.W.: Pulmonary adenocarcinoma metastatic to the adrenal gland mimicking normal adrenal cortical epithelium on fine needle aspiration. Acta cytol. 29: 994–998 (1985).

156 Miyamoto, H.; Inoue, S.; Abe, S.; Murao, M.; Yasuda, S.; Sakai, E.: Relationship between cytomorphologic features and prognosis in small-cell carcinoma of the lung. Acta cytol. 26: 429–433 (1982).

157 Modin, B.E.; Greenberg, S.D.; Buffler, P.A.; Lockhart, J.A.; Seitzman, L.H.; Awe, R.J.: Asbestos bodies in a general hospital/clinic population. Acta cytol. 26: 667–670 (1982).

158 Moloo, Z.; Finley, R.J.; Lefcoe, M.S.; Turner-Smith, L.; Craig, I.D.: Possible spread of bronchogenic carcinoma to the chest wall after a transthoracic fine needle aspiration biopsy. A case report. Acta cytol. 29: 167–169 (1985).

159 Murray, J.F.; Felton, C.P.; Garay, S.M.; Gottlieb, M.S.; Hopewell, P.C.; Stover, D.E.; Teirstein, A.S.: Pulmonary complications of the acquired immunodeficiency syndrome. Report of a National Heart, Lung, and Blood Institute workshop. New Engl. J. Med. 310: 1682–1688 (1984).

160 Mylius, E.A.; Gullvag, B.: Alveolar macrophage count as an indicator of lung reaction to industrial air pollution. Acta cytol. 30: 157–162 (1986).

161 Nash, G.: The diagnosis of lung cancer in the 80s. Will routine light microscopy suffice? Human Pathol. 14: 1021–1023 (1983).

162 Nasiell, M.: Diagnosis of lung cancer by aspiration biopsy and a comparison between this method and exfoliative cytology. Acta cytol. 11: 114–119 (1967).

163 Nasiell, M.; Roger, V.; Nasiell, K.; Enstad, I.; Vogel, B.; Bisther, A.: Cytologic findings indicating pulmonary tuberculosis. Part I. Acta cytol. 16: 146–151 (1972).

164 Nasiell, M.; Sinner, W.; Tornvall, G.; Roger, V.; Vogel, B.; Enstad, I.: Clinically occult lung cancer with positive sputum cytology and primarily negative radiological findings. Scand. J. resp. Dis. 58: 134–144 (1977).

165 Nathanson, L.; Hall, T.C.: Lung tumors. How they produce their syndromes. Ann. N.Y. Acad. Sci. VII: 367–377 (1974).

166 National Cancer Institute; National Institutes of Health; US Department of Health and Human Services: Atlas of early lung cancer (Igaku-Shoin, Tokyo 1983).
167 Naylor, B.: The shedding of the mucosa of the bronchial tree in asthma. Thorax *17:* 69–72 (1962).
168 Naylor, B.; Railey, C.: A pitfall in the cytodiagnosis of sputum of asthmatics. J. clin. Path. *17:* 84–89 (1964).
169 Ng, A.B.P.; Horak, G.C.: Factors significant in the diagnostic accuracy of lung cytology in bronchial washing and sputum samples. I. Bronchial washings. Acta cytol. *27:* 391–396 (1983).
170 Ng, A.B.P.; Horak, G.C.: Factors significant in the diagnostic accuracy of lung cytology in bronchial washing and sputum samples. II. Sputum samples. Acta cytol. *27:* 397–402 (1983).
171 Nguyen, G.-K.; Jeannot, A.: Cytopathologic aspects of pulmonary metastasis of malignant fibrous histiocytoma, myxoid variant. Fine needle aspiration biopsy of a case. Acta cytol. *26:* 349–353 (1982).
172 Nickels, J.; Koivuniemi, A.: Cytology of malignant hemangiopericytoma. Acta cytol. *23:* 119–125 (1979).
173 Nieberg, R.K.: Fine needle aspiration cytology of alveolar soft-part sarcoma. A case report. Acta cytol. *28:* 198–202 (1984).
174 Nieberg, R.K.; Gong, H., Jr.: Diagnosis of *Pneumocystis carinii* pneumonia by bronchoalveolar lavage in patients with the acquired immunodeficiency syndrome. Am. clin. Products Rev. *6:* 28–31 (1987).
175 Non, D.P., Jr.; Lang, W.R.; Patchefsky, A.; Takeda, M.: Pulmonary blastoma. Cytopathologic and histopathologic findings. Acta cytol. *20:* 381–386 (1976).
176 Nordenström, B.E.W.: Technical aspects of obtaining cellular material from lesions deep in the lung. A radiologist's view and description of the screwneedle sampling technique. Acta cytol. *28:* 233–242 (1984).
177 Nutting, S.; Carr, I.; Cole, F.M.; Black, L.L.: Solitary pulmonary nodules due to sarcoidosis. Can. J. Surg. *22:* 584–586 (1979).
178 Oho, K.: Transbronchial needle aspiration biopsy (TBAB) (Needle aspiration biopsy via the fiberoptic bronchoscope); in Sinner, Needle biopsy and transbronchial biopsy, chap. 23, pp. 118–122 (Thieme, Stuttgart 1982).
179 Oho, K.; Kato, H.; Ogawa, I.; Hayashi, N.; Hayata, Y.: A new needle for transfiberoptic bronchoscopic use. Chest *76:* 492 (1979).
180 Orenstein, M.; Weber, C.A.; Heurich, A.E.: Cytologic diagnosis of *Pneumocystis carinii* infection by bronchoalveolar lavage in acquired immune deficiency syndrome. Acta cytol. *29:* 727–731 (1985).
181 Osborn, P.T.; Giltman, L.I.; Uthman, E.O.: Trichomonads in the respiratory tract: A case report and literature review. Acta cytol. *28:* 136–138 (1984).
182 Papanicolaou, G.N.: Degenerative changes in ciliated cells exfoliating from the bronchial epithelium as a cytologic criterion in the diagnosis of diseases of the lung. N.Y. St. J. Med. *56:* 2647–2650 (1956).
183 Pearse, A.G.E.: The cytochemistry and ultrastructure of polypeptide hormone-producing cells of the APUD series and the embryologic, physiologic and pathologic implications of the concept. J. Histochem. Cytochem. *17:* 303–313 (1969).
184 Pearse, A.G.E.; Polak, J.M.: Endocrine tumours of neural crest origin. Neurolophomas, apudomas and the APUD concept. Med. Biol. *52:* 3–18 (1974).

185 Pedersen, B.; Brøns, M.; Holm, K.; Pedersen, D.; Lund, C.: The value of provoked expectoration in obtaining sputum samples for cytologic investigation. A prospective, consecutive and controlled investigation of 134 patients. Acta cytol. 29: 750–752 (1985).
186 Pilotti, S.; Rilke, F.; Gribaudi, G.; Damascelli, B.: Fine needle aspiration biopsy cytology of primary and metastatic pulmonary tumors. Acta cytol. 26: 661–666 (1982).
187 Pilotti, S.; Rilke, F.; Gribaudi, G.; Damascelli, B.; Ravasi, G.: Transthoracic fine needle aspiration biopsy in pulmonary lesions. Updated results. Acta cytol. 28: 225–232 (1984).
188 Pilotti, S.; Rilke, F.; Gribaudi, G.; Ravasi, G.L.: Sputum cytology for the diagnosis of carcinoma of the lung. Acta cytol. 26: 649–654 (1982).
189 Pilotti, S.; Rilke, F.; Gribaudi, G.; Spinelli, P.: Cytologic diagnosis of pulmonary carcinoma on bronchoscopic brushing material. Acta cytol. 26: 655–660 (1982).
190 Pilotti, S.; Rilke, F.; Lombardi, L.: Pulmonary carcinoid with glandular features. Report of two cases with positive fine needle aspiration biopsy cytology. Acta cytol. 27: 511–514 (1983).
191 Pintozzi, R.; Blecka, L.; Nanos, S.: The morphologic identification of *Pneumocystis carinii*. Acta cytol. 23: 35–39 (1979).
192 Plamenac, P.; Nikulin, A.; Kahvic, M.: Cytology of the respiratory tract in advanced age. Acta cytol. 14: 526–530 (1970).
193 Plamenac, P.; Nikulin, A.; Pikula, B.: Cytology of the respiratory tract in former smokers. Acta cytol. 16: 256–260 (1972).
194 Plamenac, P.; Nikulin, A.; Pikula, B.; Vujanic, G.: Cytologic changes of the respiratory tract as a consequence of air pollution and smoking. Acta cytol. 23: 449–453 (1979).
195 Pontiflex, A.H.; Roberts, F.J.: Fine needle aspiration biopsy cytology in the diagnosis of inflammatory lesions. Acta cytol. 29: 979–982 (1985).
196 Prolla, J.; Rosa, U.; Xavier, R.: The detection of cryptococcus neoformans in sputum cytology. Report of one case. Acta cytol. 14: 87–91 (1970).
197 Ramzy, I.: Pulmonary hamartomas. Cytologic appearances of fine needle aspiration biopsy. Acta cytol. 20: 15–19 (1976).
198 Ramzy, I.; Geraghty, R.; Lefcoe, M.S.; Lefcoe, N.M.: Chronic eosinophilic pneumonia. Diagnosis by fine needle aspiration. Acta cytol. 22: 366–369 (1978).
199 Reale, F.R.; Variakojis, D.; Compton, J.; Bibbo, M.: Cytodiagnosis of Hodgkin's disease in sputum specimens. Acta cytol. 27: 258–261 (1983)
200 Recalde, A.L.; Nickerson, B.G.; Vegas, M.; Scott, C.B.; Landing, B.H.; Warburton, D.: Lipid-laden macrophages in tracheal aspirates of newborn infants receiving intravenous lipid infusions. A cytologic study. Pediat. Pathol. 2: 25–34 (1984).
201 Reyes, C.V.; Kathuria, S.; MacGlashan, A.: Diagnostic value of calcium oxalate crystals in respiratory and pleural fluid cytology. A case report. Acta cytol. 23: 65–68 (1979).
202 Risse, E.K.J.; van't Hof, M.A.; Laurini, R.N.; Vooijs, P.G.: Sputum cytology by the Saccomanno method in diagnosing lung malignancy. Diagn. Cytopath. 1: 286–291 (1985).
203 Risse, E.K.J.; van't Hof, M.A.; Vooijs, P.G.: Relationship between patient character-

istics and the sputum cytologic diagnosis of lung cancer. Acta cytol. *31:* 159–165 (1987).
204 Risse, E.K.J.; Vooijs, P.G.; van't Hof, M.A.: The quality and diagnostic outcome of postbronchoscopic sputum. Acta cytol. *31:* 166–169 (1987).
205 Risse, E.K.J.; Vooijs, P.G.; van't Hof, M.A.: Relationship between the cellular composition of sputum and the cytologic diagnosis of lung cancer. Acta cytol. *31:* 170–176 (1987).
206 Roger, V.; Nasiell, M.; Linden, M.; Enstad, I.: Cytologic differential diagnosis of bronchiolo-alveolar carcinoma and bronchogenic adenocarcinoma. Acta cytol. *20:* 303–307 (1976).
207 Roger, V.; Nasiell, M.; Nasiell, K.; Hjerpe, A.; Enstad, I.; Bisther, A.: Cytologic findings indicating pulmonary tuberculosis. II. The occurrence in sputum of epithelioid cells and multinucleated giant cells in pulmonary tuberculosis, chronic non-tuberculous inflammatory lung disease and bronchogenic carcinoma. Acta cytol. *16:* 538–542 (1972).
208 Roggli, V.L.; Greenberg, S.D.; McLarty, J.W.; Hurst, G.A.; Heiger, L.R.; Farley, M.L.; Mabry, L.C.: Comparison of sputum and lung asbestos body counts in former asbestos workers. Am. Rev. resp. Dis. *122:* 941–945 (1980).
209 Roggli, V.L.; Vollmer, R.T.; Greenberg, S.D.; McGavran, M.H.; Spjut, H.J.; Yesner, R.: Lung cancer heterogeneity. A blinded and randomized study of 100 consecutive cases. Human Pathol. *16:* 569–579 (1985).
210 Rorat, E.; Garcia, R.L.; Skolom, J.: Diagnosis of *Pneumocystis carinii* pneumonia by cytologic examination of bronchial washings. J. Am. med. Ass. *254:* 1950–1951 (1985).
211 Rosen, P.; Melamed, M.; Savino, A.: The 'ferruginous body' content of lung tissue. A quantitative study of eighty-six patients. Acta cytol. *16:* 207–211 (1972).
212 Rosen, S.E.; Vonderheid, E.C.; Koprowska, I.: Mycosis fungoides with pulmonary involvement. Cytopathologic findings. Acta cytol. *28:* 51–57 (1984).
213 Rosenberg, M.; Rachman, R.: *Entameba gingivalis* in sputum. Its distinction from *Entameba histolytica.* Acta cytol. *14:* 361–362 (1970).
214 Rosenthal, D.L.: Cytology in the diagnosis of benign lung diseases. Clins Chest Med. *8:* 147–159 (1987).
215 Rosenthal, D.L.; Wallace, J.M.: Fine needle aspiration of pulmonary lesions via fiberoptic bronchoscopy. Acta cytol. *28:* 203–210 (1984).
216 Saba, S.R.; Espinoza, C.G.; Richman, A.V.; Azar, H.A.: Carcinomas of the lung. An ultrastructural and immunocytochemical study. Am. J. clin. Path. *80:* 6–13 (1983).
217 Saccomanno, G.: Diagnostic pulmonary cytology; 2nd ed. (American Society of Clinical Pathologists Press, Chicago 1986).
218 Saccomanno, G.; Archer, V.E.; Auerbach, O.; Saunders, R.P.; Brennan, L.M.: Development of carcinoma of the lung as reflected in exfoliated cells. Cancer *33:* 256–270 (1974).
219 Saccomanno, G.; Bechtel, J.J.; Kelley, W.A.: Transbronchial fine needle aspiration cytology of lung tumors. Acta cytol. *27:* 556 (1983).
220 Saccomanno, G.; Moran, P.G.; Schmidt, R.D.; Hartshorn D.F.; Brian, D.A.; Dreher, W.H.; Sowada, B.J.: Effects of 13-CIS retinoids on premalignant and malignant cells of lung origin. Acta cytol. *26:* 78–85 (1982).

221 Saccomanno, G.; Saunders, R.P.; Archer, V.E.; Auerbach, O.; Kuschner, M.; Beckler, P.A.: Cancer of the lung: the cytology of sputum prior to the development of carcinoma. Acta cytol. 9: 413–423 (1965).
222 Saccomanno, G.; Saunders, R.P.; Klein, M.G.; Archer, V.E.; Brennan, L.: Cytology of the lung in reference to irritant, individual sensitivity and healing. Acta cytol. 14: 377–381 (1970).
223 Said, J.W.; Nash, G.; Banks-Schlegel, S.; Sassoon, A.F.; Murakami, S.; Shintaku, I.P.: Keratin in human lung tumors. Patterns of localization of different-molecular-weight keratin proteins. Am. J. Path. 113: 27–32 (1983).
224 Said, J.W.; Nash, G.; Sassoon, A.F.; Shintaku, I.P.; Banks-Schlegel, S.: Involucrin in lung tumors. A specific marker for squamous differentiation. Lab. Invest. 49: 563–568 (1983).
225 Said, J.W.; Nash, G.; Tepper, G.; Banks-Schlegel, S.: Keratin proteins and carcinoembryonic antigen in lung carcinoma. An immunoperoxidase study of fifty-four cases, with ultrastructural correlations. Human Pathol. 14: 70–76 (1983).
226 Shaheen, K.; Oertel, Y.C.: Mycosis fungoides cells in sputum. A case report. Acta cytol. 28: 483–486 (1984).
227 Shoemaker, S.A.; Scoggin, C.H.: DNA molecular biology in the diagnosis of pulmonary disease. Clins Chest Med. 8: 161–171 (1987).
228 Shure, D.: Fiberoptic bronchoscopy. Diagnostic applications. Clins Chest Med. 8: 1–13 (1987).
229 Silverman, J.F.; Finley, J.L.; Park, H.K.; Strausbauch, P.; Unverferth, M.; Carney, M.: Fine needle aspiration cytology of bronchioloalveolar-cell carcinoma of the lung. Acta cytol. 29: 887–894 (1985).
230 Silverman, J.F.; Johnsrude, I.S.: Fine needle aspiration cytology of granulomatous cryptococcosis of the lung. Acta cytol. 29: 157–161 (1985).
231 Silverman, J.F.; Marrow, H.G.: Fine needle aspiration cytology of granulomatous diseases of the lung, including nontuberculous mycobacterium infection. Acta cytol. 29: 535–541 (1985).
232 Silverman, J.F.; Weaver, M.D.; Gardner, N.; Larkin, E.W.; Park, H.K.: Aspiration biopsy cytology of malignant schwannoma metastatic to the lung. Acta cytol. 29: 15–18 (1985).
233 Silverman, J.F.; Weaver, M.D.; Shaw, R.; Newman, W.J.: Fine needle aspiration cytology of pulmonary infarct. Acta cytol. 29: 162–166 (1985).
234 Simmons, D.H.; Chopra, S.: Fiberoptic bronchoscopy in bronchogenic carcinoma. Chest 70: 694–695 (1976).
235 Sinner, W.N.: Needle biopsy and transbronchial biopsy. With special reference to carcinoma of the lung (Thieme, Stuttgart 1982).
236 Skitarelic, K.; Haam, E. von: Bronchial brushings and washings. A diagnostically rewarding procedure? Acta cytol. 18: 321–326 (1974).
237 Smith, J.H., Frable, W.J.: Adenocarcinoma of the lung. Cytologic correlation with histologic types. Acta cytol. 18: 316–320 (1974).
238 Smith, M.J.; Kini, S.R.; Watson, E.: Fine needle aspiration and endoscopic brush cytology. Comparison of direct smears and rinsings. Acta cytol. 24: 456–459 (1980).
239 Smith, R.C.; Amy, R.W.: Adenoid cystic carcinoma metastatic to the lung. Report of a case diagnosed by fine needle aspiration biopsy cytology. Acta cytol. 29: 533–534 (1985).

240 Sobin, L.H.: The histologic classification of lung tumors. The need for a double standard. Human Pathol. *14:* 1020–1021 (1983).
241 Solcia, E.; Capella, C.; Buffa, R.; Usellini, L.; Fiocca, R.; Sessa, F.; Tortora, O.: The contribution of immunohistochemistry to the diagnosis of neuroendocrine tumors. Semin. Diagn. Pathol. *1:* 285–296 (1984).
242 Spahr, J.; Draffin, R.M.; Johnston, W.W.: Cytopathologic findings in pulmonary blastoma. Acta cytol. *23:* 454–459 (1979).
243 Spahr, J.; Frable, W.J.: Pulmonary cytopathology of an invasive thymoma. Acta cytol. *25:* 163–166 (1981).
244 Steinmann, G.; Greul, W.: Effect of methods of sample taking on the cytologic diagnosis of lung tumors. Acta cytol. *22:* 425–430 (1978).
245 Suprun, H.; Pedio, G.; Ruttner, J.R.: The diagnostic reliability of cytologic typing in primary lung cancer with a review of the literature. Acta cytol. *24:* 494–500 (1980).
246 Swank, P.R.; Greenberg, S.D.; Montalvo, J.; Hunter, N.R.; Spjut, H.J.; Estrada, R.; Winkler, D.G.; Taylor, G.R.: The application of visual cell profiles in the study of premalignant atypias in sputum. Acta cytol. *29:* 373–378 (1985).
247 Tanaka, T.; Yamamoto, M.; Tamura, T.; Moritani, Y.; Miyai, M.; Hiraki, S.; Ohnoshi, T.; Kimura, I.: Cytologic and histologic correlation in primary lung cancer. A study of 154 cases with resectable tumors. Acta cytol. *29:* 49–56 (1985).
248 Tani, E.M.; Franco, M.: Pulmonary cytology in paracoccidioidomycosis. Acta cytol. *28:* 571–575 (1984).
249 Tao, L.C.; Delarue, N.C.; Sanders, D.; Weisbrod, G.: Bronchiolo-alveolar carcinoma. A correlative clinical and cytologic study. Cancer *42:* 2759–2767 (1978).
250 Tao, L.-C.; Robertson, D.I.: Cytologic diagnosis of bronchial mucoepidermoid carcinoma by fine needle aspiration biopsy. Acta cytol. *22:* 221–224 (1978).
251 Thomas, L.; Risbud, M.; Gabriel, J.B.; Caces, W.; Chauhan, P.M.: Cytomorphology of granular-cell tumor of the bronchus. A case report. Acta cytol. *28:* 129–132 (1984).
252 Tokuoka, S.; Hayashi, Y.; Inai, K.; Egawa, H.; Aoki, Y.; Akamizu, H.; Eto, R.; Nishida, T.; Ohe, K.; Kobuke, T.; Nambu, S.; Takemoto, T.; Kou, E.; Nishina, H.; Fujihara, M.; Yonehara, S.; Tsuya, T.; Suehiro, S.; Horiuchi, K.: Early cancer and related lesions in the bronchial epithelium in former workers of mustard gas factory. Acta path. jap. *36:* 553–542 (1986).
253 Tsumuraya, M.; Kodama, T.; Kameya, T.; Shimosato, Y.; Koketsu, H.; Uei, Y.: Light and electron microscopic analysis of intranuclear inclusions in papillary adenocarcinoma of the lung. Acta cytol. *25:* 523–532 (1981).
254 Turner-Warwick, M.; Haslam, P.L.: Clinical applications of bronchoalveolar lavage. Clins Chest Med. *8:* 15–26 (1987).
255 Valicenti, J.F., Jr.; McMaster, K.R., III; Daniell, C.J.: Sputum cytology of giant cell interstitial pneumonia. Acta cytol. *23:* 217–221 (1979).
256 Variakojis, D.; Straus, F.H., II; Fennessy, J.J.; Lu, C.-T.; Bibbo, M.: Transcatheter bronchial brush and forceps biopsies. Histologic evaluation. Am. J. clin. Path. *72:* 163–166 (1979).
257 Vernon, S.E.: Cytodiagnosis of 'signet-ring'-cell lymphoma. Acta cytol. *25:* 291–294 (1981).
258 Vigorita, V.J.; Gupta, P.K.; Bargeron, C.B.; Frost, J.K.: Occurrence and identifica-

tion of intracellular calcium crystals in pulmonary specimens. Acta cytol. *23:* 49–52 (1979).
259 Walker, K.R.; Fullmer, C.J.: Progress report on study of respiratory spirals. Acta cytol. *14:* 396–398 (1970).
260 Walts, A.E.: Localized pulmonary cryptococcosis. Diagnosis by fine needle aspiration. Acta cytol. *27:* 457–459 (1983).
261 Walts, A.E.; Said, J.W.; Banks-Schlegel, S.: Keratin and carcinoembryonic antigen in exfoliated mesothelial and malignant cells. An immunoperoxidase study. Am. J. clin. Path. *80:* 671–676 (1983).
262 Walts, A.E.; Said, J.W.; Shintaku, I.P.: Epithelial membrane antigen in the cytodiagnosis of effusions and aspirates. Immunocytochemical and ultrastructural localization in benign and malignant cells. Diag. Cytopathol. *3:* 41–49 (1987).
263 Walts, A.E.; Said, J.W.; Shintaku, I.P.; Lloyd, R.V.: Chromogranin as a marker of neuroendocrine cells in cytologic material. An immunocytochemical study. Am. J. clin. Path. *84:* 273–277 (1985).
264 Walts, A.E.; Said, J.W.; Shintaku, I.P.; Sassoon, A.F.; Banks-Schlegel, S.: Keratins of different molecular weight in exfoliated mesothelial and adenocarcinoma cells. An aid to cell identification. Am. J. clin. Path. *81:* 442–446 (1984).
265 Wang, K.P.; Marsh, B.R.; Summer, W.R.; Terry, P.B.; Erozan, Y.S.; Baker, R.R.: Transbronchial needle aspiration for diagnosis of lung cancer. Chest *80:* 48–50 (1981).
266 Wang, K.P.; Terry, P.B.: Transbronchial needle aspiration in the diagnosis and staging of bronchogenic carcinoma. Am. Rev. resp. Dis. *127:* 344–347 (1983).
267 Wang, K.P.; Terry, P.; Marsh, B.: Bronchoscopic needle aspiration biopsy of paratracheal tumors. Am. Rev. resp. Dis. *118:* 17–21 (1978).
268 Wang, N.-S.; Huang, S.-N.; Thurlbeck, W.M.: Combined *Pneumocystis carinii* and cytomegalovirus infection. Archs Path. *90:* 529–535 (1970).
269 Wang, S.E.; Nieberg, R.K.: Fine needle aspiration cytology of sclerosing hemangioma of the lung, a mimicker of bronchioloalveolar carcinoma. Acta cytol. *30:* 51–54 (1986).
270 Wang, T.; Reyes, C.; Kathuria, S.; Strinden, C.: Diagnosis of *Strongyloides stercoralis* in sputum cytology. Acta cytol. *24:* 40–43 (1980).
271 Weaver, K.M.; Novak, P.M.; Naylor, B.: Vegetable cell contaminants in cytologic specimens. Their resemblance to cells associated with various normal and pathologic states. Acta cytol. *25:* 210–214 (1981).
272 Weber, W.R.; Askin, F.B.; Dehner, L.P.: Lung biopsy in *Pneumocystis carinii* pneumonia. A histopathologic study of typical and atypical features. Am. J. clin. Path. *67:* 11–19 (1977).
273 Weibel, E.R.; Knight, B.W.: A morphometric study on the thickness of the pulmonary air-blood barrier. J. Cell Biol. *21:* 367–384 (1964).
274 Weingarten, J.: Cytologic and histologic findings in a case of tracheobronchial papillomatosis. Acta cytol. *25:* 167–170 (1981).
275 Wheater, P.R.; Burkitt, H.G.; Daniels, V.G.: Functional histology (Churchill-Livingstone, Edinburgh 1979).
276 Whitaker, D.: Asbestos bodies in sputum. Acta cytol. *22:* 443–444 (1978).
277 Whitaker, D.; Sterrett, G.: *Cryptococcus neoformans* diagnosed by fine needle aspiration cytology of the lung. Acta cytol. *20:* 105–107 (1976).

278 Willie, S.; Snyder, R.: The identification of *Paragonimus westermani* in bronchial washings. Case report. Acta cytol. *21:* 101–102 (1977).
279 Woolner, L.B.; Fontana, R.S.: Pulmonary cytology in lung cancer screening, chap. 7, pp. 105–119; in Miller, Screening for cancer (Academic Press, New York 1985).
280 World Health Organization: The World Health Organization histologic typing of lung tumors; 2nd ed. Am. J. clin. Path. *77:* 123–136 (1982).
281 Yang, K.; Ulich, T.; Taylor, I.; Cheng, L.; Lewin, K.J.: Pulmonary carcinoids. Immunohistochemical demonstration of brain-gut peptides. Cancer *52:* 819–823 (1983).
282 Yesner, R.: Small cell tumors of the lung. Am. J. surg. Path. *7:* 775–785 (1983).
283 Zaharopoulos, P.; Wong, J.Y.; Lamke, C.R.: Endometrial stromal sarcoma. Cytology of pulmonary metastasis including ultrastructural study. Acta cytol. *26:* 49–54 (1982).
284 Zaharopoulos, P.; Wong, J.Y.; Stewart, G.D.: Cytomorphology of the variants of small-cell carcinoma of the lung. Acta cytol. *26:* 800–808 (1982).
285 Zajicek, J.: Aspiration biopsy cytology. I. Cytology of supradiaphragmatic organs; in Wied, Monographs in clinical cytology, vol. 4 (Karger, Basel 1974).

Subject Index

Absidia 62
Acinic cell tumors 154
Actinomyces israelii 64
Actinomycosis 64, 65
Adenocarcinoma(s)
 bronchogenic 110
 colonic 31, 130, 131, 132
 confusion with benign atypia 75, 126, 127
 cytologic features 125, 176, 177
 lung 107–110
  cytologic criteria 110–126
  diagnostic pitfalls 125–132
  differentiation 109, 110
  incidence 107
  types 111–123
 metastatic 129–139
 moderately differentiated 121, 123
 papillary 110
 poorly differentiated 98
 types 179–181
Adenoid cystic carcinoma 154
Adenovirus 82–84
AIDS 42
 with pneumocystis 67
Air-blood barrier 7
Airways, *see also* Respiratory tract
 anatomy 1, 2
 naming 1
Allergic disease, eosinophils 12
Alveolar ducts 2, 5
Alveolar interstitium 7
Alveolar lining cell hyperplasia 72
Alveolar macrophage(s) 7, 8
 bronchoalveolar lavage 22
 deep cough specimen 13, 14
 fine needle aspirates 20
 origin 3, 7

Alveolar sacs 2, 3, 6
Alveolar septa, obliteration 76
Alveoli 2, 6, 7
 capillary walls 7
 epithelium 6
Amyloid 41
APUD classification 140, 203
Asbestos bodies 36, 39, 40
Aspergillosis 58–62
 calcium oxalate crystals 60–62
 clinical course 60
Aspiration pneumonia 20
Asteroid bodies 44
Asthma 29
Atlas of Early Lung Cancer 1, 2

B cells 10
Bacterial infections 84
BAL, *see* Bronchoalveolar lavage
BALT, *see* Bronchus-associated lymphoid tissue
Basal cell hyperplasia
 diagnosis 19
 lung cancer 88
Basal cells 3, 4, 13
 changes not associated with neoplasia 34–36
 sputum samples 16
Basidiobolus 62
Basophilic inclusion bodies 84
Basophils 22
Benign cells
 metaplastic 26, 27
 sputum samples 13–17
 squamous 24, 25
Blastomas, pulmonary 148–150, 162, 184, 185, 188
 cytologic features 177

Subject Index

Blastomyces dermatitidis 52
Blastomycosis, North American 52–57
  cytologic evidence 54–56
  lung 54
  mortality 54
Bombesin 4
Breast adenocarcinoma, metastatic to lungs 131–135, 175
  small cell 144
Bronchial adenomas, lung 153, 154
Bronchial branches 2
Bronchial brushing 17, 18, 196, 208
Bronchial disease, chronic 29, *see also* specific types
Bronchial washings 12, 196, 200, 208
Bronchiectasis 150
Bronchioles, anatomy 2, 3
Bronchioli, respiratory 2
Bronchiolitis
  necrotizing 84
  obliterans 82, 84
Bronchiolo-alveolar adenocarcinoma 107, 109, 185, 187
  cell typing 124
  combine 116–118, 122, 123
  cytologic features 124, 177
  origin 124
  types 110
Bronchitis, chronic 30
Bronchoalveolar lavage 2, 20–22, 80, 208
  diagnostic accuracy 198, 199
  pneumocystitis diagnosis 67, 72
  viral infection diagnosis 73
Bronchogenic adenocarcinoma 110
Bronchogenic carcinoma 12, 92
  carcinogenesis 88
  diagnosis 96–130
Bronchopneumonia, necrotizing 60
Bronchopulmonary dysplasia 91, 92
Bronchoscopy
  accuracy 190, 192, 195–197
  cells obtained 18, 19
    invention IX, 94
  flexible vs. rigid 196
  Pneumocystis carinii 72
Bronchus (bronchi)
  anatomy 1

  epithelium 4–6
  granular-cell tumor 156
  mucus-secreting glands 3
Bronchus-associated lymphoid tissue 3, 4
Busulfan therapy 34, 102, 107

Calcific concretions 41
Calcium oxalate crystals 61, 62
Cancer, *see* Adenocarcinoma, Carcinoma, specific sites
Candida 63, 64
  albicans 64
  pathogenic 24, 25
  tropicalis 64
Candidiasis 25, 64
Carcinoid tumor, lung 153–156
  cytologic criteria 152
  diagnostic pitfalls 153
Carcinoma, *see also* Adenocarcinoma, specific sites
  amine precursor uptake decarboxylase 140
  (APUD) 140, 203
  bronchogenic 12, 96–104, 110–121
  cytopathologic categorization of sputum 91
  in situ 88
  keratinizing squamous 3
  metastatic to lung 169
  precursor states 32
  screening for occult 29, 89, 191–197, 201, 202
  staging 94, 199
Carcinosarcomas 162
  pulmonary 148–150
Cell typing 199–202
Cellular changes, *see also* specific types
  activity 23
  carcinogenesis of lung cancer 86–92
  chemotherapy 107
  mimicking adenocarcinoma of lung 126–132
  not associated with neoplasia 23–41
  radiation 106
  viral infection 74–76
Cervical adenocarcinoma, metastatic to lung 135, 136

Subject Index

Charcot-Leyden crystals 36
Chemotherapy
  cellular changes 107
  radiation 139
Chest X-ray, diagnostic accuracy 192, 193, 195
Chicken pox 80
Chromatin
  bizarre patterns 106
  changes with cancer therapy 140
  coarsened 28, 98
  oat cell carcinoma 140, 142
  pattern in adenocarcinoma 124
Cilia 5
  absence in hyperplastic cells 74, 75
  presence in benign hyperplastic cells 29
Ciliacytophthoria 16, 84
  viral attacks on cells 74
Ciliary escalator 2
Ciliated columnar cells 2, 5, 13
  changes not associated with neoplasia 28, 29
Clara cells 3, 5, 6
  bronchiolo-alveolar carcinoma 124
  changes not associated with neoplasia 32
  hyperplasia 32
Coccidioides immitis 47
Coccidioidomycosis 47-51, 53
  cytologic features 50, 51
  lung involvement 47-50
Colon adenocarcinoma, metastatic to lungs 31, 130-132
Colon-rectal carcinoma, metastatic to lungs 175
Columnar cell atypia, with viral infection 75
Columnar cells, *see also* Ciliated columnar cells, Nonciliated columnar cells
  changes not associated with neoplasia 27-33
  sputum samples 16
Concretions 40, 41
Connective tissue 7
Corpora amylacea 40
Creola bodies 29-31, 132
Cryptococcosis 51, 52
Cryptococcus neoformans 51

Curschmann's spirals 36, 38
Cystosarcoma phyllodes, metastatic to lungs 169-171
Cytomegalovirus 73, 78-81
Cytoplasmic inclusions
  cytomegalovirus 78, 80
  eosinophilic 82
  with respiratory syncytial virus 84

Diagnostic accuracy
  according to histological type and method 190
  according to examination method and location of lesion 189
  bronchoalveolar lavage 198, 199
  cell typing 199-202
  fiberoptic bronchoscopy 195-197
  fine needle aspiration of lung 197, 198
  pulmonary cytology 189, 190
    historic background 191
  refining 179-185
  sputum cytology 191-195
Dirofilariasis 85
DNA hybridization techniques 80
DNA probes 206
  accuracy 199
  viral infection diagnosis 74
Dysplasia (atypical metaplasia) 89-92

Early Lung Cancer Project 88
  diagnostic methods 195
  establishment 192
  screening programs 193
Echinococcus 85
Electron microscopy 199, 203, 206
  criteria in lung cancer diagnosis 204, 205
  diagnosis of large cell undifferentiated carcinoma 96, 150, 151
  diagnosis of 'oat cell' carcinoma 96
  diagnosis of squamous carcinoma 97
Emphysema, goblet cell hyperplasia 30
Endobronchial biopsy 199
Endometriosis 162-166
Entamoeba gingivalis 85
Eosinophilia, pulmonary 12
Eosinophilic debris, granular 83

Subject Index

Eosinophils 12
  in lavage fluid 22
Epidermoid carcinoma, *see also*
  Squamous carcinoma
  cytologic criteria 90, 91, 103
Epithelioid sarcoma, soft tissue 107
Epithelium
  alveolar 6
  nasal cavity 1
  upper respiratory tract 1, 2
Esophageal squamous carcinomas 107
Esophagitis, herpetic 78
Exfoliated cells 13, 18, 19

Ferruginous bodies 36, 39, 40
Fiberoptic bronchoscopy 94
  accuracy 189, 190, 195–197
  benign cells obtained 18, 19
Fibrosis, interstitial 84
Fine needle aspiration(s)
  coccidioidomycosis 50
  diagnostic accuracy 189, 190, 197, 198
  misinterpretation 18, 19
  samples 19, 20
  transbronchial 197
  transthoracic 80, 197, 198
  viral infection diagnosis 74
Fluoroscopy 94
FNA, *see* Fine needle aspiration(s)
Fungi, *see also* specific fungi
  granuloma-producing 44
  hyperkeratosis and squamous metaplasia associated with 24, 25
  pneumonia-producing 56–62
  variably disease-producing 62–72

Gas exchange, pulmonary alveoli 6, 7
Gas-blood barrier 6, 7
Giant cell(s)
  multinucleated 8, 14, 56, 82
  pneumonia 16, 82, 83
Giant histiocytes 20
Giant interstitial pneumonia 16
Glandular cell atypia 32, 33
GMS stain procedure 211, 212
GMST stain 67
Goblet cell hyperplasia 5, 30

Goblet cells 5, 13
  nasal cavity 1
  nonciliated 30
  sputum samples 16
Granular-cell tumor, bronchus 156
Granulated cells, dense-core 4
Granuloma(s) 12
  aspirated, cytologic features 43, 44
  blastomycosis 54
  coccidioidomycosis 50, 51
Granulomatous disease 14, 20
  fungi-producing 44–56
Grocott's methenamine silver stain (GMA) procedure 211, 212

Hamartomas, pulmonary 162, 166
Hamman-Rich syndrome 32
Helminthic infections 12
Hemangioma, sclerosing 132
Hematoporphyrin
  derivative 92
  fluorescence 92, 94
  localization of lesion 94, 105, 194
Hemorrhagic infarct 60
Hemosiderin 16
Herpes (type I) virus 76–79
  cytologic features 73
  prevalence 73
Herpes zoster 80
Herpetic tracheobronchitis 76, 78
Histiocytic proliferation 47
Histoplasma capsulatum 46
Histoplasmomas 47
Histoplasmosis 46–48
  chronic 47
  disseminated 47
Hodgkin's disease 80, 156, 159
Hyaline membranes 72
  cytomegalovirus 79
  herpes virus type I 76
  varicella-zoster infections 80
Hyperkeratinization 24, *see also* Keratinization
Hyperkeratosis 13
Hyperplasia
  alveolar lining cells 72
  basal cell 19, 88

Subject Index

benign lymphoid 159
Clara cells 32
glandular 32
misinterpretation 19
nonciliated goblet cells 30
reserve cell 34-36
Hypersensitivity reactions 12
Hypopharynx 1, 2

Immune response 7
Immune system, study 20-22
Immunochemistry 132, 205, 206
Immunocompromise
  bronchoalveolar lavage 199
  chemotherapy 107
  children 82
  cytomegalovirus 78
  increasing incidence 72, 73
  pneumocystis 67
Infectious disease 42, *see also* specific diseases
  bacterial 84
  fungal 44-71
  incidence 42
  rare 85
  viral 72-84
Inflammation
  lung response 23
  neutrophils 8
Inflammatory response 75, 76
Inflammatory stimuli
  neutrophils 8
  macrophages 7
Influenza virus 84
Intermediate cells 3, 5
Interstitial plasma cell pneumonia 72
Interstitium, alveolar 7
Intra-alveolar edema 84
Intranuclear inclusions
  adenocarcinoma 110
  adenoviral infections 83, 84
  basophilic 79, 84
  Cowdry type A 78, 84
  cytomegalovirus 79, 81
  eosinophilic 82
  herpes virus 76, 77
  varicella-zoster infection 82

Keratin
  epithelial cells 203, 205
  squamous cell carcinoma 100
Keratinization 2, 3, 13, *see also* Hyperkeratinization
  classic squamous carcinoma 97-100
Killer cells 10
Kulchitsky cells 3, 152

Langhans' type giant cells 43
Large cell lymphoma 158, 159
Large cell undifferentiated carcinoma 150, 153, 177
  cytologic criteria 150, 151
  diagnostic pitfalls 152
  types 178, 179
Larynx 1
  mucus-secreting glands 3
Laser treatment 94, 105, 194
Leukemia 156-162
  aspergillosis 58
  diagnosis 16
Leukoplakia 13, 24
Lipid pneumonia 14
Lung
  neoplasms, *see* Lung cancer, Lung tumors, specific types
  open biopsy 67
  respiratory unit 2
  tissue response to environment 23
Lung cancer
  classification 95-169
  comparative cytologic criteria 168-188
  diagnostic approach 95
  electron microscopic criteria in diagnosis 204, 205
  mortality 93
  preneoplastic lesions 86-92
  screening 93, 94
    programs 86, 89, 93, 192-195
  survival rates 93
Lung tumors
  accuracy of cell-typing 199-202
  adenocarcinoma 125
  APUD classification 140, 203
  bronchiolo-alveolar carcinoma 134
  classification 95-169

Lung tumors, classification (cont.)
  future 206
  comparative cytologic criteria 169–188
  small cell undifferentiated carcinoma 146
  squamous carcinoma 103
Lymph nodes 3
Lymphatics, alveolar 7
Lymphocytes 10
  bronchoalveolar lavage 22
  cytotoxic 10
  mitogen-stimulated 8
  vs. oat cell tumor cells 142–144
  sputum samples 16
Lymphoepithelium 4
Lymphoid hyperplasia, benign 159
Lymphoid tissue 3, 4
Lymphokines 8
Lymphoma(s) 183, 185
  cytologic features 160–162, 177
  diagnosis 16
  large cell 158, 159
  lung involvement in 156–162
  metastatic to lungs 175
Lymphoreticular aggregates 4

Macrophages
  alveolar 3, 7, 8, 13, 14, 20, 22
  bronchoalveolar lavage identification 22
  phagocytosis of dust 4
  pulmonary 7–11
Mast cells 7
May-Grünwald-Giemsa stain 177, 211
Measles virus 82
Meat fibers 41
Megakaryocyte nuclei 36
Melanoma, metastatic to lung 162, 163, 175
  spindle cell variant 164, 166
Mesopharynx 1
Mesothelial cells, microscopic appearance 19, 20
Metaplasia 5
  benign 26, 27
  causes 104
  squamous 101–105

Metaplastic atypia
  carcinogenesis 88, 89
  cytologic criteria 90
Microvilli, blunt 6
Mouth epithelium 2
Muco-epidermoid carcinoma 154
Mucor 62
Mucormycosis 62
  metaplasia 5
Multinucleated histiocytes 20, 21
Multinucleation
  ciliated columnar cells 21, 28, 29
  giant cells 8, 14, 82
    blastomycosis 56
  large cell undifferentiated carcinoma 151
  respiratory epithelial cells 29
Mycelia 60
  aspergillosis 58, 59
  nocardia 67
Mycetoma 50, 62, 105
  vs. squamous carcinoma 102, 105, 106

Nasal cavity 1
Nasopharynx epithelium 2
Necrotic debris
  mycetoma 50, 105
  oat cell carcinoma 150
  tumor diathesis 102
  squamous cell carcinoma 100
Neutrophils 8–10
Nocardia 65, 67
Nocardiosis 65, 67
Noncellular elements 36, 38–41
Nonciliated columnar cells 5
Nonciliated goblet cells 30
Non-Hodgkin's lymphoma 156
North American blastomycosis, see Blastomycosis, North American
Null cells 10

Oat-cell carcinoma 34, 188
  small cell 132, 139–150
    accuracy of cell typing 200
    cytologic criteria 140–142, 146, 185, 188
    diagnostic pitfalls 142–150
    endocrine production 140, 203

Subject Index

Oral cavity 1
Oropharynx epithelium 2

Pancreas adenocarcinoma, metastatic to lung 135, 137
Papanicolaou stain
    fungi 44-67
    pneumocysts 67
    procedure 208-211
    viral infection diagnosis 74
Papillary adenocarcinoma of the lung 110
Papillomatosis, tracheobronchial 156
Paracoccidioidomycosis 85
Paragonimus westermani 85
Peribronchial connective tissue 7
Periodic acid-Schiff stain 52
Phagocytosis 7
Pharynx 1
Phycomycosis 62
Pleomorphic adenoma 154
Pleural connective tissue 7
Pneumococcal pneumonia 10
Pneumoconiosis 14
Pneumocystis 68-71
Pneumocystis carinii 67-72
Pneumocytes 34, 37
    changes not associated with neoplasm 34
    fusion of type 2 82
    herpes virus 76
    type 1 3, 6
    type 2 3, 6
Pneumonia
    acute 64
        interstitial 80
        necrotizing 67
    adenovirus 82, 83
    aspiration 20
    blastomycosis 54
    chronic progressive 48
    giant cell 16, 82, 83
    herpetic 76, 78, 79
    immunocompromised hosts 66
    interstitial 16, 72, 80
    invasive fungal 56-62
        diagnosis 56, 58
    measles 82

    mortality rate 82
    segmental 52
    viral 73
Pneumonic processes 126-132
Pollen 40, 41
Pollutants, diagnosis of reactions 20
Postbronchoscopy sputa 191, 192, 196
Postcapillary venules 4
Preneoplastic lesions 86-92
Preparatory procedures 207-212
Prostate-specific antigen 132
Psammoma bodies 41
    adenocarcinoma 110
Pseudostratified epithelium 4
Pulmonary alveoli 6, 7
Pulmonary aspergillosis 60
Pulmonary blastoma/carcinosarcoma 148, 149
Pulmonary cytology
    diagnostic accuracy 189-202
    future 203-206
Pulmonary disease, chronic obstructive 30, *see also* specific diseases
Pulmonary dust sumps 4
Pulmonary eosinophilia 12
Pulmonary infarction 126
Pulmonary lymphomas 156-162
Pulmonary macrophages 7-9, 11
    ingestion of neutrophils 10
Pulmonary parenchyma 2
Pulmonary squamous carcinoma, *see* Squamous carcinoma, lung
Pulmonary surfactant, and type 2 pneumocytes 6

Radiation
    reaction 102, 106, 107
Reactive processes 126-132
Repair cells 25, 26, 50, 150
    atypical 27, 104
    changes not associated with neoplasia 25, 26
Reserve cell(s)
    hyperplasia 34-36, 146
    vs. oat cell tumor cells 144
Respiratory bronchioles, division 5, 6
Respiratory epithelial cells 20

Subject Index

Respiratory epithelium 4–6
Respiratory syncytial virus 82, 84
Respiratory tract
  anatomy 1, 2
  cell types 3–12
  epithelium 4–6
    response to irritants 24–41
  histology 2–12
  non-disease-producing organisms 85
  upper 1, 2
Rhizopus 62
RSV, *see* Respiratory syncytial virus

Saccomanno sputum method 193, 194
Salivary gland tumors, metastatic to lung 154, 175
Sarcoidosis 43–45
  diagnosis 16
Scar adenocarcinoma 32
Schaumann bodies 44
Schwannoma, lung 168, 169
Sclerosing hemangioma 132
Seminoma 147, 148, 184, 185
  cytologic features 177
  metastatic to lungs 175
  vs. oat cell tumor cells 144
Small cell oat cell carcinoma, *see* Oat cell carcinoma, small cell
Smoking
  epithelial cell changes 26, 27
  globlet cell hyperplasia 30
  lung cancer pathogenesis 86, 93
  macrophage numbers 10
Smudge cells 83, 84
Spindle cell sarcoma, metastatic to lung 166, 167
Sputum
  accuracy of cytology 191–195
  benign cells 13–17
  concretions 40, 41
  deep cough 13, 14
  processing 207
  screening program 193, 194
Squamous carcinoma 20
  distinguishing cell features 103, 176
  esophageal 107
  head and neck 107
  keratinizing 108, 109
  location 96, 97
  lung 96–98
    cytologic criteria 98–101
    diagnostic pitfalls 101–107
    differentiation 97, 98
    misinterpretation 128–130
    nonkeratinizing 101
    theory for development 86
    treatment 96
Squamous cells, *see also* Squamous carcinoma, Squamous metaplasia
  cancer precursor, 86
  dysplastic, 60–62
  mouth, 24
  response, to irritants, 24, 25
  vacuolated, 92, 128
Squamous metaplasia 28, 49
  carcinogenesis 88, 89
  cytologic criteria 90, 91
  lung cancer 88
  precursor to squamous carcinoma 101–105
Staining procedures 207–212, *see also* specific procedures
Stress, cellular response 24–41
Strongyloides stercoralis 85
Submucosal glands 3
Surfactant 6, 7

T cells 10
T-helper cells 10
T-suppressor cells 10
Talc 41
TB, *see* Tuberculosis
Testicular carcinoma, embryonal, metastatic to lungs 165, 166
Thoracotomy 201
  pneumocystis 67
  viral infection diagnosis 74
Thymomas 162
  metastatic to lungs 101, 175
  spindle cell 172, 173
Thyroid papillary carcinoma, metastatic to lungs 138, 139
Trachea 1
  epithelium 4–6

Subject Index

Tracheobronchial lesions 156
Tracheobronchial papillomatosis 92, 156
Tracheobronchitis, herpetic 76
    pathogenesis 78
Transbronchial biopsy
    diagnostic accuracy 196
    penumocystis 67
    sarcoidosis 44
Transbronchial needle aspirates 19, 80, 197
Transitional cell carcinoma, metastatic to lungs 173, 174
Transthoracic needle aspirates 19, 80, 197
Trichomonads 85
Tuberculosis 6, 42–44
    diagnosis 16
Tumor cells, metastatic 10
Tumor diathesis 102, 150–152

Tumors *see also* Adenocarcinoma, Carcinoma, Lung cancer, Lung tumors
    acinic cell 154
    carcinoid 153–156
    metastatic to lung 96, 162–169

Valley fever 47, 48
Varicella-zoster virus 80–82
Vascular disease 12
Vegetable material concretions 41
Viral infections 72–76
    benign cellular response 28
    cytologic changes 74, 75
    diagnosis 73, 74
    immunocompromise 72, 73
    inflammatory response 75, 76
    specific types 76–84